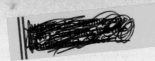

Applied
Pharmacology
for the Dental
Hygienist

Applied Pharmacology
for the Dental Hygienist

Barbara Requa-Clark,
Pharm.D.

Professor of Dentistry (Pharmacology),
University of Missouri-Kansas City, School of
Dentistry, Kansas City, Missouri

Sam V. Holroyd,
B.S., D.D.S., M.S. (Pharmacology),
M.S. (Periodontics), F.A.C.D., F.I.C.D.

Professor and Chairman, Department of Periodontics,
Professor of Pharmacology,
Washington University School of Dental Medicine,
St. Louis, Missouri

SECOND EDITION

Illustrated

The C.V. Mosby Company

ST. LOUIS • PHILADELPHIA • BALTIMORE • TORONTO   1989

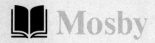 Mosby

Editor: Robert W. Reinhardt
Assistant Editor: Maureen Slaten
Project Manager: Mark Spann
Production: Editing, Design & Production, Inc.
Design: Liz Fett

SECOND EDITION

Copyright © 1989 by The C.V. Mosby Company

Previous edition copyrighted 1982
Printed in the United States of America

The C.V. Mosby Company
11830 Westline Industrial Drive, St. Louis, Missouri 63146

Library of Congress Cataloging-in-Publication Data

Applied pharmacology for the dental hygienist/[edited by] Barbara
   Requa-Clark, Sam V. Holroyd. — 2nd ed.
     p. cm.
     Rev. ed. of: Applied pharmacology for the dental hygienist
   Barbara S. Requa, Sam V. Holroyd, 1982.
     Includes bibliographical references and index.
     ISBN 0-8016-4266-3
     1. Dental pharmacology.   2. Dental hygiene.
     I. Requa-Clark,
   Barbara.   II. Holroyd, Samuel V., 1931-
     [DNLM: 1. Dental Hygienists.   2. Pharmacology, Clinical.   QV 50
   A652]
RK701.R46   1989   615'.7'0246176—dc19
   DNLM/DLC
   for Library of Congress   88-39037
                                                                  CIP

C/MV/MV   9 8 7 6 5 4 3

Contributors

Ronald D. Baker, D.D.S., M.A. (Ed.), F.A.C.D.

Professor and Chairman, Department of Oral and Maxillofacial Surgery, The University of North Carolina at Chapel Hill, School of Dentistry, Chapel Hill, North Carolina

Stewart A. Bergman, D.D.S., M.S.

Associate Professor, Department of Oral and Maxillofacial Surgery, Department of Pharmacology, Baltimore College of Dental Surgery, Dental School, University of Maryland at Baltimore, Baltimore, Maryland

William K. Bottomley, D.D.S., M.S.

Professor and Chairman, Department of Oral Diagnosis, Georgetown University, School of Dentistry, Washington, D.C.

Sherry Burns, R.D.H., M.S.

Associate Professor of Dentistry, University of Missouri-Kansas City, School of Dentistry, Kansas City, Missouri

Tommy W. Gage, D.D.S., Ph.D., F.A.C.D.

Professor and Chairman, Department of Pharmacology, Baylor College of Dentistry, Dallas, Texas

J. Max Goodson, D.D.S., M.S., Ph.D.

Head, Department of Pharmacology, Forsyth Dental Center, Boston, Massachusetts

Sam V. Holroyd, B.S., D.D.S., M.S. (Pharmacology), M.S. (Periodontics), F.A.C.D., F.I.C.D.

Professor and Chairman, Department of Periodontics, Professor of Pharmacology, Washington University School of Dental Medicine, St. Louis, Missouri

James L. Matheny, Ph.D.

Professor, Department of Oral Health Science, University of Kentucky, College of Dentistry, Lexington, Kentucky

Norbert R. Myslinski, Ph.D.

Associate Professor, Oral-Facial Neuroscience Group, Department of Physiology, Baltimore College of Dental Surgery, Dental School, University of Maryland at Baltimore, Baltimore, Maryland

Barbara S. Requa-Clark, Pharm.D.

Professor of Dentistry (Pharmacology), University of Missouri-Kansas City, School of Dentistry, Kansas City, Missouri

Barbara F. Roth-Schechter, B.S., Ph.D.

Professeur Conv. Pharmacology, Université Louis Pasteur, Laboratoire de Pharmacodynamie, Strasbourg, France

Martha J. Somerman, D.D.S., Ph.D.

Associate Professor, Department of Periodontics, Department of Pharmacology, Baltimore College of Dental Surgery, Dental School, University of Maryland at Baltimore, Baltimore, Maryland

Richard L. Wynn, M.S., Ph.D.

Associate Professor and Chairman, Department of Pharmacology, Baltimore College of Dental Surgery, Dental School, University of Maryland at Baltimore, Baltimore, Maryland

Samuel L. Yankell, Ph.D., R.D.H.

Research Professor, Department of Periodontics, University of Pennsylvania, School of Dental Medicine, Philadelphia, Pennsylvania

Preface

After using the first edition of this textbook in teaching several classes of dental hygiene students and talking with others that have used the book, the main comment we received was that it was too detailed. We realized that, given the time that the student has to spend on pharmacology, a reduction in the size of the book was in order. We believe that this edition still provides the dental hygiene students and practitioners with the necessary information related to pharmacology and therapeutics. We have attempted to minimize the references, excluding footnotes referring to facts that are common knowledge. We would expect students who desire more in-depth information to use the Index to Dental Literature or Medline to search for specific topics or for current journal articles.

This textbook can be used to learn basic pharmacology as it pertains to the practice of dental hygiene or it may be used to review the subject. The drugs used in dentistry are discussed in more detail than the drugs that the patient may be taking.

Drug groups are presented in sections, while the differences within groups are mentioned only if they are significant. It is easier to master the general properties of a drug group than to learn those properties independently for each individual drug.

At the end of each chapter, there is a set of review questions for student use. These questions can assess whether the content of the chapter has been mastered. By reviewing the questions, the student can determine areas of strength as well as areas of potential weakness and review these areas.

The Appendix lists the 200 most commonly prescribed drugs and the chapter(s) in which each of these drugs is discussed. Using this alphabetical listing to improve the history-taking function during patient visits will make the medical history in the dental records more accurate.

We encourage our readers—students, faculty, and practitioners—to provide suggestions for improving this textbook. Any input regarding ways in which it can be made more useful would be appreciated. Please don't hesitate to let us hear your comments, for they are the most valuable feedback we have for improvement for future editions.

We wish to express our sincere appreciation to our chapter contributors. Without their beginnings and continuing interest, this textbook would not have been written.

My appreciation to Dean Reed for his support and to the library staff and my student assistant, Sai Chu, for their tireless attention to detail. Last, but not least, we thank our families without whose support this endeavor would not have been possible or nearly as meaningful.

Barbara Requa-Clark
Sam V. Holroyd

Contents

9 **Local anesthetics**

Barbara S. Requa-Clark
Sam V. Holroyd

10 **Antianxiety agents**

Richard L. Wynn
Barbara S. Requa-Clark
Stewart A. Bergman
Barbara F. Roth-Schechter
Sam V. Holroyd

11   General anesthetics

Tommy W. Gage
Barbara S. Requa-Clark
Ronald D. Baker

12   Fluorides

Sherry Burns
Samuel L. Yankell

13   Vitamins and minerals

Richard L. Wynn
Barbara S. Requa-Clark

14   Oral conditions and their treatment

Barbara S. Requa-Clark
William K. Bottomly
Sam V. Holroyd

SECTION III
DRUGS THAT MAY ALTER DENTAL TREATMENT

15   Cardiovascular drugs

Tommy W. Gage
Barbara S. Requa-Clark

Applied Pharmacology

for the Dental
Hygienist

Chapter 1

Introduction

Pharmacology is the study of drugs. When one considers that a **drug** may be broadly defined as any chemical substance that affects biologic systems, the scope of this discipline is obvious.

HISTORY

Pharmacology had its beginning when our ancestors began to notice that chewing certain plant roots or leaves altered one's awareness or function. The first pharmacologist was a person who became more astute in observing and remembering which plant products produced predictable results. From this beginning a huge industrial and academic community concerned with the study and development of drugs has evolved. The agents discovered are then prescribed and dispensed through the practice of medicine, dentistry, and pharmacy.

PHARMACOLOGY AND THE DENTAL HYGIENIST

The American Dental Hygienists' Association (ADHA) has analyzed the tasks performed by the dental hygienist and enumerated the courses essential for each task. The knowledge of pharmacology is imperative for several functions performed by the dental hygienist. As the laws controlling the dental hygiene profession are modified, it is likely that more responsibility will be given to the dental hygienist and a greater knowledge of pharmacology will become necessary.

The dental hygienist will require the knowledge of principles of pharmacology in the following situations:

1. Obtaining the health history. In order to obtain a complete and useful health history, a knowledge of the drugs commonly prescribed is required. Patients with systemic diseases unrelated to their dental health often have medication prescribed by their physician. An understanding of the action, indications, adverse reactions, and therapeutic uses of these drugs can help the dental hygienist to determine their effect on dental treatment.

2. Administering drugs in the office. Since both the dental hygienist and the dentist administer certain drugs in the office, knowledge of these agents is imperative. The hygienist commonly applies fluoride, and in some states both the dentist and the hygienist administer local anesthetics and nitrous oxide. Because of their frequent use, an in-depth knowledge of these agents is required.

3. Handling emergency situations. The ability to recognize and assist in the treatment of emergency situations requires the knowledge of certain drugs. The indications for these drugs and their adverse reactions must be considered.

4. Planning appointments. Patients taking medication for systemic diseases may require special handling in the dental office. For example, asthmatic patients should have afternoon appointments, whereas diabetic patients usually have

fewer problems with a morning appointment.

5. Choosing self-medication. The dental hygienist will have occasion to self-medicate various minor conditions. The study of pharmacology will assist the hygienist in an intelligent selection of an appropriate over-the-counter (OTC) product.

6. Discussing drugs prescribed by the dentist. Drugs prescribed by the dentist can cause adverse effects. Patients often ask the hygienist questions about drugs prescribed for them. A knowledge of the terms used to describe adverse reactions can facilitate discussions with the dentist, or physician as needed.

When the dental hygienist takes a health history and lists the drugs the patient is taking, treatment should not begin until the nature of those drugs is elucidated. Since it is impossible to remember all the drug names and their actions, and since new drugs are always being discovered, an appropriate reference source should be consulted.

SOURCES OF INFORMATION

There are four general types of books related to the subject of pharmacology. The books are useful for different purposes and provide information helpful in different situations. They include basic pharmacology textbooks, publications sponsored by medical, dental, or pharmaceutical associations, reference sources, and manufacturing standards. The uses of these books and their relative merits are as follows:

1. Pharmacology textbooks. A pharmacology textbook provides the necessary background for understanding the effects, adverse reactions, and use of each group of drugs. A few of these textbooks have some application to dentistry. A list is provided in the references.[1-6]

2. Association-related publications

a. *Accepted Dental Therapeutics*, ed. 40, Chicago, 1984, American Dental Association (ADA) Council on Dental Therapeutics. The ADA is no longer planning to publish this book, which provided information on dentally related drugs.

b. *AMA Drug Evaluations*, ed. 6, Chicago, 1986, American Medical Association Council on Drugs. This book contains unbiased information for commonly prescribed drugs. It also discusses disease states for which the drugs are indicated.

c. *American Hospital Formulary Service—Drug Information*, Bethesda, Md., 1988, American Society of Hospital Pharmacists, Inc. This detailed reference tool provides an unbiased guide to drug information. It is updated yearly, and quarterly supplements are also provided. It discusses all aspects of a drug's properties.

d. *Handbook of Nonprescription Drugs*, ed. 8, Washington, D.C., 1986, American Pharmaceutical Association. This book provides a monograph on many groups of OTC drugs. It also contains comparison charts that include the ingredients contained in these products. Sections included are oral health products and contraceptive methods.

3. Reference sources. Reference books provide information about brand name and generic products that are prescribed for patients. They do not cover basic pharmacology or explain terms used in them. They do include the drug's mechanism of action, indications for use, contraindications, precautions, doses, and preparations available.

a. Kastup, E.K., and Olin, B.R., editors: *Facts and Comparisons*, St. Louis, 1988, J.B. Lippincott Co. This reference tool includes most prescription drug products available in the United States. It also includes many OTC products. Since it is arranged by pharmacologic class, drugs with similar indications are listed together. Charts also facilitate the comparison among several drugs in one class. One disadvantage of *Facts and Comparisons* is its cost, but student rates are available. It is available in a hardcover book, or in a loose-leaf binder with monthly supplements.

b. *Physicians' Desk Reference* (PDR), ed. 42, Oradell, N.J., 1988, Medical Economics Co. This annually published book lists some products from a variety of manufacturers. Manufacturers purchase space in the PDR to advertize their higher volume products. The drugs are organized alphabetically by brand name within each section by manufacturer, and each manufacturer's section is listed alphabetically. Two advantages of the PDR are its relatively inexpensive price, owing to sub- sidy by the manufacturers, and its picture section (colored pictures of selected drug dosage forms). In general, the information in the PDR is the same as the package insert required for each product. This is not necessarily current or com- plete.

c. *United States Pharmacopeia—Drug Infor- mation* (USP-DI), ed. 8, Rockville, MD., 1988, United States Pharmacopeial Convention, Inc. This detailed reference book is a two-volume set. Volume I is entitled Information for the Health Care Provider, and Volume II is called Informa- tion for the Patient, presented in lay language. A complex advisory panel system derived from a cross-section of health care providers assures that this book is unbiased. The American Medical As- sociation (AMA) uses this source to prepare their patient medication instruction (PMI) sheets.

4. Manufacturing standards. *The United States Pharmacopeia—National Formulary,* Rockville, MD, 1980, U.S. Pharmacopeial Convention, Inc. This compendium includes manufacturing stan- dards for the quality of drugs available.

The dental office should have at least one ref- erence tool that lists the names of prescription and OTC drugs. A standard textbook of pharma- cology is helpful in understanding the use of the reference tool. Because of the release of new drugs, a recent edition of a reference book is needed.

The practicing pharmacist can be another source of information about new drugs. It is important for the dental professional to estab- lish a professional relationship with a local pharmacist. They may assist the dentist or hy- gienist in understanding a new drug's effect on the dental patient.

DRUG NAMES

Since the dental hygienist must be able to discuss drugs with the patient, the patient's physician, and the dentist, it is important to understand the ways in which a drug can be named. The ability to do this is complicated by the fact that all drugs have at least two names and often more.

When a drug is being investigated by a com- pany, it is identified by its **chemical name,** which is determined by its chemical structure. If the structure is unknown at the time of investigation, a code name, usually a combination of letters and numbers, is assigned to the product.

After a compound has been found to be useful and it is determined that it will be marketed com- mercially, the pharmaceutical company gives the drug a **trade name** or **proprietary name.** This trade name, registered as a trademark under the Federal Trade-Mark Law, is the property of the registering company. The trade name is usually chosen so that it can be easily remembered and promoted commercially. It is capitalized. Al- though the **brand name** technically is the name of the company marketing the product, it is often used interchangeably with trade name. The trade name is protected by the Federal Patent Law for 17 years.

Before any drug is marketed, it is given a **ge- neric name** that becomes the "official" name of the drug. There is only one generic name se- lected by the U.S. Adopted Name Council. This council selects a generic name that does not con- flict with other drug names. The generic name is not capitalized.

An example of the many names a product can have is provided by lidocaine, a local anesthetic commonly used in dentistry.

Chemical name: 2-diethylamino-2,6
                -acetoxylidide
Generic name: lidocaine
Trade names: Xylocaine
             Octocaine

After the original manufacturer's patents have expired other companies can market the generic drug under their trade name. When lidocaine first appeared on the market, it was made by As- tra and available only as Xylocaine, but when its patent expired, other companies started making lidocaine and each company gave it their own brand name (for example, Octocaine). When a pa- tient states an allergy to Xylocaine, the hygienist must be aware that lidocaine is the generic name of this drug and that the patient should not be given lidocaine under another trade name, such as Octocaine.

Drugs prescribed by physicians cause a similar problem. Patients often know these drugs by the trade name. If a patient reports an allergic reaction to Valium (the trade name) the hygienist must be aware that this patient should not take other brands of diazepam (the generic name).

Since there is only one generic name for each drug, this book will use generic names when discussing drugs. Trade names will appear in parentheses after the generic name.

A problem occurs in naming multiple-entity drugs (drugs with several ingredients). These drugs are difficult to discuss by their generic names because they contain several different ingredients.

Drug substitution. When discussing generic and trade names, the question of generic equivalence and substitution arises. Are different generic products equivalent? After 17 years the patent of the original drug expires, and other companies may market the same compound under a generic name. In 1984 Congress passed the Drug Price Competition and Patent Term Restoration Act. This allowed generic drugs to receive expedited approval. The Food and Drug Administration still requires that the active ingredient of the generic product enters the bloodstream at the same rate as the trade name product. The variation allowed for the generic name product is the same as for the reformulations of the brand name product. For a very few drugs that are difficult to formulate and have narrow therapeutic indices, differences may exist between the trade name and the generic product. But, for all dental drugs, generic substitution is suitable. Drugs can be judged similar in several ways. When two formulations of a drug meet the chemical and physical standards established by the regulatory agencies, they are termed *chemically equivalent*. If they produce similar concentrations of the drug in the blood and tissues, they are termed *biologically equivalent*. If they prove to have an equal therapeutic effect in a clinical trial, they are termed *therapeutically equivalent*. Preparations can be chemically equivalent and yet not biologically or therapeutically equivalent. These products are said to differ in their bioavailability.

Top 200 drugs

Appendix A lists the 200 drugs most frequently prescribed in 1987 and their pharmacologic group. Both generic and trade names appear on the list, depending on how the prescription is written. The dental hygienist must become familiar with the names of these drugs because patients may know the names of drugs they are taking but not know how the names are spelled. By referring to the list of the top 200 drugs, the hygienist can record the patient's medications accurately. Throughout this textbook an attempt is made to discuss the agents included in this list.

FEDERAL REGULATORY AGENCIES

Many agencies are involved in regulating the production, marketing, advertising, labeling, and prescribing of drugs.

Food and Drug Administration

The Food and Drug Administration (FDA) of the Department of Health and Human Services determines what drugs can be marketed in the United States. Data relative to safety and effectiveness of drug entities and physical and chemical standards for specific products are considered. The FDA requires quality control in drug manufacturing plants and determines what drugs may be sold only by prescription. It also regulates the labeling and advertising of prescription drugs. Because the FDA is frequently more stringent than regulatory bodies in other countries, drugs are often marketed in Europe and South America before they are available in the United States.

Federal Trade Commission

The Federal Trade Commission (FTC) regulates the trade practices of drug companies and prohibits the false advertising of foods, nonprescription drugs, and cosmetics.

Drug Enforcement Administration

The Drug Enforcement Administration (DEA) of the Department of Justice administers the Controlled Substances Act of 1970. This federal agency regulates the manufacture and distribution of substances that have a potential for abuse, including narcotics (opiods), stimulants, and sedatives.

REVIEW QUESTIONS

1. Define the term "pharmacology."
2. Explain why the dental hygienist should have a knowledge of pharmacology.
3. Name two reference publications that are useful for looking up brand names of drugs. Explain the advantages and disadvantages of these two sources.
4. State the number and type of reference books that an up-to-date dental office should have.
5. Define and give an example of the following terms:
   a. Chemical name
   b. Trade name
   c. Brand name
   d. Generic name
6. Explain why a list of the top 200 drugs should be available in every dental office. Explain the term "rank order."
7. Name three federal regulatory agencies and state the major responsibility of each.

REFERENCES

1. Clark, W.G., Brater, D.C., and Johnson, A.R.: Goth's medical pharmacology, ed. 12, St. Louis, 1988, The C.V. Mosby Co.
2. Csaky, T.Z., and Barnes, B.A.: Cutting's handbook of pharmacology: the actions and uses of drugs, ed. 7, New York, 1984, Appleton and Lange.
3. DiPalma, J.R., editor: Basic pharmacology in medicine, ed. 2, New York, 1981, McGraw-Hill Book Co.
4. Gerald, M.C.: Pharmacology: an introduction to drugs, New York, 1981, Appleton and Lange.
5. Gilman, A.G., Goodman, L.S., and Gilman, A.: Goodman and Gilman's The pharmacologic basis of therapeutics, ed. 7, New York, 1985, Macmillan Publishing Co., Inc.
6. Katzung, B.G.: Basic and clinical pharmacology, ed. 3, Los Altos, Calif., 1987, Lange Medical Publications.

Chapter 2

Drug action and handling

In order to discuss the drugs used in dentistry or those that patients may be taking when they come to the dental office, the dental hygienist must be familiar with some basic principles of pharmacology. This chapter discusses the methods of drug administration and action of drugs in the body. Chapter 3 considers the problems or adverse reactions these drugs can cause. By understanding how drugs work, what effects they can have, and what problems they can cause, the dental hygienist can communicate better with the patient and the dentist about medications the patient may be taking or may need to have prescribed for dental treatment.

Drugs are broadly defined as chemical substances used for the diagnosis, prevention, or treatment of disease or for the prevention of pregnancy. Most drugs are differentiated from inert chemicals and chemicals necessary for the maintenance of life processes (such as vitamins) by their ability to act selectively in biologic systems to accomplish a desired effect. Historically, drugs were discovered by randomly searching for active components among plants, animals, minerals, and the soil. Today the search for new drugs involves a different approach—systematic screening techniques. Also organic synthetic chemistry researchers have developed thousands of new synthetic drugs. Parent compounds that exhibit known pharmacologic activity are chemically modified to produce congeners or analogs—agents of a similar chemical structure with a similar pharmacologic effect. This technique of modifying a chemical molecule to provide more useful therapeutic agents has evolved from studies of the relationship between the chemical structure and the biologic structure (structure-activity relationship or SAR).

CHARACTERIZATION OF DRUG ACTION

Drugs can be classified as follows:
1. Biochemical action (such as hypoglycemic or blood sugar–lowering agents)
2. Physiologic effects (such as antihypertensive or blood pressure–lowering agents)
3. Organ systems involved (such as central nervous system stimulants)

Log dose-effect curve

When drugs exert an effect on biologic systems, the effect can be related quantitatively to the dose of the drug given. If the dose of the drug is plotted against the intensity of the effect, a curve will result (Fig. 2-1). If this curve is replotted using the log of the dose versus the response, another curve is produced from which the potency and efficacy of a drug's action may be determined (Fig. 2-2).

Potency

The potency of a particular drug is shown by the location of that drug's curve along the log dose axis (x axis). In Fig. 2-3 the curve for drug B (meperidine) is to the right of the curve for drug A (morphine). This indicates that a higher dose of drug B would be necessary to obtain an equal effect. The potency of different drugs that elicit similar effects can be compared by observing the dose that gives 50% of the total or maximum effect. The maximum effect is the effect produced at a certain dose of the drug that cannot be increased with a higher dose of the drug. If drug A requires a smaller dose than drug B to produce 50% of the maximum effect, drug A is more potent than drug B. However, since potency is a relative term, this indicates merely that the less potent drug must be administered in higher doses

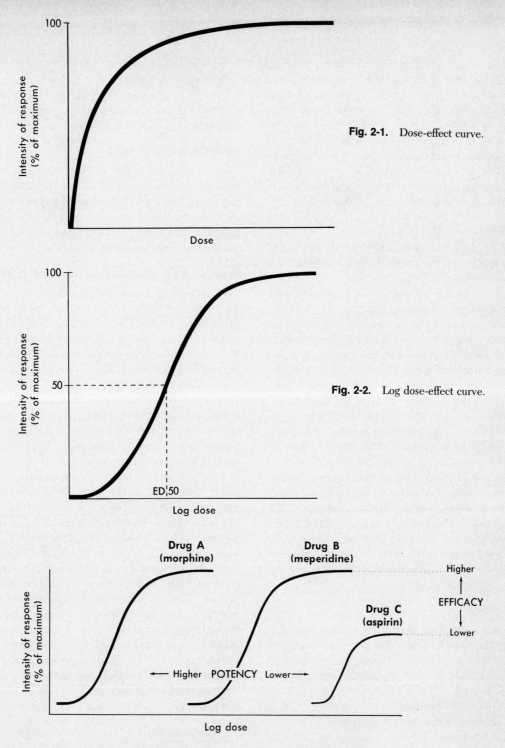

Fig. 2-1. Dose-effect curve.

Fig. 2-2. Log dose-effect curve.

Fig. 2-3. Comparison of log dose-effect curves.

to obtain the same effect. The absolute potency of a drug is immaterial as long as an appropriate dose is used. For example, both meperidine and morphine have the ability to treat severe pain, but approximately 100 mg of meperidine would be required to produce the same action as 10 mg of morphine. Thus the absolute potency of morphine is 10 times that of meperidine, or meperidine is ¹⁄₁₀ as potent as morphine, even though both agents can relieve intense pain (equal efficacy).

Efficacy

Efficacy is the maximum intensity of effect or response that can be obtained when sufficient drug is administered. In Fig. 2-3 drug A and drug B possess equal efficacy and unequal potency, while drug C is less efficacious. This value is illustrated by the plateau of the curve. The efficacy of any drug is a major descriptive characteristic indicating its action. For example, the efficacy of drug B (meperidine) and drug A (morphine) is about the same, since both drugs relieve severe pain. Other analgesics, such as drug C (aspirin), are less efficacious since they relieve only mild to moderate pain. It can be seen that the efficacy of a drug is **not** related to its potency. The dose of a drug required to produce a specific intensity of effect in an individual is regarded as the effective dose for that individual. The efficacy can also be expressed in terms of the median effective dose, or ED50. The ED50 is the dose of a drug required to produce a specified intensity of effect in 50% of the test animals given the drug. If death is the endpoint, the median effective dose becomes the median lethal dose (LD50).

Variations

When a given dose of a drug is administered to many individuals, variations in response and effect will occur. These variations in individual response may be caused by, among other factors, the following:

1. Route of administration
2. Passage across body membranes
3. Absorption
4. Distribution
5. Molecular mechanisms of action
6. Metabolism
7. Excretion

These processes are discussed as they relate to variations in individual drug response and the time course of drug action.

PHARMACOKINETICS

Pharmacokinetics is the study of how a drug enters the body, circulates within the body, and leaves the body and what factors influence these movements. The four major steps in the body's handling of a drug are absorption, distribution, metabolism, and excretion (ADME).

Routes of administration and dosage forms

The route of administration of a drug affects both the onset and duration of response. Onset refers to the time it takes for the drug to begin to have its effect. Duration is the length of a drug's effect. The routes of administration can be classified as **enteral** and **parenteral**. Drugs given enterally are placed directly into the gastrointestinal tract by oral or rectal administration. Parenteral administration bypasses the gastrointestinal tract and includes various injection routes, inhalation, and topical administration. In practice, the term parenteral usually refers to an injection.

Although oral administration is considered the safest, least expensive, and most convenient route, the parenteral injection of a drug has certain advantages. The injection results in fast absorption, which produces a rapid onset and a more predictable response than oral administration. The parenteral route is useful for emergencies, unconsciousness, lack of cooperation, or nausea. Some drugs must be administered by injection to remain active. The disadvantages of the parenteral route include that asepsis must be maintained to avoid infection, an intravascular injection can occur by accident, administration by injection is more painful, and self-medication is difficult. Parenteral therapy is also more dangerous and more expensive than oral medication.

Enteral routes

Oral route. The oral (PO) route of administration is the simplest way to introduce a drug into the body. It allows the use of many different dosage forms to obtain the desired results; tablets, capsules, and liquids are conveniently given. An advantage of this route is the large absorbing area present in the small intestine. Oral administration produces a slower onset of action than parenterally administered agents. One disadvantage of this route is that stomach and intestinal irritation may result in nausea and vomiting. Another disadvantage is that certain drugs such as insulin are inactivated by gastrointestinal tract acidity or enzymes. When drugs are given orally, they initially pass through the hepatic (liver) portal circulation, which inactivates some drugs. This inactivation by the liver is termed the first-pass effect.

The blood levels obtained after oral administration are less predictable than those obtained parenterally. The presence of food in the stomach, pathologic conditions of the gastrointestinal tract, the effects of gastric acidity, and passage through the hepatic portal circulation can alter blood levels. The oral route necessitates greater patient cooperation.

Rectal route. Drugs may be given rectally as suppositories, creams, or enemas. Rectal administration can be used if a patient is vomiting or unconscious. This route may be used for either a local (e.g., hemorrhoids) or a systemic (e.g., antiemetic) effect. Because most drugs are poorly and irregularly absorbed rectally, this route is not frequently used to achieve a systemic drug effect. Also, patient acceptance of this route is poor.

Parenteral routes

Intravenous route. Intravenous (IV) administration produces the most rapid drug response, with an almost immediate onset of action. Because the injection is made directly into the blood, the absorption phase is bypassed. Another advantage of the IV route is that it produces a more predictable response than oral administration because factors that affect drug absorption have been eliminated. It is also the route of choice for an emergency situation. The disadvantages of IV administration include phlebitis caused by local irritation, drug irretrievability, al-

lergy, and side effects related to high plasma concentrations of the drug.

Intramuscular route. Absorption of drugs injected into the muscle occurs because of the high blood flow through skeletal muscles. Somewhat irritating drugs may be tolerated if given by the intramuscular (IM) route. This route may also be used for injection of suspensions to provide a sustained effect. Injections are usually made in the deltoid region or gluteal mass.

Subcutaneous route. The subcutaneous (SC, SQ) route involves the injection of solutions or suspensions of drugs into the subcutaneous areolar tissue to gain access to the systemic circulation. If irritating solutions are injected, sterile abscesses may result. Insulin is commonly administered by this route.

Intradermal route. Small amounts of drugs such as local anesthetics can be injected into the epidermis of the skin to provide local anesthesia. The tuberculosis skin test is performed using the intradermal (ID) route.

Intrathecal route. Intrathecal (IT) administration involves the injection of solutions into the spinal subarachnoid space. This may be used for spinal anesthesia or for the treatment of certain forms of meningitis.

Intraperitoneal route. Injections may be made into the peritoneal cavity where absorption of the drug occurs through the mesenteric veins.

Inhalation route. Gaseous, microcrystalline, and volatile drugs may be administered by inhalation. They are then absorbed through the pulmonary endothelium in the alveoli to gain access to the systemic circulation. General anesthetics such as ether, halothane, and nitrous oxide (laughing gas) are given by this route. Drugs in solution may be aerosolized so that the fine droplets can be inhaled into the lungs. Finely powdered drugs may also be inhaled to be absorbed through the mucous membranes of the respiratory tract. This route of administration is commonly used in the treatment of asthma.

Topical route. The topical route of administration includes local application to oral mucous membranes, the skin, and other epithelial surfaces. Topical application may be used to obtain either local or systemic effects. A local anesthetic may be applied topically to the mucous membranes of the oral cavity to provide anesthesia before an injection.

Since most drugs do not penetrate intact skin, application to the skin is generally used for local effects. However, some highly lipid-soluble substances such as organophosphate insecticides can produce toxicity if they come in contact with the skin. Rarely, systemic side effects can occur from topical administration of corticosteroids. Systemic effects are more likely if an occlusive dressing is applied, a large area is treated topically, or the skin is abraded or denuded. Drugs that frequently produce allergic reactions such as penicillin should not be applied topically, since sensitization occurs more readily.

For systemic effects an ointment containing nitroglycerin is available for topical application. When applied to the intact skin of the arm or chest, it is absorbed systemically and produces an effect on the blood vessels of the heart.

Drugs can be applied locally to the vagina as suppositories or creams. Drugs can also produce local effects when instilled into the ear and eye as solutions or suspensions. Some extremely toxic drugs may be safely administered to the eye to cause a local effect with little systemic effect.

Although solutions or sprays may be applied to the throat or nose for their local effects, occasionally systemic effects can result. For example, when certain local anesthetic sprays such as tetracaine are applied to the mucous membranes, they can achieve systemic blood levels equivalent to those after intravenous injection.

SUBLINGUAL AND BUCCAL ROUTES. The mucous membranes of the oral cavity provide a convenient absorbing surface for the systemic administration of drugs, which can be placed under the tongue (sublingual) or on other areas of the oral mucosa (buccal pouch). Absorption of many drugs into the systemic circulation occurs rapidly. An example of this effect is the fast onset of action of nitroglycerin sublingual tablets to treat acute anginal pain. Drugs that are susceptible to degradation by the gastrointestinal tract and even the

liver, such as testosterone, are safely administered as sublingual tablets.

TRANSDERMAL PATCH. Transdermal drug delivery systems (drug patches) are designed to provide continuous controlled release of medication through a semipermeable membrane over a given period after application of drug to the intact skin. This eliminates the need for repeated oral dosing. There are four currently marketed patch systems: scopolamine (Transderm-Scop), nitroglycerin (Transderm-Nitro, Nitrodisc, Nitro-Dur), clonidine (Catapres-TTS), and estradiol (Estraderm). The patch itself comprises four layers. Proceeding from the visible surface toward the surface attached to the skin, these are (1) a tan-colored backing layer that is impermeable to the drug; (2) a drug reservoir in which the drug is absorbed on lactose, colloidal silicone dioxide, and silicone medical fluid; (3) a polymer membrane permeable to the drug; and (4) a layer of hypoallergenic silicone adhesive. Before use a protective strip is removed from the adhesive surface.

Dermatologic reactions have occurred from the adhesive of the patch, and a new generation of patches is under development. These new breathable (air-permeable) patches can remain in place for 1 week to 1 month with fewer dermatologic side effects than the other patches. Agents being tested for use as transdermal patches include contraceptives, nonsteroid antiinflammatory analgesics, opioid analgesics, and antihypertensive drugs.

Dosage forms

Table 2-1 lists the usual dosage forms. The most commonly used dosage forms in dentistry are the tablet and capsule. Sometimes drugs are given in solution or suspension when a liquid form is desired. For injection the drug may be in solution such as a local anesthetic, or it may be in a suspension such as procaine penicillin G when a longer duration of action is desired. Mouthwashes containing alcohol are also recommended by dental hygienists.

Table 2-1. Dosage forms

Form	Definition	Example
Tablet	Molded or compressed medicinal substance with inert binder included to make a hard mass	Aspirin tablet
Capsule	Gelatin shell that disintegrates in water to administer solids or lipids	Tetracycline capsule
Pill	Globular or ovoid dosage form made by incorporating medicinal agents with other binders to make a plastic mass; obsolete	Ferrous carbonate pill
Lozenge, troche	Flavored dosage form, often round, designed to be held in the mouth to dissolve or disintegrate slowly	Cough drop
Suppository	Single dosage medication in waxy or fatty conical or ovoid shape that liberates active ingredient after insertion into the rectum or vagina for local or systemic effects	Glycerin suppository
Solution	One-phase system of two or more chemical components	Saline water
Elixir	Sweetened hydroalcoholic solution containing flavoring materials	Diphenhydramine elixir
Syrup	Nearly saturated aqueous solution of sugar	Senna syrup
Tincture	Alcoholic or hydroalcoholic solution of drugs	Iodine tincture
Spirit	Solution of volatile substance in alcohol	Aromatic ammonia spirit
Emulsion	Preparation of two immiscible liquids, usually water and oil, one dispersed as small globules in the other	Liquid petrolatum emulsion
Suspension	Dispersion containing finely divided insoluble material suspended in a liquid medium	Penicillin suspension
Ointment	Semisolid preparation for external use that is of a consistency that can be applied by rubbing	Hydrocortisone ointment, A and D Ointment
Transdermal patch	A permeable polymer membrane backed with a drug reservoir designed to provide controlled release of medication over a given period after application to the intact skin	Nitroglycerine, scopolamine

Passage across body membranes

The amount of drug passing through a body membrane and the rate at which a drug moves are important in describing the time course of action and the variation in individual response for a drug. Before a drug is absorbed, transported, and distributed to body tissues, metabolized, and subsequently eliminated from the body, it must pass through various membranes such as the blood capillary membranes, cellular membranes, and intracellular membranes. Although these membranes have variable functions, they share certain physicochemical characteristics that influence the passage of drugs across their borders. These membranes are composed of lipids (fats), proteins, and carbohydrates. The membrane lipids make the membrane relatively impermeable to ions and polar molecules. Membrane proteins function as enzymes in the transport process and also make up the structural components of the membrane. Membrane carbohydrates are combined with either proteins or lipids. The lipid molecules orient themselves so that they form a fluid bimolecular leaflet structure, with the hydrophobic ends of the molecules shielded from the surrounding aqueous environment and the hydrophilic ends in contact with the water. The various proteins are embedded in and layered onto this fluid lipid bilayer, forming a mosaic (Fig. 2-4). Studies of the ability of substances to penetrate this membrane have indicated the presence of a system of pores or holes through which lower molecular weight and smaller size chemicals can pass.

The physicochemical properties of drugs that influence their passage across biologic membranes are lipid solubility, degree of ionization, and molecular size and shape. The mechanism of drug transfer across biologic membranes is by passive transfer and specialized transport.

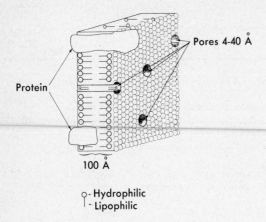

Fig. 2-4. Membrane structure.

Passive transfer

Lipid-soluble substances move across the lipoprotein membrane by a passive transfer process called **simple diffusion**. This type of transfer is directly proportional to the concentration gradient (difference) of the drug across the membrane and the degree of lipid solubility. For example, a highly lipid-soluble compound will attain a higher concentration at the membrane site and will readily diffuse across the membrane into an area of lower concentration.

Water-soluble molecules small enough to pass through the membrane pores may be carried through the pores by the bulk flow of water. This process of **filtration** through single-cell membranes may occur with drugs having molecular weights of 200 or less. However, drugs with molecular weights of 60,000 can "filter" through capillary membranes.

Specialized transport

Certain substances are transported across cell membranes by the following processes, which are more complex than simple diffusion or filtration:

1. **Active transport** is a process by which a substance is transported against a concentration gradient or electrochemical gradient. This action is blocked by metabolic inhibitors. Active transport is believed to be mediated by transport "carriers" that furnish energy for the transportation of the drug.
2. **Facilitated diffusion** does not move against a concentration gradient. This phenomenon involves the transport of some substances such as glucose into cells. It is also blocked by metabolic inhibitors. It has been suggested that the process of pinocytosis may explain the passage of macromolecular substances into the cells.

Fig. 2-5 shows the passage of drugs across body membranes in diagrammatic form. The various aspects of this figure are discussed now, beginning with absorption.

Absorption

Absorption is the process by which drug molecules are transferred from the site of administration in the body to the circulating fluids. This process requires the drug to pass through biologic membranes.

The following factors influence the rate of absorption of a drug:

1. The physicochemical factors discussed previously.
2. The site of absorption, which is determined by the route of administration. For example, one advantage of the oral route is the large absorbing area presented by the gastrointestinal mucosa.
3. The drug's solubility. Drugs in solution are more rapidly absorbed than are insoluble drugs.

Effect of ionization

Drugs that are weak electrolytes dissociate in solution into a nonionized form and an ionized form. The nonionized or uncharged portion acts like a nonpolar, lipid-soluble compound that readily traverses body membranes. The ionized portion, being less lipid soluble, will traverse these membranes with greater difficulty. Thus the more the compound is ionized, the less absorption will occur, and vice versa (Fig. 2-6).

The pH of the tissues at the site of administra-

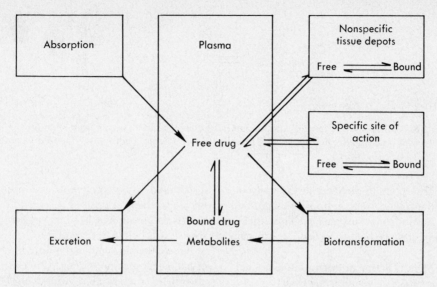

Fig. 2-5. Absorption and fate of a drug. (From Holroyd, S.V.: Clinical pharmacology in dental practice, ed. 4, St. Louis, 1987, The C.V. Mosby Co.)

tion and the dissociation characteristics of the drug will determine the amount of ionization of any weak electrolyte.

1. For **weak acids,** the higher the pH (more alkaline), the greater the degree of ionization.

$$H^+ + A^- \rightleftharpoons H \cdot A$$

2. For **weak bases,** the lower the pH (more acid), the greater the ionization.

$$\diagdown N \diagup + H^+ \rightleftharpoons -N^+ -H$$

The dissociation characteristics of a weak electrolyte are given by the dissociation constant (pKa), which is an indication of the electrolyte's tendency to ionize. When the pKa is the same as the pH, half of the compound will be ionized and half will be nonionized. For example, aspirin, which has a pKa of 3.5, will be 50% ionized when the pH is 3.5. Since aspirin is a weak acid, de-

creasing the pH below 3.5 would decrease ionization to less than 50%. This would result in an increase in the amount of nonionized aspirin, and absorption would increase. Conversely, increasing the pH above 3.5, as would occur in the intestine or if the gastric contents were alkalinized with antacid, would increase the ionization of aspirin above 50% and subsequently decrease the amount absorbed. Increasing the pH also facilitates dissolution. This increases aspirin's absorption.

This principle can also explain the fact that in infection the acidity of the tissue increases (lower pH) and the action of local anesthetics decreases. For weak bases such as the local anesthetics, the lower pH would result in greater ionization. This increased ionization could result in a decreased penetration of the membrane and a decreased clinical effect.

Oral absorption

The dosage form of a drug is an important factor influencing absorption by the oral route of administration. Unless the drug is administered as a so-

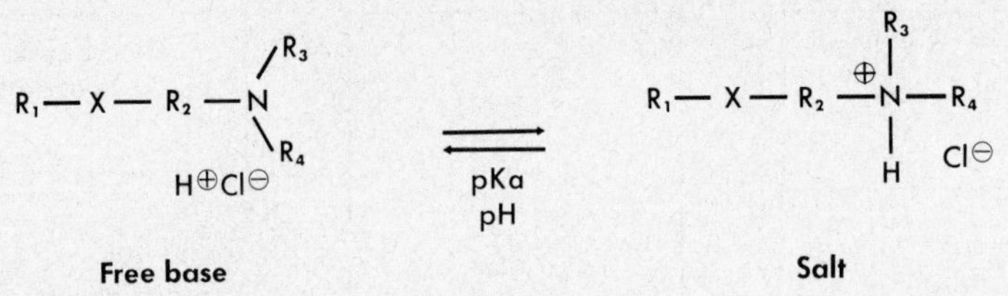

Fig. 2-6.   Dissociation of ionized and nonionized forms. The free base is fat soluble (lipophilic), nonionized (uncharged), and nonpolar. The salt is water soluble (hydrophilic), ionized (charged), and polar (see Fig. 12-1). *X*, ester or amide.

lution, the absorption of the drug in the gastrointestinal tract involves a release from a dosage such as a tablet, capsule, or suspension. This release requires several steps before absorption can take place:

1. Disruption. The initial disruption of a tablet coating or capsule shell is necessary.
2. Disintegration. The tablet or capsule contents must disintegrate (break apart).
3. Dispersion. The concentrated drug particles must be dispersed (spread) throughout the stomach or intestines.
4. Dissolution. The drug must be dissolved (in solution) in the gastrointestinal fluid.

Absorption from injection site

The absorption of a drug from the site of injection depends on the solubility of the drug and the blood flow at that site. For example, drugs with low water solubility such as some penicillin salts are absorbed very slowly after intramuscular injection. Absorption at injection sites is also affected by the dosage form. Drugs in suspension are absorbed much more slowly than those in solution. Certain insulin preparations are formulated in suspension form to decrease their absorption rate and prolong their action.

Distribution

For a drug to exert its activity, it must be made available to its site of action in the body. The mechanism by which this is accomplished is distribution: the passage of drugs into various body fluid compartments such as plasma, interstitial fluids, and intracellular fluids. The way a drug is distributed in the body will determine how rapidly it produces a desired response, the duration of that response, and in some cases whether a response will be elicited at all.

Drug distribution allows a drug to reach its site of action in specific tissues. However, drugs are also distributed to areas where no action is desired (nonspecific tissues), which serve as storage depots (see Fig. 2-5). Some drugs, because of their characteristics, are poorly distributed to certain regions of the body. Other drugs are distributed and then redistributed from one tissue site to another.

Distribution by plasma

After a drug is absorbed from its site of administration, it is distributed to its site of action by the blood plasma (see Fig. 2-5). Therefore the biologic activity of a drug is related to the concentration of the free or unbound drug in the plasma. Drugs are bound reversibly to plasma proteins such as albumin and globulin. The drug that is bound to the protein does not contribute to the intensity of the drug action, since only the unbound form is biologically active. The bound drug is considered a storage site. If one drug is highly bound, another drug may displace it from its plasma protein binding sites, increasing the effect of the first drug.

Tissue distribution

The distribution by the plasma eventually places the drug in organ tissue sites. These sites may be either specific or nonspecific. The specific site elicits the therapeutic response desired, whereas the nonspecific site elicits either no response or an undesirable one. When drugs are distributed to the tissues from the plasma, the process involves the passage of drugs across cell membranes. Drugs are also bound to components inside the cells.

The biologic **half-life** ($t_\frac{1}{2}$) of a drug is the time necessary for the body to eliminate half of the drug present in the circulation at any given time. This figure determines the duration of any drug's effect; the longer the half-life, the longer the action of a drug.

The tissue sites of distribution should be considered before administration. For example, in order for drugs to penetrate the central nervous system they must cross the **blood-brain barrier**. The passage of a drug across this barrier is related to the drug's lipid solubility and degree of ionization. Thiopental, a highly lipid-soluble, nonionized drug, easily penetrates the barrier to gain access to the cerebrospinal fluid and induce sleep within seconds after IV administration. In contrast, a highly ionized compound such as hexamethonium would be unlikely to cross this barrier and therefore would produce few effects on the brain.

The passage of drugs across the **placenta** involves simple diffusion in accordance with their degree of lipid solubility. Nonionized drugs with high lipid solubility cross the placenta quickly. The placenta may act as a selective barrier against a few drugs.

Redistribution

Duration of action of a drug can be greatly affected by redistribution of the drug from one organ to another. If redistribution occurs between specific sites and nonspecific sites, a drug's action will be terminated. For example, thiopental produces sleep within seconds, but the effect subsides in a few minutes. This is because the drug is first distributed to the central nervous system, subsequently redistributed through the plasma to the muscle, and finally reaches the fat depots of the body. The rapid termination of the hypnotic activity of thiopental results from its redistribu-

tion from the brain to muscle and finally to adipose tissue. A drug may also be redistributed to other tissues.

Mechanisms of action

Once drugs have been distributed to their site of action, they can elicit a pharmacologic effect by interacting at receptor sites.

Drug-receptor interactions

The general concept of drug-receptor interactions is that drugs interact with specific macromolecular components (**receptors**) of an organism to cause a modulation in function of the organism. Drugs do not impart a new function to the organism. Many of these actions are associated with enzymatic and regulatory processes that result in modulation of cell function only after a series of reactions, not just a single reaction of drug combining to receptor. For example, many receptors respond to drug binding by stimulating or inhibiting adenylate cyclase. Intracellular receptors for steroids, such as estrogen, respond to drug binding by inducing the synthesis of specific proteins that bind to nuclear chromatin and enhance the transcription of genetic material. Also, receptors for several types of endogenous chemicals such as acetylcholine and γ-aminobutyric acid (GABA), and maybe for selected drugs, are the actual ion channels in the cell membrane. These channels open in response to the drug to control the membrane potential of the cell and influence its composition.

Most drug receptors are cellular proteins and are involved in transport processes, metabolic pathways, and regulatory pathways. Many of these proteins normally function to act as receptors for endogenous substances such as hormones, neurotransmitters (acetylcholine and norepinephrine), autocoids (kinins and prostaglandins), and the morphine-like neuropolypeptides (enkephalins and endorphins).

When a drug combines with a receptor to cause a modulation in function, enhancement or inhibition of the organism results. Drugs are called **agonists** when they cause effects by directly altering the functional properties of the receptors with which they interact. Drugs can also cause effects by inhibiting the action of an agonist drug by competing for the agonist's binding sites on the receptor. These drugs usually have no intrinsic activity of their own and are called **antagonists**. Although certain antagonists interact with receptors to inhibit the action of an agonist while initiating no effect themselves, the inhibition can be overcome by increasing the concentration of the agonist. This type of inhibition is termed **competitive** and occurs when the antagonist binds reversibly to a receptor. A **noncompetitive** antagonist prevents the agonist from producing effects, no matter what the concentration of the agonist, and usually results from the irreversible binding of the antagonist to the receptor.

Physicochemical action

The mechanism by which some drugs may act involves the alteration of the structure of essential macromolecules. This action may characterize agents such as general anesthetics that act at the cellular level through physicochemical rather than purely chemical means.

Metabolism (biotransformation)

A mechanism for termination of drug action must exist, since most drugs have a limited duration of action in the body. The processes of metabolism or biotransformation and elimination provide termination of drug action.

Many drugs undergo metabolic transformation or change in the body. The metabolic product (metabolite) formed is usually more polar (ionized) and less lipid soluble than its parent compound. This means that renal tubular reabsorption of the metabolite will be reduced, since this process favors lipid-soluble compounds. Metabolites are also less likely to bind to plasma or tissue proteins and less likely to be stored in fat tissue. Decreased renal tubular reabsorption, decreased binding to the plasma or tissue proteins, and decreased fat storage cause the metabolite to be excreted more easily.

Drug metabolism is an enzyme-dependent process that has developed through evolution. Although this process results in the formation of compounds of a more polar nature, these products are not always biologically inactive. Enzymatic change (metabolism) of a parent drug can result in three patterns:

1. An inactive parent drug may be transformed into an active compound. The inactive compound is then called a **prodrug**.
2. An active parent drug may be converted to a second active compound that is then converted to an inactive product. This can prolong the action of a drug.
3. An inactive compound may be formed from an active parent drug. This type of reaction is the most common in drug biotransformation.

Although the rates and pathways of drug metabolism may vary, most studies indicate that drug biotransformation in laboratory animals is similar to that in humans. Many synthetic mechanisms of drug metabolism occur in the body to form metabolites. Table 2-2 summarizes these mechanisms and indicates some of the compounds that are detoxified by each mechanism and the active compound responsible for the donation of a molecule for metabolism.

Conjugation

The body can convert a lipid-soluble drug to a more polar compound through the synthesis of a conjugated compound. This is achieved by the attachment of a molecule of an acid present in the body to the drug being conjugated. Either the parent drug or the metabolites formed in the body can be conjugated—a process mediated by enzymes called **transferases**.

Glucuronic acid, one of the acids involved in the conjugation process, is a substance normally occurring in the body. It may be transferred to a drug molecule with an appropriate functional group to accept it. Functional groups that may be involved include ethers, alcohols, aromatic amines, and carboxylic acid.

Table 2-2. Synthetic mechanisms of drug metabolism

Mechanism	Compounds detoxicated	Active donor compound
Glucuronic acid conjugation	Compounds having: 　Phenolic OH 　Alcoholic OH 　COOH 　Aromatic amines	Glucuronic acid as uridine diphosphoglucuronic 　acid (UDPGA)
Acetylation	Aromatic amines	Acetyl CoA
Mercapturic acid formation	Aromatic hydrocarbons Halogenated aromatic hydrocarbons Halogenated nitrobenzenes	Activated glutathione
Sulfuric acid ester formation	Aromatic OH Aliphatic OH	3′-Phosphoadenosine-5′-phosphosulfate (PAPS)
Glutamine conjugation	Aromatic acids	CoA derivative of the acid to be conjugated
Methylation	Compounds having: 　Two phenolic OH 　>NH 　—NH$_2$	S-Adenosylmethionine

From Holroyd, S.V.: Clinical pharmacology in dental practice, ed. 4, St. Louis, 1987, The C.V. Mosby Co.

Oxidation

When a drug does not possess the appropriate functional group suitable for conjugation, the body has a more difficult problem detoxifying that drug. An enzyme system responsible for the oxidative metabolism of many drugs is located in the liver. The enzymes are located in the endoplasmic reticulum and are termed **microsomal enzymes,** since they are found in the microsomal fraction as prepared from liver homogenates. A variety of oxidative reactions, such as hydroxylation or incorporation of oxygen into the substrate molecule, occur in these hepatic microsomes. The specific metabolic reactions include the following:

Aromatic ring and side-chain hydroxylation
N-dealkylation and O-dealkylation
Sulfoxide formation
N-oxidation and N-hydroxylation
Deamination of primary and secondary amines

Oxidative processes involving enzymes other than those of the hepatic microsomal system may take place. Some compounds are oxidatively deaminated by enzymes located in the liver, kidney, and nervous tissue. Other agents are detoxified by specific oxidative enzymes.

Hydrolysis

Some ester compounds are metabolized by hydrolysis. Hydrolytic enzymes, found in the plasma and in a variety of tissues, break up esters and add water. The ester local anesthetics are inactivated by plasma cholinesterases.

Reduction

Many reduction reactions are mediated by the enzymes found in the hepatic microsomes.

Hepatic microsomal enzyme drug metabolism

It has been well documented that the activity of the hepatic microsomal enzymes is increased when certain drugs are administered. This is caused by an increase in the concentration of an enzyme protein—a phenomenon referred to as **enzyme induction**. Drugs that cause enzyme induction can decrease the pharmacologic response to certain agents metabolized in the liver. For example, phenobarbital stimulates the production of microsomal enzymes that normally metabolize the anticoagulant warfarin. Thus phenobarbital decreases the anticoagulant response by increasing the metabolism of the anticoagulant.

Some drugs can also stimulate their own metabolism. The tolerance that patients develop to certain drugs can be explained, at least in part, by an increased ability to metabolize the drug because of stimulation of microsomal enzymes.

Excretion

Although drugs may be excreted by any route that has direct access to the environment, renal (kidney) excretion is the most important. Extrarenal routes include the lungs, bile, gastrointestinal tract, sweat, saliva, and milk. Drugs may be excreted unchanged or as metabolites.

Renal route

Elimination of substances in the kidney can occur by three routes:

1. Glomerular filtration. Either the unchanged drug or its metabolites are filtered through the glomeruli and concentrated in the renal tubular fluid. This filtration process depends on the amount of plasma protein binding and the glomerular filtration rate. Bound drugs cannot be filtered and remain in the systemic circulation.

2. Active tubular secretion. Active secretion transports the drug from the bloodstream across the renal tubular epithelial cells and into the renal tubular fluid. Glomerular filtration and active tubular secretion are relatively nonselective, and several compounds, both exogenous and naturally occurring, can compete for transport.

3. Passive tubular diffusion. With most drugs, passive tubular diffusion plays a part in regulating the amount of drug in the tubular fluid. This is also termed passive reabsorption. This process favors the reabsorption of nonionized, lipid-soluble compounds. Since more ionized, less lipid-soluble metabolites have more difficulty in penetrating the cell membranes of the renal tubules, they are more likely to be retained in the tubular fluid and eliminated in the urine. This process is also influenced by the urinary pH, which affects the amount of ionized and nonionized drug in the tubular fluid. By altering the pH of the urine, drug excretion can be favored in cases of poisoning or can be inhibited when a prolongation of the drug effect is desired. Weakly ionized acids or bases are excreted in the following fashion:

a. Alkaline urine. When the tubular urinary pH is more alkaline than the plasma, weak acids are excreted more rapidly and weak bases are excreted more slowly.

b. Acid urine. When tubular urine is more acid, weak acids are excreted more slowly and weak bases are excreted more rapidly.

Extrarenal routes

Certain drugs may be partially or completely eliminated by the lungs. For example, gases used in general anesthesia are excreted across the lung tissue by a process of simple diffusion. This fact is used when testing the breath for the presence of alcohol.

Biliary excretion is the major route by which systemically absorbed drugs enter the gastrointestinal tract and are eliminated in the feces. Drugs excreted in the bile may also be reabsorbed from the intestines. This is termed **enterohepatic** circulation and prolongs a drug's action.

Two minor routes of elimination are excretion in the milk and sweat. The excretion of drugs in milk may be a potential source of undesirable effects for the nursing infant.

Salivary drug secretion is of interest in dentistry. After drugs are excreted in the saliva, they are usually swallowed and their fate is the same as that of drugs ingested orally. The following drugs have been detected at significant levels in saliva after oral ingestion: aspirin, phenytoin, ampicillin, diazepam, penicillin VK, and phenobarbital. Present evidence suggests that most drugs that are secreted in the salivary glands enter saliva by simple diffusion, and their passage depends mainly on the lipid solubility of the drug.

Thus a drug with high lipid solubility at plasma and salivary pH will readily enter saliva from plasma.

Drug levels in saliva can be used to monitor therapy with certain agents. For example, antiepileptic drug monitoring is essential for the rational treatment of the epilepsies, and the measurement of these drugs in plasma is now routine. Assay of salivary concentrations of these drugs has been shown to be a reliable, noninvasive method of predicting plasma levels.

Drugs may also be excreted in the gingival crevicular fluid (GCF). Drugs excreted in the GCF may be useful in treating periodontal disease.

FACTORS THAT ALTER DRUG EFFECTS

When a drug is administered, the following factors may influence or modify a drug's effect:

1. Patient compliance. Through either lack of understanding or lack or motivation, patients often take medication incorrectly or not at all. Sometimes this may result from faulty communication or inadequate patient education.

2. Placebo effect. A placebo effect is the effect associated with the taking of an inert compound. The magnitude of this effect depends on the patient's perception, and there is large individual variation. The placebo effect can be used to advantage to achieve an improved therapeutic result.

3. Tolerance. A patient may exhibit tolerance to many drugs, including the sedative-hypnotics and the opioids. Drug **tolerance** is defined as the need for an increasingly larger dose of the drug to obtain the same effects as with the original dose, or the decreased effect produced after repeated administration of a given dose of the drug. When a patient becomes tolerant to one drug, **cross-tolerance** develops to the action of other drugs with a similar pharmacologic activity. If tolerance does develop, a normal sensitivity to the drug's effect may be restored by ceasing administration of the drug. **Tachyphylaxis** is the very rapid development of tolerance, often within hours.

4. Pathologic state. Diseased patients may respond to the administration of medication differently from other patients. For example, patients with hyperthyroidism are extremely sensitive to the toxic effects of epinephrine. Hepatic or renal disease influences the metabolism and excretion of drugs, potentially leading to an increased duration of drug action.

5. Time of administration. The time a drug is administered, especially in relation to meals, alters the response to that drug. Certain drugs with a sedative action are best administered at bedtime.

6. Route of administration. The effect of the route of administration on the onset and duration of action of a drug was discussed previously.

7. Sex. The sex of the patient can alter a drug's effect. Women may be more sensitive to certain drugs than men, perhaps because of their smaller size. Pregnancy alters the effect of certain drugs.

8. Genetic variation. Many differences in patient response to drugs have been identified with variations in ability to metabolize certain drugs. This difference may account for the fact that certain populations have a higher incidence of adverse effects to some drugs—a genetic predisposition.

9. Drug interactions. A drug's effect may be modified by previous or concomitant administration of another agent. There are many mechanisms by which drug interactions may modify a patient's treatment, as discussed in Chapter 25.

10. Age and weight. The amount of drug administered to a patient depends partially on the age and weight of the patient. Because the age of a patient is only roughly proportional to the patient's weight, age is rarely used to determine the dosage of a drug for children.

Calculation of children's dosage

The patient's weight is the usual basis for determining drug dosage, although not the ideal method. Table 2-3 gives various methods of determining the child's dose based on the adult's dose.

Table 2-3. Children's dosage calculations

1. *Clark's rule:*
$$\frac{\text{Weight (lb)} \times \text{Adult dose}}{150} = \text{Infant dose}$$

2. *Fried's rule:*
$$\frac{\text{Age (mo)} \times \text{Adult dose}}{150} = \text{Infant dose}$$

3. *Young's rule:*
$$\frac{\text{Age (yr)} \times \text{Adult dose}}{\text{Age (yr)} + 12} = \text{Child dose}$$

4. *Cowling's rule:*
$$\frac{\text{Age (at next birthday)} \times \text{Adult dose}}{24} = \text{Child dose}$$

5. *Surface area rule:*
$(0.7 \times \text{weight in lb}) + 10 = \%$ Adult dose
$(1.5 \times \text{weight in kg}) + 10 = \%$ Adult dose

Since weight may vary in children of the same age, a better method of calculating a child's or infant's dose is based on body surface area (Table 2-3). This method requires the use of a table or nomogram from which the body surface of the child can be determined. The surface area formula is convenient and more accurate than formulas based on age or weight of the child.

Another method for determining the child's dose is to follow a suggested pediatric dosage schedule prepared by the manufacturer. These are usually given in terms of drug per pound or kilogram of body weight per 24 hours. This is especially common for antibiotic agents. It is important to note that the 24-hour dose must be divided into doses given at several administration times. The manufacturer's recommendations probably provide the most accurate suggestions.

REVIEW QUESTIONS

1. Define and differentiate between the potency and efficacy of a drug.
2. Describe the dose-response curve using the terms "ED50" (effective dose) and "LD50" (lethal dose).
3. Define the term "pharmacokinetics." Name the four categories involved.
4. Define the major routes of drug administration including the following:
   a. Oral
   b. Intravenous
   c. Inhalation
   d. Topical
5. State the dosage forms most frequently used in dentistry.
6. Describe the mechanism of drug transfer across biologic membranes.
7. Explain the influence of pH on the dissociation characteristics of weak acids and weak bases. Describe one dental example of each for absorption and excretion.
8. Explain each of the steps involved in oral absorption including the following:
   a. Disruption
   b. Disintegration
   c. Dispersion
   d. Dissolution
9. Define the $t_{1/2}$ or half-life of a drug and state its significance.
10. Define the following terms:
    a. Agonist
    b. Antagonist
    c. Partial agonist
    d. Competitive antagonist
11. Describe the importance of the hepatic microsomal enzymes in relation to drug metabolism.
12. State the major route of drug excretion and describe the three processes by which it occurs.
13. When given a child's weight (20 kg) and the usual adult dose of a drug (100 mg), determine the child's dose using the best method.

Chapter 3

Adverse reactions

Although drugs may act on biologic systems to accomplish a desired effect, they lack absolute specificity in that they can act on many different organs or tissues. This lack of specificity is the reason for undesirable or adverse drug reactions. No drug is free from producing some adverse effects in a certain number of patients. It has been estimated that about 5% of the patients hospitalized annually in the United States are admitted because of adverse reactions to drugs,[1] with some hospitals reporting an incidence as high as 20%.[2] A minimum of 15% of hospitalized patients experience at least one adverse drug reaction.[3]

The dental hygienist is in a good position to observe any adverse reactions or undesirable effects caused by drugs administered in the dental office. Adverse reactions to drugs prescribed by the patient's physician can be identified in the health history. The side effects of drugs that affect the oral cavity can also be noted. A knowledge of adverse drug reactions can help dental office personnel to minimize or prevent them. Because of the rapport between a patient and the dental hygienist, the patient will often reveal important facts about the health history or ask questions concerning medications prescribed. The dental hygienist must know the terms used to describe an adverse reaction in order to discuss a drug's undesirable effect accurately with other health professionals. For example, the word "allergy," refers to a specific type of reaction to a drug.

DEFINITIONS AND CLASSIFICATIONS

Unfortunately, every drug has more than one action. The clinically desirable actions are termed **therapeutic effects,** and the undesirable reactions are termed **adverse effects.** This division of a drug's effects into two categories will depend on the use of the drug. For example, if an antihistamine used to relieve hay fever causes drowsiness, that can be considered an adverse effect. However, if the antihistamine were being used to induce sleep, drowsiness would be considered a therapeutic effect.

An adverse drug reaction is a response to a drug that is not desired, is potentially harmful, and that occurs at usual therapeutic doses. It may be an exaggeration of the desired response, an expected but not desired response, an allergic or cytotoxic reaction, or it may affect the fetus. Often adverse drug reactions are divided into the following categories:

1. Toxic reaction. This adverse drug reaction is an extension of the pharmacologic effect resulting from a drug's effect on the target organs. In this instance, the amount of the desired effect is excessive.

2. Side effect. A side effect is a dose-related reaction that is not related to the desired therapeutic outcome. It occurs when a drug acts on nontarget organs producing undesirable effects. Although not strictly correct, often the terms "side effect" and "adverse reaction" are used interchangably.

3. Idiosyncratic reaction. An idiosyncratic reaction is a genetically related abnormal drug response. Certain populations, because of their genetic constitution, are more susceptible to certain adverse reactions to specific drugs.

4. Drug allergy. A drug allergy is an immunologic response to a drug resulting in a reaction such as rash or anaphylaxis.

5. Interference with natural defense mecha-

nisms. Certain drugs, such as steroids, can reduce the body's ability to fight infection.

The importance of distinguishing between different types of adverse effects can be seen from an example of penicillin G. Penicillin's two different types of adverse reactions vary greatly in their incidence, with its toxicity being low since it has practically no effect on body tissues, whereas its allergenic potential is high. These differences are significant and become pertinent when discussing an adverse reaction with another health professional. Fig. 3-1 describes the types of adverse reactions and notes whether they are predictable and/or dose dependent.

CLINICAL MANIFESTATIONS OF ADVERSE REACTIONS
Exaggerated effect on target tissues

One type of adverse reaction may be caused by an exaggerated effect of a drug on its target organ or tissue. This is considered to be an extension of the therapeutic effect caused by an overreaction of a sensitive patient or by a dose of the drug that is too large. For example, a patient may experience exaggerated hypoglycemia when given a therapeutic dose of a hypoglycemic agent for the treatment of diabetes. The patient's blood sugar may fall too low, either because of an unusual sensitivity to the drug or because the dose administered was too high for that patient. Occasionally, this type of adverse reaction may result from liver or kidney disease. Because the disease interferes with the drug's metabolism or excretion the drug's action may be enhanced or prolonged.

Effect on nontarget tissues

The effect on nontarget organs or tissues is caused by the nontherapeutic action of the drug. These reactions can occur at usual doses, but they appear more frequently at higher doses. For example, aspirin may produce gastric upset in usual therapeutic doses, but with higher doses salicylism, characterized by tinnitus, disturbances in acid-base balance, and confusion, can result. These toxic reactions can affect many parts of the body. A reduction in the dose of a drug usually reduces these adverse reactions.

Effect on fetal development (teratogenic effect)

The word "teratogenic" comes from the Greek prefix *terato-*, meaning monster and the suffix *-genic* meaning producing, or producing a malformed fetus. Since 1941 when the relationship between German measles and birth defects was noticed, the relationship between drugs and congenital abnormalities has been recognized. In 1961 thalidomide, an over-the-counter (OTC) drug in Europe, was found to produce phocomelia, or short limbs, in exposed infants. This incident reinforced the lack of sufficient studies to make drugs safe for the pregnant woman. Even though more information is now available about the safety of drugs in the pregnant woman, sufficient information is still lacking.

The Food and Drug Administration (FDA) has attempted to address concerns about the lack of adequate knowledge of drugs by devising five FDA pregnancy categories—A, B, C, D, and X, ranked from least to most risk. Table 24-1 discusses the meaning of these categories.

Although no drug can be considered "safe" for administration to a pregnant woman, many of the drugs used in dentistry are considered among the safest including penicillin, lidocaine, and erythromycin, but even these drugs should be admin-

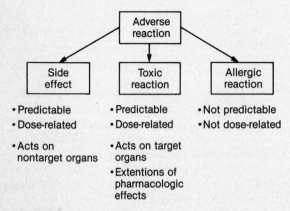

Fig. 3-1. Diagram of classification of adverse drug reactions.

istered only if there is a clear need. Elective dental procedures should be conservatively addressed. Drugs that are used in dentistry that are contraindicated include tetracycline, nonsteroidal antiinflammatory agents, and the benzodiazepines. The teratogenic potential for drugs are discussed in Chapter 24.

Many drug manufacturers, especially those that produce some of the older drugs, continue to place in their package inserts such statements as the following:

1. "There are no adequate and well-controlled studies in pregnant women."
2. "Risks must be balanced against the uncontrolled disease."
3. "Safety during pregnancy has not been established; use requires that potential benefits be weighed against its possible hazard to the mother and child."
4. "Animal reproductive studies are not always indicative of human effects."

Encouraging changes in the information provided, especially for newer agents, have resulted in more information about usage during pregnancy such as the following statements:

1. "Pregnancy category D"
2. "Shown to decrease fetal birth weight . . . when given at 50 times the dose recommended for humans"
3. "No evidence of birth abnormalities or impaired fertility in doses 2 times the usual human dose"

In regard to teratogenesis, it is important to remember that the risk to the fetus must always be considered when considering the benefit to the mother. Also dental patients do not always announce that they are pregnant, so it is important to ask any woman of childbearing age if she is pregnant so that problem drugs can be avoided as early as possible during the pregnancy.

Local effect

Local reactions are characterized by local tissue irritation. Occasionally, injectable drugs can produce irritation, pain, and tissue necrosis at the site of injection. Topically applied agents can produce irritation at the site of application. Drugs taken orally can produce gastrointestinal symptoms such as nausea or dyspepsia because of their local actions on the gastrointestinal tract.

Effect of drug interactions

The influence of one drug on the effectiveness of another drug may result in an undesirable drug effect and in some cases a toxic result. Drug interactions are discussed in Chapter 25.

Allergic reaction (hypersensitivity)

For a drug to produce an allergic reaction, it must act as an antigen and react with an antibody in a previously sensitized patient. This reaction is neither dose dependent nor predictable. For an allergic reaction to occur, an ingested drug must be metabolized to a reactive metabolite known as the **hapten.** This hapten can act as an antigen after combining with proteins in the body. The antigen formed then stimulates the production of an antibody. With subsequent exposure to the drug, the antigen formed will react with the antibody previously produced and elicit an antigen-antibody reaction. This reaction triggers a series of biochemical and physiologic events that can be life-threatening.

Drug allergy (hypersensitivity) can be divided into four types of reactions, depending on the type of antibody or cell mediating the reaction. Type I reactions are mediated by immunoglobulin E (IgE) antibodies. When a drug antigen binds to IgE antibody, histamine, leukotrienes, and prostaglandins are released producing vasodilation, edema, and the inflammatory response. The targets of this reaction are the vasculature, resulting in anaphylactic shock; the respiratory system, resulting in rhinitis and asthma; and the skin, resulting in urticaria and dermatitis. Because these reactions can occur relatively quickly after drug exposure, they are known as immediate hypersensitivity reactions. Anaphylaxis is an acute, life-threatening allergic reaction characterized by hypotension, bronchospasm, laryngeal edema, and cardiac arrhythmias that can occur within a few minutes after drug administration. Drugs used in dentistry that have produced fatal anaphylaxis include the penicillins, local anesthetics, and aspirin. Unexpected anaphylaxis may occur, such as the death of a patient medicated with a benzocaine-containing throat lozenge.

Type II, or cytolytic, reactions are complement-dependent reactions involving either immunoglobulin G (IgG) or immunoglobulin M (IgM) antibodies. The antigen-antibody complex is then fixed to a circulating blood cell resulting in lysis. Examples of this reaction are penicillin-induced hemolytic anemia and methyldopa-induced autoimmune hemolytic anemia.

Type III, or Arthus, reactions are mediated by IgG. In this reaction, the drug antigen-antibody complex fixes complement and deposits in the vascular endothelium. The reaction is manifested as serum sickness and includes urticarial skin eruptions, arthralgia, arthritis, lymphadenopathy, and fever. This reaction can be caused by the penicillins and sulfonamides.

Type IV, or delayed-hypersensitivity, reactions are mediated by sensitized T-lymphocytes and macrophages. When the cells contact the antigen an inflammatory reaction is produced by lymphokines, neutrophils, and macrophages. An example is allergic contact dermatitis caused by topical application of drugs. Both topical benzocaine and penicillin can produce this type of reaction. Another example is the dermatitis resulting from poison oak or ivy.

Idiosyncrasy

An idiosyncratic reaction is a genetically determined abnormal reaction to a drug. For example, about 10% of black males can develop severe hemolytic anemia when given the antimalarial drug, primaquine. This is due to a deficiency in an enzyme, glucose-6-phosphate dehydrogenase.

Interference with natural defense mechanisms

A drug's effect on the body defense mechanisms can result in an adverse reaction. Antibiotics have been shown to cause an overgrowth of the intestinal flora with abnormally occurring bacteria and fungi. Long-term systemic administration of corticosteroids can result in decreased resistance to infection.

TOXICOLOGIC EVALUATION OF DRUGS

Optimally, evaluations of the toxic effects of drugs are based on experiments with lower animals and clinical trials in humans. Animal experiments can frequently elicit adverse drug reactions that could occur in humans, but unfortunately, drug reactions in animals do not always predict reactions in humans. The lethal dose (LD50), one measure of the toxicity of a drug, is the dose of a drug that kills 50% of the treated animals. The median effective dose (ED50) is the dose required to produce a specified intensity of effect in 50% of the animals. Fig. 3-2 plots the dose of a drug against the percentage of maximum response (sleep or death) in animals. A dose-response curve is then obtained. The value on the dose axis that corresponds to the 50% intensity level on the response axis can be read directly from the curve. This figure is the ED50 or LD50.

Since all drugs are toxic at some dose, the LD50 is meaningless unless the ED50 is also known. The ratio LD50:ED50 is the therapeutic index of a drug.

$$\text{Therapeutic index} = \frac{LD50}{ED50}$$

This figure gives some measure of how far a therapeutic dose may be exceeded before toxic effects are elicited. It is also an indication of the "safety" of a drug. A therapeutic index of greater than 10 is usually needed to produce a therapeutically useful drug.

The LD50 and the therapeutic index derived from animal studies are merely two measurements of many that are obtained for the evaluation of any drug. The following tests are necessary to evaluate drug safety:

1. Toxicity tests. Before clinical trials, a drug must undergo tests for acute and chronic toxicity. Certain special studies, such as carcinogenicity, teratogenicity, potentiation with other drugs, and biotransformation, may be indicated by these early preclinical tests.

2. Clinical trials. Before a drug is approved for clinical trials, an Investigational New Drug (IND) application must be approved by the FDA. Clinical trials are conducted in four phases, and the

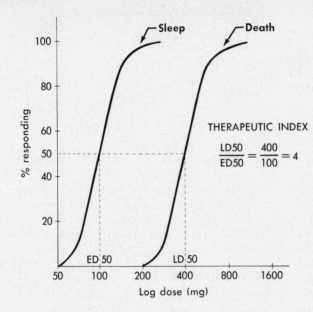

Fig. 3-2. Dose-response curve and therapeutic index.

THERAPEUTIC INDEX

$$\frac{LD50}{ED50} = \frac{400}{100} = 4$$

first three phases must be completed in order for a New Drug Application (NDA) to be approved by the FDA. Phase I is the first human administration of the drug and uses small numbers of volunteers. This phase determines the biologic effects, metabolism, and safe dosage range in humans, as well as toxic effects of the drug. Phase II involves testing of the drug to determine the potential therapeutic usefulness and later, the final dose ranges. Phase III is the broad clinical trial phase involving a large sample of specified patients to determine drug safety and efficacy. The drug is evaluated in this phase under conditions that may exist when the drug is marketed. During these three clinical phases, some long-term animal studies may be conducted simultaneously, such as chronic toxicity and teratogenic studies. If the FDA approves the NDA on the basis of the three clinical phases, the drug is allowed to be marketed initially to limited numbers of patients. In this phase IV study, patients are given the drug under specified supervision, and the drug's efficacy is monitored. Ultimately the drug is allowed to be used in large numbers of patients when it is shown to be safe and effective

for its intended use. Phase IV trials end when the FDA eventually approves the drug for unlimited marketing. It takes 6 to 8 years to complete the first three phases of clinical testing, including the chronic toxicity animal studies.

REVIEW QUESTIONS

1. Name four classifications of adverse drug reactions.
2. Describe the problem with identifying teratogenic agents (see also Chapter 24).
3. Describe the types of toxic reactions.
4. Explain the mechanism by which an allergic reaction occurs.
5. Give the formula for the therapeutic index and describe its usefulness.
6. Explain the various stages of testing through which a drug must pass before it is marketed for the general public.

REFERENCES

1. Azarnoff, D.L.: Application of metabolic data to the evaluation of drugs, J.A.M.A. **211:**1691, 1970.
2. Miller, L.C.: How good are our drugs? Am. J. Hosp. Pharm. **27:**367, 1970.
3. International Conference on Adverse Reactions Reporting System, Washington, D.C., 1970: Adverse reactions reporting systems: report, Washington, D.C. National Academy of Sciences, 1971.

Chapter 4

Prescription writing

The dental hygienist needs to become familiar with the basics of prescription writing for several reasons. In some cases, after the dentist has written a prescription, the hygienist may be expected to explain the regimen of therapy to the patient. The patient may feel more at ease or have more opportunity to discuss the prescription with the hygienist than with the dentist. The hygienist needs to understand any questions that the patient might have about the prescription in order to answer them. Also, knowledge of the proper prescription format can assist the hygienist in providing a double check on the prescriber.

Prescription writing formerly was a rather complex and pretentious art. Prescriptions were written in Latin and embellished by the hieroglyphics of the apothecaries' system of weights and measures. Early prescriptions were compounded from numerous constituents. In more recent years several changes have simplified prescription writing:

1. The pharmaceutical manufacturers provide drugs in most dosage forms needed. Therefore complicated compounding instructions can be omitted.
2. Prescriptions are no longer written in Latin (although currently used abbreviations are generally derived from Latin).
3. The metric system of weights and measures is replacing the more confusing apothecaries' system in prescription writing.
4. The use of abbreviations is being discouraged because of the potential for errors.

METRIC SYSTEM

Scientific calculations employ a base of 10. Consequently the metric system, which is based on 10, is the language of scientific measurement. Only metric units should be used in prescription writing.

The basic metric unit for the measurement of weight is the kilogram (kg). The basic metric unit for volume is the liter (L). One milliliter (ml), 1/1000 of a liter, is exactly 1 cubic centimeter (cc). Since the various units of the metric system are based on multiples of 10, several prefixes can apply to units of both weight and volume (Table 4-1.)

Solid drugs are dispensed by weight (milligrams, mg) and liquid drugs by volume (milliliters, ml). It is rarely necessary to use units other

Table 4-1. Metric weight and volume

Weight		Volume	
1 *kilo*gram (kg) =	1000 grams (gm or Gm)		
1 gram (gm) =	10 *deci*grams (dg)	1 liter (L) =	10 *deci*liters (dl)
	100 *centi*grams (cg)		100 *centi*liters (cl)
	1000 *milli*grams (mg)		1000 *milli*liters (ml)
	1,000,000 *micro*grams (μg, mcg)		1,000,000 *micro*liters (μl)

than the milligram or the milliliter in prescription writing. Although the apothecary system is cumbersome, some practitioners continue to use it. Table 4-2 shows the approximate equivalents between the metric and apothecaries' systems.

ABBREVIATIONS

Abbreviations are used in prescription writing to save time. They also make alteration of a prescription by the patient more difficult. In some cases they are necessary to get all the required information into the space on the prescription form. Some abbreviations that may be useful are shown in Table 4-3. If abbreviations are used on a prescription, they should be clearly written.

HOUSEHOLD MEASURES

Although the clinicians will direct the pharmacist to dispense a liquid preparation in milliliters, it is generally converted by the pharmacist to a convenient household measurement in directions to the patient. The teaspoonful contains 5 ml and the tablespoonful contains 15 ml. When accuracy is important, such as pediatric dosing, the pharmacist will recommend a calibrated oral syringe or dropper.

Table 4-2. Approximate equivalents of metric and apothecaries' systems

Metric	Apothecary
Weight	
60 mg	1 gr (grain)
1 gram (gm or Gm)	15 gr
30 gm	1 ounce (oz, ℥)
1 kilogram (kg)	2.2 pounds (lb)*
Volume	
30 ml	1 fluidounce (fl oz, fl ℥)
500 ml	1 pint (pt)
1000 ml	1 quart (qt)

*This unit of weight is avoirdupois, not apothecary.

PARTS OF THE PRESCRIPTION

The parts of the prescription have been named and defined classically as follows:
 1. Superscription: Patient's name, address, and age; date; and the symbol ℞ (L. *recipe,* "[you] take" or "take thou of")
 2. Inscription: Name of drug, dose form, and amount
 3. Subscription: Directions to the pharmacist
 4. Transcription (or signature): Directions to the patient

Since the classic categorization serves no particularly useful purpose, it is more practical to consider the prescription as consisting of the following three parts (Fig. 4-1).

Heading

 Name,* address,* and telephone number of the prescriber
 Name,* address,* age, and telephone number of the patient
 Date*

The name, address, and telephone number of the prescriber are important when the pharmacist must contact the prescribing clinician for verification or questions. The date is particularly important because it allows the pharmacist to intercept prescriptions that may not have been filled at the time of writing. The age of the patient enables the pharmacist to check for the proper dose. The dental hygienist can check a prescription for the presence of this information.

Body

 The symbol ℞*
 Name and dosage size or concentration (liquids) of the drug*
 Amount to be dispensed*
 Directions to the patient

The first entry after the ℞ symbol is the name of the drug being prescribed. This is followed by the size (mg) of the tablet or capsule desired. In the case of liquids the name of the drug is followed by its concentration (mg/ml). The second entry is

*Required by law.

Table 4-3. Common abbreviations

Abbreviation	English
a or $\bar{a}$	before
ac	before meals
bid	twice a day
$\bar{c}$	with
cap	capsule
d	day
disp	dispense
gm	gram
gr	grain
gtt	drop
h	hour
hs	at bedtime
$\bar{p}$	after
pc	after meals
PO	by mouth
prn	as required, if needed
q	every
qid	4 times a day
$\bar{s}$	without
sig	write (label)
stat	immediately (now)
tab	tablet
tid	3 times a day

the quantity to be dispensed, that is, the number of capsules or tablets or milliliters of liquid. This should be preceded by "Dispense:" or "Disp:."

℞
    Ibuprofen 400 mg
    Dispense: 12 (twelve)/tablets
or
℞
    Penicillin VK suspen, 125 mg/5 ml
    Dispense: 120 ml

In the case of tablets and capsules, the word "dispense" is frequently replaced with #, the symbol for a number. When writing prescriptions for opioids or other controlled substances, the prescriber should add in parentheses after the Arabic number of tablets or capsules the number written out longhand or in Roman numerals. This prevents the possibility of an intended 8 becoming an 18 or 80 at the discretion of an enterprising patient. Directions to the patient are preceded by the abbreviation "Sig:" (L. *signa*, "write"). The directions to the patient must be completely clear and explicit and should include the amount of medication and the time, frequency, and route of

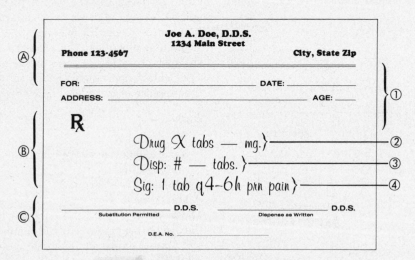

Fig. 4-1. Typical prescription blank.
    A. Heading   1. Superscription
    B. Body   2. Inscription
    C. Closing   3. Subscription
                  4. Transcription

administration. The pharmacist will transcribe Latin abbreviations into English on the label when the prescription is filled.

The body of the prescription will look like this:

 ℞ Ibuprofen 400 mg tablets
  Dispense: 12 (twelve) tablets
   (or 12 [XII] tablets)
  Sig: Take 2 tablets every 4 hours if needed
   for pain.

or, if abbreviations are used:

 ℞ Ibuprofen 400 mg tablets
  Disp: #12 (XII)
  Sig: 2 tabs q4h prn pain

Closing

 Prescriber's signature*
 DEA number, if required
 Refill instructions
 "Label"

After the body of the prescription, space is provided for the prescriber's signature. In this area there should also be space for the Drug Enforcement Administration (DEA) number and refill instructions (Fig. 4-1).

When the word "Label" is printed on a prescription blank the prescription bottle will contain the name of the medication. This allows easy identification by other practitioners or in emergency situations.

PRESCRIPTION WRITING AND HANDLING

Although the dental hygienist will not be writing prescriptions, he or she should be able to answer the patient's questions about the prescription. The dental hygienist should make sure that the patient knows how to take the medication prescribed (how long and when), what precautions to observe (drug interactions, possible side effects, driving limitations), and the reason for taking the medication. By informing the patient about the medication, the likelihood that the patient will comply with the prescription instructions increases. The dental office should either keep a copy of each prescription written in the patient's record or record the medication, dose, and num-

---

*Required by law.

ber prescribed. A patient should never get home and not know which drug is the antibiotic (for infection) and which is the analgesic (for pain). Side effects, such as drowsiness, should be noted on the label. The hygienist plays an important role in reinforcing the instructions to the patient.

Drug abusers are always "shopping" for a dental office that will provide them with prescriptions for controlled substances or for prescription blanks that they can forge themselves. Every dental office should keep prescription blanks in a secure place. The prescriber's DEA number should not be printed on the prescription blanks but should be written in only when needed. The dental hygienist can watch to see that the prescription blanks are not scattered around the office.

DRUG LEGISLATION

The Food and Drugs Act of 1906 was the first federal law to regulate interstate commerce in drugs. It was rewritten and reenacted to become the Food, Drug and Cosmetic Act of 1938. This law and its subsequent amendments prohibit interstate commerce in drugs that have not been shown to be safe and effective.

The Durham-Humphrey Law of 1952 is a particularly important amendment to the Food, Drug and Cosmetic Act because it requires that certain types of drugs be sold by prescription only. This law requires that these drugs be labeled "Caution: Federal law prohibits dispensing without prescription." This law also prohibits the refilling of a prescription unless directions to the contrary are indicated on the prescription.

The Drug Amendments of 1962 (Kefauver-Harris Bill) made some major changes in the Food, Drug and Cosmetic Law. Under these amendments manufacturers were required to demonstrate the effectiveness of drugs, to follow strict rules in testing, and to submit to the FDA any reports of adverse effects from drugs already on the market. Manufacturers were also required to list drug ingredients by generic name in labeling and advertising and to state adverse effects, contraindications, and efficacy of a drug.

The Drug Abuse Control Amendments of 1965 required accounting for drugs with a potential for

Table 4-4. Schedules of controlled substances

Schedule	Abuse potential	Examples	Handling
I	Highest	Heroin, LSD, marijuana, hallucinogens	No accepted medical use, experimental use, only in research
II	High	Morphine, meperidine, amphetamine, secobarbital	Prescriber's written prescription only; no refills
III	Moderate	Codeine mixtures, "weaker" stimulants and sedatives	Prescriptions may be telephoned; no more than 5 refills in less than 6 months
IV	Less	Diazepam (Valium), dextropropoxyphene (Darvon)	
V	Least	Some codeine-containing cough syrups	Can be bought over the counter in some states

abuse such as the barbiturates and amphetamines.

The **Harrison Narcotic Act** of 1914 and its amendments provided federal control over narcotic drugs and required registration of all practitioners prescribing narcotics.

The **Controlled Substances Act** of 1970 replaced the Harrison Narcotics Act and the Drug Abuse Control Amendments to the Food, Drug and Cosmetic Act. The Controlled Substances Act is extremely important, since it sets current requirements for writing prescriptions for drugs frequently prescribed in dental practice. The federal law divides controlled substances into five schedules according to their abuse potential (Table 4-4). The requirements for methods of prescribing these agents, telephoning prescriptions to the pharmacist, and refilling prescriptions differ with the schedule in which the agent is listed. Drug entities are continually being evaluated and added to schedules or moved from one schedule to another.

The current requirements for prescribing controlled drugs are as follows (Controlled Substance Act of 1970):

1. Any prescription for a controlled substance requires a DEA number.
2. All Schedule II through IV drugs require a prescription.
3. Any prescription for Schedule II drugs must be signed in ink by the prescriber and cannot be telephoned to the pharmacist or refilled (except in emergencies).
4. Prescriptions for Schedule III and IV drugs may be telephoned to the pharmacist and may be refilled no more than five times in 6 months, if so noted on the prescription.

REVIEW QUESTIONS

1. List the information required in a prescription.
2. Perform the following conversions:
   a. Grains to milligrams and milligrams to grains (approximate). For example,
      ½ gr equals how many milligrams?
      5 mg equals how many grains?
   b. Pounds to kilograms and kilograms to pounds. For example,
      25 lb equals how many kilograms?
      1.6 kg equals how many pounds?
   c. Milliliters to cubic centimeters and cubic centimeters to milliliters. For example,
      15 ml equals how many cubic centimeters?
      40 cc equals how many milliliters?
   d. Teaspoonfuls to milliliters and milliliters to teaspoonfuls. For example,
      2 tsp equals how many milliliters?
      5 ml equals how many teaspoonfuls?
3. Given a prescription, written using Latin abbreviations, state the directions to the patient in English. For example,
   Ibuprofen 400 mg
   Disp: 20 (twenty)
   Sig: 1–2 tabs q4h prn pain
4. Explain two precautions that should be taken in the dental office to discourage drug abusers.
5. List the components of the Controlled Substances Act and explain how it affects the dental office.

Chapter 5

Autonomic drugs

The dental hygienist should become familiar with the autonomic nervous system (ANS) drugs for three reasons. First, some ANS drugs are used in dentistry. For example, the vasoconstrictors in local anesthetic solutions and drugs used to reduce salivary flow are ANS drugs. Second, some ANS drugs produce oral adverse reactions. For example, the anticholinergics produce xerostomia. Third, drugs in other groups have effects similar to the ANS drugs. Antihypertensives and antipsychotics are drugs with autonomic effects. An understanding of the effects of the autonomic drugs will facilitate an understanding of the action of other drug groups that have autonomic effects.

AUTONOMIC NERVOUS SYSTEM

The autonomic nervous system functions largely as an automatic modulating system for many bodily functions including the regulation of blood pressure, heart rate, gastrointestinal tract motility, salivary gland secretions, and bronchial smooth muscle. This system relies on specific neurotransmitters and a variety of receptors to initiate functional responses in the target tissues. Before ANS pharmacology is discussed, the anatomy and physiology of this system will be reviewed.

Anatomy

The ANS has two divisions, the sympathetic autonomic nervous system (SANS) and the parasympathetic autonomic nervous system (PANS). Each consists of afferent (sensory) fibers, central inte-

grating areas, efferent (peripheral) motor preganglionic fibers, and postganglionic motor fibers.

The preganglionic neuron (Fig. 5-1, *1*) originates in the central nervous system (CNS) and passes out to form the ganglia *(2)* at the synapse *(3)* with the postganglionic neuron *(4)*. The space between the preganglionic and postganglionic fibers is termed the synaptic cleft. The postganglionic neuron originates in the ganglia and innervates the effector organ or tissue *(5)*.

Parasympathetic nervous system

Cell bodies in the CNS give rise to the preganglionic fibers of the parasympathetic division. They originate in the nuclei of the third, seventh, ninth, and tenth cranial nerves (C3, C7, C9, C10), as well as the second through the fourth sacral segments (S2 to S4) of the spinal cord. The preganglionic fibers of the PANS are relatively long and extend near to or into the innervated organ. The distribution is relatively simple for the third, seventh, and ninth cranial nerves, whereas the tenth or vagus nerve has a complex distribution. There is usually a low ratio of synaptic connections between preganglionic and postganglionic neurons, which leads to a discrete response when the PANS is stimulated. The postganglionic fibers, originating in the ganglia, are usually short and terminate on the innervated tissue.

Sympathetic nervous system

The cell bodies that give origin to the preganglionic fibers of the SANS are located in the tho-

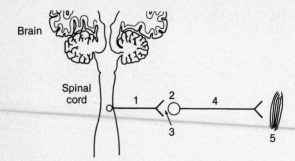

Fig. 5-1. Typical nerve. The preganglionic fiber *(1)* and the postganglionic fiber *(4)* are separated by the synapse *(3)*. Many of these synapses make up a ganglion *(2)*. The response occurs in the effector organ or tissue *(5)*.

racic (T1) and lumbar (L2-3) portion of the spinal cord. The preganglionic fibers exit the cord to enter the sympathetic chain located along each side of the vertebral column. Once a part of the sympathetic chain, preganglionic fibers form multiple synaptic connections with postganglionic cell bodies located up and down the sympathetic chain. Thus a single SANS preganglionic fiber often synapses with numerous postganglionic neurons. The postganglionic fibers then terminate at the effector organ or tissues.

The adrenal medulla is also innervated by the sympathetic preganglionic fibers. It functions much like a large sympathetic ganglion, with the glands in the medulla representing the postganglionic component. When the SANS is stimulated, the adrenal medulla releases primarily epinephrine and a small amount of norepinephrine into the systemic circulation. A diffuse response is produced when the SANS is stimulated because of the high ratio of synaptic connections between the preganglionic and postganglionic fibers and because epinephrine is released by the adrenal medulla when stimulated.

Functional organization

In general the two divisions of the ANS, the parasympathetic and the sympathetic, tend to act in opposite directions. The sympathetic division is designed to cope with sudden emergencies such as the "fright and flight" or "fight and flight" situation. In contrast, the parasympathetic division is concerned with the conservation of body processes. In most, but not all, instances the actions produced by each system are opposite—one increases the heart rate and the other decreases it, one dilates the pupils and the other constricts them.

Almost all body tissues are innervated by the ANS, with many organs receiving both parasympathetic and sympathetic innervation. The response of a specific tissue at any one time will be equal to the sum of the excitatory and inhibitory influences of the two divisions if a tissue receives both innervations. Table 5-1 summarizes the responses of the major tissues and organ systems to the ANS.

In addition to the dual innervation of tissues, there is another way in which the two divisions of the ANS can interact. Sensory fibers in one division can influence the motor fibers in the other.

Thus, although in an isolated tissue preparation the stimulation of one of the divisions would produce a specific response, in the patient a more complex and integrated response can be expected. The net effect would be a combination of the direct and indirect effects.

Neurotransmitters

Nerve-to-nerve or nerve-to-effector tissue communication takes place by release of chemical neurotransmitters across the synaptic cleft. Neurotransmitters are released in response to the nerve action potential (or pharmacologic agents in certain cases) to interact with a specific membrane component, the receptor. Receptors are usually found on the postsynaptic tissue but may be located on the presynaptic membrane as well (see Fig. 15-3). The interaction between neurotransmitter and receptor is specific, and rapidly terminated by disposition of the neurotransmitter substance. Disposition occurs most frequently by either enzymatic breakdown of the transmitter or reuptake into the presynaptic nerve terminal.

Table 5-1. Responses of major tissues and organ systems to the autonomic nervous system

Effector organ or tissue	Response to cholinergic (parasympathetic) impulse*	Adrenergic (sympathetic) impulse	
		Receptor type	Response*
Eye			
Iris	Miosis + + +	α	Mydriasis + +
Ciliary muscle (accommodation)	Contraction for near vision + + +	β	Relaxation for distant vision +
Heart			
SA node	Decreased heart rate + + +	β_1	Increased heart rate + +
Arterioles (vessels)			
Skin and mucosa	Dilation	α	Constriction + + +
Skeletal muscle	Dilation +	α	Constriction + +
		β_2	Dilation + +
Abdominal viscera	—	α	Constriction + + +
		β_2	Dilation +
Salivary glands	Dilation + +	α	Constriction + + +
Lungs			
Bronchial muscle	Contraction + +	β_2	Relaxation +
Stomach, intestine, urinary bladder			
Motility and tone	Increase + + +	β_2	Decrease +
Sphincters	Relaxation (usually) + to + +	α	Contraction (usually) + to + +
Secretion (GI tract)	Stimulation + + to + + +	·	Inhibition (?)
Skin			
Pilomotor muscles	—	α	Contraction + +
Adrenal medulla	Secretion of epinephrine and norepinephrine		—
Liver	Glycogen synthesis +	α, β_2	Glycogenolysis, gluconeogenesis + + +
Sex organs,			
male	Erection + + +	α	Ejaculation + + +
Glands			
Salivary secretion	Potassium and water secretion + + +	α_1	Potassium and water secretion +
		β	Amylase secretion +
Lacrimal, bronchial, nasopharyngeal	Secretion + + to + + +		—
Sweat	Secretion + + +	α	Palms of hands +

Adapted from Goodman, L.S., and Gilman, A.: The pharmacological basis of therapeutics, ed. 7, New York, 1985, Macmillan Publishing Co., Inc.
*Relative importance of adrenergic and cholinergic influence on tissue (graded + to + + +).

Nerves in the ANS contain the necessary enzyme systems and other metabolic processes to synthesize, store, and release neurotransmitters. Thus drugs can modify ANS activity by altering any of the events associated with neurotransmitters: (1) synthesis, (2) storage, (3) release, (4) receptor interaction and (5) disposition. The specificity of the neurotransmitters and receptors dictate the tissue response.

The locations and identities of the ANS neurotransmitters in the PANS and SANS divisions are as follows (Fig. 5-2):

1. Between the preganglionic and postganglionic nerves
    a. The neurotransmitter substance of the synapse (ganglia) formed between the preganglionic and postganglionic nerves is acetylcholine. Nerves that release acetylcholine are termed **cholinergic.** Because this synapse is also stimulated by nicotine, it is also termed **nicotinic** in response (Fig. 5-2, *C*).

2. Between postganglionic nerves and the effector tissues
    a. PANS. The neurotransmitter released from the postganglionic nerve terminal is acetylcholine and as before it is also termed **cholinergic.** Because the postsynaptic tissue responds to muscarine it is identified as **muscarinic** (Fig. 5-2, *B*). Thus the cholinergic synapses are distinguished from one another.
    b. SANS. Norepinephrine is the transmitter substance released by the postganglionic nerves and is designated as **adrenergic** (Fig. 5-2, *A*).

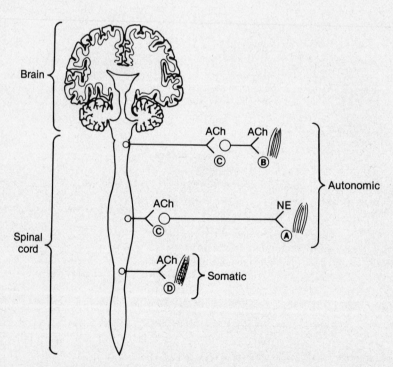

Fig. 5-2. Location of the neurotransmitters acetylcholine *(ACh)* and norepinephrine *(NE).* The synapses are as follows: *A,* adrenergic; *B,* muscarinic cholinergic; *C,* nicotinic cholinergic; *D,* cholinergic somatic.

3. For comparison purposes, the neurotransmitter released at the neuromuscular junction of skeletal muscle (somatic system) is acetylcholine and is also termed **cholinergic** (Fig. 5-2, *D*). However, the neuromuscular junction is not part of the ANS and drug actions on the somatic system must be separated from the ANS.

DRUG GROUPS

Four groups of drugs exert their effects primarily on the ANS. Some groups have several names and divisions, but basically the following agents are available:

1. **Cholinergic** agents or parasympathomimetics mimic the effects of the parasympathetic nervous system.
2. **Anticholinergic** agents, parasympatholytics, or cholinergic blocking agents block the effects of the parasympathetic nervous system.
3. **Adrenergic** agents or sympathomimetics mimic the effects of the sympathetic nervous system.
4. **Adrenergic** or sympathetic **blocking agents,** or sympatholytics, block the effects of the sympathetic nervous system.

Parasympathetic nervous system

Acetylcholine has been identified as the principal mediator in the PANS. When an action potential travels along the nerve, it causes the release of the stored acetylcholine from the synaptic storage vesicles and, if sufficient acetylcholine is released, it will initiate a response in the postsynaptic tissue. If the postsynaptic tissue is a postganglionic

nerve, depolarization with generation of an action potential occurs in that neuron. In the postganglionic parasympathetic fibers, the postsynaptic tissue is an effector organ and the response will be that of that organ.

The action of the released acetylcholine is terminated by acetylcholinesterase hydrolysis to yield the inactive metabolites choline and acetic acid.

Some postsynaptic tissues respond to acetylcholine and not to other mediators, suggesting that acetylcholine possesses certain characteristics that cause the tissues to respond. Acetylcholine must physically and chemically fit a specific site called the receptor in order to be an effective mediator. It has been shown that atropine can block the action of acetylcholine at the postganglionic endings (Fig. 5-2, *B*) but not at the neuromuscular junction (Fig. 5-2, *D*). In contrast, curare blocks the response of skeletal muscle to acetylcholine (Fig. 5-2, *D*) but does not block its effect on tissues such as the salivary gland (Fig. 5-2, *B*). Hexamethonium blocks the action of acetylcholine at the ganglia (Fig. 5-2, *C*). This information implies that different types of receptors that have acetylcholine as a neurotransmitter are located in anatomically different synapses (Table 5-2). Other factors such as the amount of acetylcholine released, the size of the synaptic cleft, and the tissue penetrability of a drug may also account for differences in the receptor response to drugs at the acetylcholine-mediated junctions.

Cholinergic (parasympathomimetic) agents

The cholinergic (parasympathomimetic) agents are classified as direct acting and indirect acting,

Table 5-2. Types of cholinergic receptors

Receptor site	Location*	Neurotransmitter	Stimulating agent	Blocking agent
Muscarinic	*B*	Acetylcholine	Muscarine	Atropine
Nicotinic	*C*	Acetylcholine	Nicotine	Hexamethonium
Somatic-skeletal muscle	*D*	Acetycholine	Nicotine	*d*-Tubocurarine (curare)

*See Fig. 5-2.

depending on their mechanism of action (Table 5-3). The direct-acting agents include the choline derivatives and pilocarpine. The choline derivatives include both acetylcholine and other, more stable choline derivatives. These derivatives of acetylcholine possess activity similar to PANS stimulation but have a longer duration of action and are more selective.

The indirect-acting parasympathomimetic agents or cholinesterase inhibitors act by inhibiting the enzyme cholinesterase. When this enzyme, which normally destroys acetylcholine, is inhibited, the concentration of acetylcholine builds up, resulting in action that resembles PANS stimulation.

Pharmacologic effects

1. Cardiovascular effects. The cardiovascular effects associated with the cholinergic agents are the result of both direct and indirect action. The **direct** effect on the heart produces a negative chronotropic and inotropic action. There is also a decrease in cardiac output associated with these agents. The cholinergic agents' effect on vessels results in smooth muscle relaxation and a decrease in the total peripheral resistance (TPR). The **indirect** effect of these agents is an increase in heart rate and cardiac output. Since the direct and indirect effects of these agents on the heart rate and cardiac output are opposite, the resulting effect will depend on the concentration of the drug present. Generally, there is bradycardia and a decrease in blood pressure and cardiac output.

2. Gastrointestinal effects. The cholinergic agents excite the smooth muscle of the gastrointestinal tract, producing an increase in activity and secretion. In the intestine this can produce diarrhea or even cramping. Increased secretions can cause salivation, lacrimation, sweating, and increased stomach acid production.

3. Effects on the eye. The cholinergic agents produce miosis and cause a "spasm of accommodation" so that the eye becomes focused for near vision. Since intraocular pressure is also decreased, these agents are useful in the treatment of glaucoma.

Table 5-3. Cholinergic (parasympathomimetic) agents

Classification and drug name	Therapeutic use
Direct acting	
Choline esters	
Acetylcholine	Experimental
Bethanechol (Urecholine)	Urinary retention
Carbachol	Glaucoma
Other	
Pilocarpine	Glaucoma
Indirect acting (cholinesterase inhibitors)	
Reversible agents	
Alkaloids	
Physostigmine (eserine)	Some drug overdoses, glaucoma
Synthetics	
Neostigmine (Prostigmin), edrophonium (Tensilon), pyridostigmine (Mestinon), ambenonium (Mytelase)	Myasthenia gravis
Irreversible organophosphates	
Isoflurophate (DFP, Floropryl), echothiophate (Phospholine)	Very long acting; glaucoma
Malathion, parathion	Agricultural insecticides
Sarin (GB), Tabun	Extremely potent "nerve gases"; chemical warfare

Adverse reactions

The adverse reactions associated with the cholinergic agents are essentially extensions of their pharmacologic effects. When large doses of these agents are ingested, the resultant toxic effects are described by the acronym SLUD: salivation, lacrimation, urination, and defecation. With even larger doses, neuromuscular paralysis can occur as a result of the effect on the neuromuscular junction. CNS effects such as confusion can be seen if toxic doses are administered.

The treatment of an overdose of cholinesterase inhibitors such as the insecticides or organophosphates includes a combination of pralidoxime (2-PAM, Protopam) and atropine. Pralidoxime regenerates the receptor sites bound by the inhibitors, and atropine blocks the muscarinic effects of the excess acetylcholine present.

Contraindications

The contraindications to the use of the cholinergic agents result from these agents' pharmacologic effects and adverse reactions. They include the following:

1. Bronchial asthma
2. Hyperthyroidism
3. Mechanical obstruction of the gastrointestinal or urinary tract
4. Severe cardiac disease
5. Myasthenia gravis treated with neostigmine (These patients should not be given an irreversible cholinesterase inhibitor, since neostigmine would occupy the enzyme and the irreversible agent could not function.)
6. Peptic ulcer

Uses

The direct-acting agents are used primarily in the treatment of glaucoma, a condition in which the intraocular pressure is elevated. Occasionally, they are used to treat myasthenia gravis, a disease resulting in muscle weakness. The urinary retention that occurs after surgery is also treated with the choline esters (Table 5-3). An attempt to use these agents in the treatment of xerostomia has met with a limited degree of success. Oral administration of pilocarpine has been employed for this purpose.

The indirect-acting agents, the cholinesterase inhibitors, are divided into groups based on the degree of reversibility with which they are bound to the enzyme. Edrophonium is rapidly reversible, whereas physostigmine and neostigmine are slowly reversible. These agents are used to treat glaucoma or myasthenia gravis. The cholinesterase inhibitors developed for use as insecticides and chemical warfare agents are essentially nonreversible.

Physostigmine has been used to treat reactions caused by several different kinds of drugs. Delirium associated with the benzodiazepines, such as diazepam, have been treated with physostigmine. Although physostigmine has been used as a treatment for CNS depression produced by the benzodiazepines, its use is controversial because it is nonspecific and has potential toxicity. Also, acute toxicity from the anticholinergic agents (such as atropine), the phenothiazines, the tricyclic antidepressants, and the antihistamines has been treated with physostigmine.

Anticholinergic (parasympatholytic) agents

The anticholinergic agents prevent the action of acetylcholine at the postganglionic parasympathetic endings. The release of acetylcholine is not prevented, but the receptor site is competitively blocked. Thus the anticholinergic drugs block the action of acetylcholine on smooth muscle, glandular tissues, and the heart. These agents could be called antimuscarinic agents, since they block the muscarinic receptors and not the nicotinic receptors (Fig. 5-2).

Pharmacologic effects

1. CNS effects. Depending on the dose administered, CNS stimulation or depression may occur. For example, scopolamine in usual therapeutic doses more frequently causes sedation, whereas atropine in high doses can cause stimulation. Also, the tertiary agents (Table 5-4), which are more lipid soluble and nonionized, can penetrate the brain tissue more easily and therefore are more likely to cause CNS effects than the qua-

Table 5-4. Anticholinergic (parasympatholytic) agents

Agent	Usual oral dose (mg)	Route of administration
Tertiary agents		
Natural alkaloids		
Atropine	0.5	PO, injection, ophthalmic
Scopolamine (L-hyoscine)	0.5	PO, injection, ophthalmic
L-Hyoscyamine (Levsin)	0.125	PO, injection
Synthetic esters		
Cyclopentolate (Cyclogyl)	—	Ophthalmic
Dicyclomine (Bentyl)	20.0	PO, injection
Quaternary synthetics		
Esters		
Methantheline (Banthine)	50.0	PO
Propantheline (Pro-Banthine)	15.0	PO, injection
Methscopolamine (Pamine)	2.5	PO, injection
Glycopyrrolate (Robinul)	1.0–2.0	PO, injection
Nonesters		
Isopropamide (Darbid)	5.0	PO
Tridihexethyl (Pathilon)	25.0	PO

Adapted from Meyers, F.H., Jaevetz, E., and Goldfien, A.: Review of medical pharmacology, ed. 6, Los Altos, Calif., 1978, Lange Medical Publications.

ternary agents. Atropine and scopolamine are tertiary agents, and propantheline (Pro-Banthine) and methantheline (Banthine) are quaternary agents.

2. Effects on exocrine glands. The anticholinergic drugs affect the exocrine glands by reducing their secretion. These glands are located in the respiratory, gastrointestinal, and genitourinary tracts. This effect is used therapeutically in dentistry to decrease salivation and create a dry field for certain dental procedures.

3. Effects on smooth muscle. Anticholinergic agents relax the smooth muscle in the respiratory and gastrointestinal tracts. This effect on gastrointestinal motility has given rise to the name "spasmolytic" agents. If these drugs are used repeatedly, constipation can result. The smooth muscle

in the respiratory tract is relaxed by the anticholinergic agents, causing bronchial dilation.

4. Effects on the eye. The parasympatholytic agents have two effects on the eye, mydriasis and cycloplegia. Cycloplegia refers to paralysis of accommodation so that the lens can focus only for distance vision and near vision is blurred. Both cycloplegia and mydriasis can be useful for ophthalmologic examinations. These effects occur whether the drug is given topically or systemically.

5. Cardiovascular effects. With large therapeutic doses, the anticholinergic agents can produce vagal blockade resulting in tachycardia. This effect has been used therapeutically to prevent cardiac slowing during general anesthesia. With small doses bradycardia predominates. This variable response in the heart rate occurs because heart rate is a function of both direct (sympathetic) and indirect (parasympathetic) effects.

Adverse reactions

The adverse reactions associated with the anticholinergic agents are essentially extensions of their pharmacologic effects. These can include xerostomia, blurred vision, photophobia, tachycardia, fever, and urinary and gastrointestinal stasis. Hyperpyrexia and hot, dry, flushed skin caused by a lack of sweating are also seen. Hyperpyrexia is treated symptomatically.

Anticholinergic toxicity can cause signs of CNS excitation including delirium, hallucinations, convulsions, and respiratory depression.

Contraindications

Specific contraindications or cautions to the use of the anticholinergic agents include the following:

1. Glaucoma. Anticholinergic drugs can cause an acute rise in intraocular pressure in patients with narrow-angle glaucoma. These drugs can precipitate an acute attack in unrecognized cases of this rare condition. In contrast, the patient with wide-angle glaucoma who is currently receiving treatment with eye drops can be given one dose of the anticholinergic agents with impunity.

2. Prostatic hypertrophy. Because the anticholinergic agents can exacerbate urinary retention, patients with prostatic hypertrophy who already have difficulty urinating should be given these agents only with great caution.

3. Intestinal or urinary obstruction or retention. Constipation or acute urinary retention can be precipitated by the use of these agents in susceptible patients.

4. Cardiovascular disease. Since anticholinergic agents have the ability to block the vagus nerve, resulting in tachycardia, patients with cardiovascular disease should be given these agents cautiously.

Uses

1. Preoperative medication. The anticholinergic agents are used preoperatively for two reasons. First, they inhibit the secretions of saliva and bronchial mucus that can be stimulated by general anesthesia. Second, they have the ability to block the vagal slowing of the heart that results from general anesthesia.

2. Treatment of gastrointestinal disorders. Many types of gastrointestinal disorders associated with increased motility or acid secretion have been treated with anticholinergic agents. For example, patients with gastric ulcers are commonly treated with the anticholinergic agents, even though there is little proof of their effectiveness. Both nonspecific diarrhea and hypermotility of the colon have also been treated with these agents. In the doses used, it is difficult to prove that the anticholinergic agents are effective for this purpose.

3. Ophthalmologic examination. Because of the ability of anticholinergic agents to cause mydriasis and cycloplegia, they are commonly used before examinations of the eye. Mydriasis is helpful for full visualization of the retina. Cycloplegia is useful to relax the lens so that the proper prescription for eyeglasses may be determined.

4. Reduction of parkinson-like movements. Before the advent of levodopa, the anticholinergic agents were commonly used to reduce the tremors and rigidity associated with Parkinson's disease. Patients treated with these agents predicta-

bly experienced the side effects of dry mouth and blurred vision. At present anticholinergic agents are only occasionally used in combination with levodopa for the treatment of Parkinson's disease. The phenothiazines, used to treat psychoses, can produce extrapyramidal (parkinson-like) side effects. Anticholinergic agents such as trihexyphenidyl (Artane) and benztropine (Cogentin) are often administered concurrently with the phenothiazines to reduce rigidity and tremor.

5. Motion sickness medication and over-the-counter (OTC) sleep aids. Scopolamine, because of its CNS depressant action, has been used in the past to treat motion sickness and induce sleep. It has largely been replaced for these purposes by the antihistamines.

6. Dentistry. Anticholinergic agents can be used to produce a dry field before some dental procedures. The most commonly used agents, atropine, methantheline, and propantheline, as well as others, are listed in Table 5-4 with their usual oral doses. This dose should be administered between 1 and 2 hours before the dental appointment and may be repeated if no results are obtained within 1 hour. Given in appropriate oral doses, for example, 0.5 mg atropine or 50 mg methantheline, these agents produce approximately equivalent results.

Drug interactions

The most important drug interaction associated with the anticholinergic agents is an additive anticholinergic effect. Other agents that have anticholinergic effects, such as the phenothiazines, antihistamines, and tricyclic antidepressants, can be additive with the parasympatholytics. Mixing more than one drug group possessing anticholinergic effects can lead to symptoms of anticholinergic toxicity including urinary retention, blurred vision, acute glaucoma, and even paralytic ileus. Dental office personnel must pay careful attention to the medications the patient is taking in order to rule out excessive anticholinergic effects. Patients receiving methotrimeprazine (Levoprome) concurrently with scopolamine have reported extrapyramidal (parkinson-like) symptoms. Also, patients taking haloperidol (Haldol) for the treatment of schizophrenia have noted a decreased therapeutic effect when the anticholinergics trihexyphenidyl or benztropine were administered. This underlines the problem of using anticholinergics routinely with antipsychotic agents. If a patient is taking a cholinesterase inhibitor, particularly neostigmine, atropine could interfere with its cholinergic effect.

SYMPATHETIC NERVOUS SYSTEM

The major neurotransmitters in the SANS are norepinephrine and epinephrine. Both are synthesized in the neural tissues and stored in synaptic vesicles. Norepinephrine is the major transmitter substance released at the nerve endings, and epinephrine is released from the adrenal medulla on stimulation and distributed throughout the body by the general circulation (bloodstream).

The term "catecholamine" refers to a specific structure (catechol = 1,2-dihydroxybenzene) associated with some of the sympathomimetic agents. Norepinephrine, epinephrine, and dopamine are endogenous catecholamines, and isoproterenol (Isuprel) is an exogenous catecholamine. The endogenous catecholamines act as neurotransmitters.

The adrenergic drugs can be classified by their mechanism of action as follows:

1. Direct action. Epinephrine, norepinephrine, and isoproterenol produce their effects directly on the receptor site by stimulating the receptor.

2. Indirect action. These agents, such as amphetamine, release endogenous norepinephrine, which then produces a response. Depletion of the endogenous norepinephrine with reserpine diminishes the response to these agents.

3. Mixed action. These agents, such as ephedrine, can either stimulate the receptor directly or release endogenous norepinephrine to cause a response.

Norepinephrine's action is terminated primarily by reuptake into the presynaptic nerve terminal by an amine-specific pump. The norepinephrine taken up in this manner is stored for reuse. In addition, two enzyme systems, monoamine oxidase (MAO) and catechol-O-methyltransferase (COMT), are involved in the metabolism of a portion of both epinephrine and norepinephrine.

Sympathetic nervous system receptors

As early as 1948, the existence of at least two types of adrenergic receptors, termed alpha (α) and beta (β), was recognized. The activation of α-receptors causes a different response than the activation of β-receptors. More subreceptor types are now known. Fig. 15-3 pictures the α- and β-receptors at the nerve endings.

α-Receptors. Stimulation of the α-receptors results in smooth muscle excitation or contraction, causing vasoconstriction. Since α-receptors are located in the skin and skeletal muscle, vasoconstriction of the skin and skeletal muscle follows stimulation. Drugs that block the action of neurotransmitters on the α-receptors are called α-adrenergic blocking agents.

β-Receptors. There are at least two types of β-receptors, β_1 and β_2. β_1-receptor excitation causes stimulation of the heart muscle, resulting in a positive chronotropic effect (increased rate) and a positive inotropic effect (increased strength). Other actions thought to be associated primarily with β_1-receptor stimulation include metabolic effects on glycogen formation (glycogenolysis).

The stimulation of the β_2-receptors results in smooth muscle inhibition or relaxation. Because the blood vessels of the skeletal muscle are innervated by β_2-receptors, stimulation causes vasodilation. Relaxation of the smooth muscles of the bronchioles, also containing β_2-receptors, results in bronchodilation. Drugs with this effect have been used in the treatment of asthma. The type of receptor found in a given tissue determines the effect adrenergic agents will produce on that tissue (Table 5-1).

Agents that block β-receptor effects are called β-adrenergic blocking agents. Some (such as propranolol) are nonspecific, blocking both β_1- and β_2-receptors, whereas others are more selective blocking primarily β_2-receptors.

Table 5-5. Some adrenergic (sympathomimetic) agents

Primary use	Route of administration	Receptor
Bronchodilating effect		
Isoproterenol (Isuprel, Medihaler-Iso)	Inhalation	β
Metaproterenol (Alupent, Metaprel)	PO, inhalation	$\beta_2 >> \beta_1$
Terbutaline (Brethine, Bricanyl)	PO, injection	$\beta_2 >>> \beta_1$
Isoetharine (Bronkosol, Bronkometer)	Inhalation	$\beta_2 > \beta_1$
Decongestant (vasoconstricting) effect		
Pseudoephedrine (Sudafed)	PO	α, β
Phenylpropranolamine (PPA)	PO	α
Nose sprays		
Phenylephrine (Neo-Synephrine)		
Naphazoline (Privine)	Drops and spray	α
Oxymetazoline (Afrin, Duration)		
Xylometazoline (Neo-Synephrine II Long-Acting, Otrivin)		
Both effects		
Epinephrine (Adrenalin, Medihaler-Epi, Primatene Mist)	Drops, injection, inhalation	α, β
Ephedrine	PO	α, β

Adrenergic (sympathomimetic) agents
Pharmacologic effects

When discussing the pharmacologic effects associated with the adrenergic drugs, it is important to note the proportion of α- and β-receptor activity each possesses. Table 5-5 lists some common adrenergic agents and the receptors they stimulate; Epinephrine has both α- and β-receptor activity, norepinephrine and phenylephrine stimulate primarily α-receptors, and isoproterenol acts mainly on β-receptors. Although the effects of these agents depend on their ability to stimulate various receptors, the general actions of the adrenergic agents are discussed with specific reference to α- or β-receptor effects as applicable.

1. CNS effects. The sympathomimetic agents such as amphetamine produce CNS excitation or alertness. With higher doses anxiety, apprehension, restlessness, and even tremors can occur.

2. Cardiovascular effects

a. Heart. The general effect of sympathomimetics such as epinephrine is to increase the force and rate of contraction (a positive chronotropic and inotropic response). Norepinephrine, with its more pronounced α-receptor effects, will elevate blood pressure and reflexly slow the heart rate. The effects of isoproterenol on the heart resemble those of epinephrine. Table 5-6 shows the net effect on cardiac rate or normal sinus rhythm.

b. Vessels. The vascular responses observed with the sympathomimetics depend on the location of the vessels and whether they are innervated by α-receptors or β-receptors, or both. Agents with α-receptor effects will produce vasoconstriction primarily in the skin and mucosa (innervated with α-receptor fibers), whereas agents with β-receptor effects will produce vasodilation of the skeletal muscle (innervated with β-receptor fibers). The resultant effect on the total peripheral resistance is an increase with an α-receptor agent and a reduction with a β-receptor agent (Table 5-6).

c. Blood pressure. The sympathomimetic effect on the blood pressure can be seen in Table 5-6. With epinephrine, which has both α- and β-stimulating properties, there is a rise in systolic pressure and a decrease in diastolic pressure. With norepinephrine there is a rise in both systolic and

Table 5-6. Cardiovascular response to sympathomimetic amines.*

	α Phenyl- ephrine	α β Epi- nephrine	β Isopro- terenol
Vascular resistance (tone)			
Cutaneous, mucous membranes (α)	↑ ↑	↑ ↑	0
Skeletal muscle (β$_2$, α)	↑	↓	↓ ↓
Renal (α)	↑	↑	↓
Splanchnic (α)	↑ ↑	↓ or ↑ †	↓
Total peripheral resistance	↑ ↑ ↑	↓ or ↑ †	↓ ↓
Venous tone	↑	↑	↓
Cardiac			
Contractility (β$_1$)	0 or ↑	↑ ↑ ↑	↑ ↑ ↑
Heart rate (predominantly β$_1$)	↓ ↓ (vagal reflex)	↑ or ↓	↑ ↑ ↑
Stroke volume	0, ↓, ↑	↑	↑
Cardiac output	↓	↑	↑ ↑
Blood pressure			
Mean	↑ ↑	↑	↓
Diastolic	↑ ↑	↓ or ↑ †	↓ ↓
Systolic	↑ ↑	↑ ↑	0 or ↓
Pulse pressure	0	↑ ↑	↑ ↑

Reproduced, with permission, from Katzung, B.G.: Basic and clinical pharmacology, ed. 2, Los Altos, Calif., 1984, Lange Medical Publications.
*(↑ = increase; ↓ = decrease; 0 = no change.)
†Small doses decrease, large doses increase.

diastolic pressure. With isoproterenol there is little change in systolic pressure but a decrease in diastolic pressure.

3. Effects on the eye. The sympathomimetic agents have at least two effects on the eye: a decrease in intraocular pressure, which makes them useful in the treatment of glaucoma, and mydriasis.

4. Bronchioles—respiratory effects. These agents cause a relaxation of the bronchiolar smooth muscle owing to their β-adrenergic effect. This has made them useful in the treatment of asthma and anaphylaxis.

5. Metabolic effects. The hyperglycemia resulting from β-stimulation can be explained on the basis of increased glycogenolysis and decrease in insulin release. Fatty acid mobilization, lipolysis, and gluconeogenesis are stimulated, and the basal metabolic rate is increased.

6. Effects on the salivary glands. The mucus-secreting cells of the submaxillary and sublingual glands are stimulated by the sympathomimetic agents to release a small amount of thick, viscous saliva. Since the parotid gland has no sympathetic innervation (only parasympathetic) and the sympathomimetics produce vasoconstriction, the flow of saliva is often reduced, resulting in xerostomia.

Adverse reactions

The adverse reactions associated with the adrenergic drugs are extensions of their pharmacologic effects. Anxiety and tremors may occur, and the patient may have palpitations. Serious arrhythmias can result. Agents with an α-adrenergic action can also cause a dramatic rise in blood pressure.

Cautions

The sympathomimetic agents should be used with caution in patients with angina, hypertension, or hyperthyroidism.

Uses

1. Vasoconstriction

a. Prolonged action. The sympathomimetic agents are used in dentistry primarily because of their vasoconstrictive action on the blood vessels. Agents with an α-effect (vasoconstriction) are frequently added to local anesthetic solutions. These vasoconstrictors prolong the action of the local anesthetics and reduce their potential for systemic toxicity.

b. Hemostasis. The adrenergic agents have been used in dentistry to produce hemostasis. Epinephrine can be applied topically or infiltrated locally around the bleeding area. Epinephrine, used to stop bleeding and to retract the gingiva before taking an impression, has the potential for producing problems because it can cause systemic toxicity. Epinephrine is quickly absorbed after topical application if the tissue is injured. The total amount of epinephrine given by all routes must be noted to prevent an overdose.

c. Decongestion. Sympathomimetic agents are often incorporated into nose drops or sprays (see Table 5-5) to treat nasal congestion. These agents provide symptomatic relief by constricting the vessels and reducing the swelling of the mucous membranes of the nose. Within a short period of time the congestion can return, a condition called "rebound congestion." With repeated local use systemic absorption can cause problems even greater than rebound congestion. Systemic decongestants are now preferred.

2. Cardiac effects

a. Treatment of shock. The value of the adrenergic agents in the treatment of shock is controversial. These drugs will elevate a lowered blood pressure, but correcting the cause of shock is more important. Some agents with both α- and β-effects (such as dopamine) are used.

b. Treatment of cardiac arrest. The sympathomimetic agents, especially epinephrine, are used to treat cardiac arrest.

3. Bronchodilation. The use of the sympathomimetic agents in the treatment of respiratory disease stems from their action as bronchodilators. Patients with asthma or emphysema are frequently treated with adrenergic agents to provide bronchodilation. In the treatment of anaphylaxis, when bronchoconstriction is predominant, epinephrine is the drug of choice.

4. CNS stimulation. The amphetamine-like agents such as dextroamphetamine (Dexedrine), phenmetrazine (Preludin) and benzphetamine (Didrex) have been used and abused as prescription "diet pills". Over-the-counter diet pills (Dexatrim-15) contain the orally effective adrenergic agent phenylpropanolamine, also used as a decongestant. There is no scientific proof that these agents have any lasting effect on weight loss. Methylphenidate (Ritalin) and pimoline (Cylert), and occasionally the amphetamines are sympathomimetics used to treat attention deficit disorder in children. These agents, given to hyperactive children, tend to reduce impulsivity and increase the attention span.

Specific adrenergic agents

Epinephrine. Epinephrine may be administered by a variety of parenteral routes including intravenous (IV) and subcutaneous (SC). It is the drug of choice for acute asthmatic attacks and anaphylaxis. It is also used in patients with cardiac arrest. It is added to local anesthetic solutions to delay absorption and reduce systemic toxicity.

Epinephrine should be stored in amber-colored containers placed out of the reach of sunlight, since light causes deterioration. It first turns pink, then brown, and finally precipitates. Solutions of epinephrine with any discoloration shoule be discarded immediately.

Norepinephrine and phenylephrine. Norepinephrine and phenylephrine cause primarily α receptor-stimulation, which produces vasoconstriction in the cutaneous vessels. This leads to an increase in total peripheral resistance and systolic and diastolic pressures. A reflex vagal bradycardia also results.

Phenylephrine is used as a mydriatic and in nose sprays or drops to relieve congestion. Both agents are used as additives to local anesthetic solutions.

Levonordefrin. Levonordefrin (Neo-Cobefrin), a derivative of norepinephrine, is a vasoconstrictor frequently added to local anesthetic solutions. Although claims made for this drug include less CNS excitation and cardiac stimulation, the dosage required to produce vasoconstriction equal to that caused by epinephrine is higher. Therefore it is difficult to distinguish levonordefrin's effects from those of other vasoconstrictors. Its effects resemble those of α-receptor stimulation.

Isoproterenol. Isoproterenol (Isuprel) is a synthetic catecholamine whose action is limited to the β-receptors. It is used in the treatment of bronchial asthma, where it can be administered by either inhalation or injection to provide bronchodilation. Excessive use can produce tachycardia, arrhythmias, palpitations, and hypotension. β-blocking agents (propranolol) interfere with the action of isoproterenol.

Ephedrine. In contrast to the catecholamines, ephedrine is effective when taken orally and has a longer duration of action. It has both α- and β-receptor activity. Its mechanism of action is mixed; that is, it has both direct and indirect action. It is often used in combination with other agents for patients with bronchial asthma. It is also present in many OTC products designed for the symptomatic treatment of the common cold or allergies. An isomer of ephedrine, pseudoephedrine (Sudafed) is used in the same manner as ephedrine.

Dopamine. Dopamine (Intropin) is a neurotransmitter in parts of the CNS. It is an α- and β-agonist employed primarily in the treatment of shock. Dopamine first acts on the β-receptors of the heart, producing a positive chronotropic and inotropic effect. In higher doses it stimulates the α-receptors, producing vasoconstriction. However, it exerts an unusual vasodilating effect in certain vessels and produces an increase in blood flow to the renal, splanchnic, cerebral, and coronary vessels. Ventricular arrhythmias and hypotension can occur.

Dipivefrin (Propine). Dipivefrin (Propine) and epinephrine are sympathomimetic ophthalmics that are used to treat glaucoma. They decrease the production of aqueous humor (β-receptor effect), increase its outflow (β-effect), and produce mydriasis (primarily α-effect). Dipivefrin, a prodrug, is metabolized in vivo to epinephrine. It may produce fewer side effects than epinephrine because it penetrates into the eye better. These patients are being treated for chronic open-angle glaucoma.

Amphetamine and amphetamine-like adrenergics. The amphetamines and other agents with similar actions are used for their CNS effects. Legitimate medical uses for these agents include narcolepsy and attention deficit disorder in children. Patients with epilepsy or Parkinson's disease are occasionally given these agents to counteract the sedation produced by the other medication they are taking. In the past, amphetamines have been used to treat obesity and mental depression. These indications are no longer considered appropriate for these products. With prolonged use, these agents can produce physical dependence and withdrawal, and may evoke suicidal tendencies. Chapter 26 discusses the abuse of these agents.

Methylphenidate (Ritalin) and pemoline (Cylert) have CNS stimulant actions similar to the amphetamines and are used to treat attention deficit disorder in children. They can manage distractibility, emotional lability, short attention span, hyperactivity, and impulsivity. Nervousness and insomnia, blood pressure and pulse changes, and anorexia have been seen. Children using these agents may not be completely controlled, leading to increased motor activity in a dental setting.

α-Adrenergic blocking agents. The α-adrenergic blocking agents competitively inhibit the vasoconstricting effects (α-receptor effects) of the adrenergic agents. They also block the mydriasis that these agents normally cause. If epinephrine (which is both an α- and a β-agonist) is given to a patient previously treated with an α-blocker, vasodilation (β-receptor effect) would predominate. This effect is termed **epinephrine reversal.**

The α-adrenergic blockers are used in the treatment of peripheral vascular disease when vascular spasm is a common feature (such as Raynaud's disease) and in the diagnosis and treatment of pheochromocytoma, a catecholamine-secreting tumor of the adrenal medulla. Some examples of α-adrenergic blocking agents are tolazoline (Priscoline) and phentolamine (Regitine).

β-Adrenergic blocking agents. In the same fashion as the α-blockers, the β-blockers competitively block the adrenergic agents' effect on the β-receptors.

Since the β-receptors produce vasodilation, bronchodilation, and hyperglycemia and stimulate the heart (increase force and rate), β-blockers can competitively block these effects. The effect of a pure β-agonist such as isoproterenol would be blocked by a β-blocker, but in the presence of an agonist with both α- and β-receptor effects such as epinephrine, the α-receptor effects would predominate.

Propranolol (Inderal) is a β-blocker that depresses the heart (negative chronotropic and inotropic effect), produces bronchoconstriction, and can cause hypoglycemia. It is used in the treatment of arrhythmias (for its quinidine-like effect), angina, hypertension, and migraine headache prophylaxis. Diseases in which tachycardia occurs, such as hyperthyroidism and pheochromocytoma, can be symptomatically treated with propranolol. β-blockers are discussed in Chapter 15.

α- and β-Blocking agents. Labetalol (Normodyne, Trandate) has both α- and β-blocking action. Note the ending *-alol* rather than *-olol*. It is a selective α$_1$-blocker and nonselective β-blocker. It is indicated for the treatment of hypertension. It produces a fall in blood pressure without reflex tachycardia.

REVIEW QUESTIONS

1. Compare and contrast the anatomic and functional organization of the parasympathetic and sympathetic nervous systems.
2. State the responses of the major tissues and organ systems to the adrenergic (sympathetic) and cholinergic (parasympathetic) nervous systems.
3. State the location(s) of acetylcholine and norepinephrine, the two major neurotransmitter substances.
4. Describe the major methods by which the actions of acetylcholine and norepinephrine are terminated.
5. State the sites of the muscarinic and nicotinic receptors and describe an agent that blocks each of these sites.
6. Explain the difference in mechanism of action between the direct-acting and indirect-acting cholinergic agents.

7. Describe the pharmacologic effects of the cholinergic agents on the heart, gastrointestinal tract, and eye.
8. State two major uses of the cholinergic agents.
9. Describe a unique dental use for pilocarpine.
10. State a use for physostigmine in the treatment of an overdose.
11. Describe the pharmacologic effects of the anticholinergic agents on the exocrine glands, smooth muscle, and eye.
12. Explain the adverse reactions associated with the anticholinergic agents.
13. State the contraindications and cautions to the use of anticholinergic agents and explain their relationship to the pharmacologic effects of these agents.
14. State the major therapeutic uses of the anticholinergics.
15. Discuss the relative α- and β-receptor effects possessed by epinephrine, norepinephrine, and isoproterenol. Include the effects of these agents on the blood pressure, heart rate, and blood vessels.
16. State the pharmacologic effect of the adrenergic agents on the eye, bronchioles, and salivary glands.
17. State the therapeutic uses of the adrenergic agents, especially the uses these agents have in dentistry.
18. Explain the limits to the accepted medical uses of the amphetamine-like agents.
19. Name the pharmacologic class to which propranolol (Inderal) belongs. Describe the effects that make it useful in the treatment of arrhythmias, angina, and hypertension.
20. Differentiate between "selective" and "nonselective" β-blockers. Name a difference important to the dental hygienist (drug interaction).

Chapter 6

Nonopioid (nonnarcotic) analgesics

9/8/93

Pain control is of great importance in dental practice. It is often pain that brings the patient to the dental office. Conversely, pain can be the factor that keeps the patient from seeking dental care at the appropriate time. Thus dental treatment is often rendered on the inflamed, hypersensitive tissues of a patient who suffers from mental fatigue after long endurance of pain.

The dental hygienist must be able to recognize and evaluate a patient's need for medication to control pain. Because pain is such a complex phenomenon, the entire patient must be considered before the type of medication that may be needed is determined.

PAIN AND ANALGESIC THERAPY

The sensation of pain is the means by which the body is made urgently aware of the presence of tissue damage. Pain represents a protective reflex for self-preservation. Just as the hand is quickly removed from a hot object, a painful dental abscess brings the patient to the dental office seeking professional assistance for its resolution. Pain is a diagnostic symptom of an underlying pathologic condition. Although the relief of pain is an immediate objective, only by treatment of the underlying cause is the ultimate resolution achieved.

Since there are two components of pain, **perception** and **reaction,** the treatment of pain differs considerably from other types of therapy. Although individuals are surprisingly uniform in their perception of pain, they vary greatly in their reaction to it. A predisposition toward a greater reaction to pain has been associated with emotional instability, fatigue, youth, Latin Americans and Southern Europeans, women, and fear and apprehension.[1] As a result, analgesic therapy must be selected for the individual. A level of discomfort that may not require drug treatment in one person may demand extreme therapy in another. Although some patients undergoing routine exodontia require no postoperative medication, even the strongest analgesics will not completely control postoperative extraction pain in other persons. For the same reason, the effectiveness of a placebo response in the treatment of dental pain cannot be ignored. Some dental patients require only a placebo for their postoperative pain. We are just beginning to learn the mechanism of the placebo response. Thus, to obtain maximum analgesic effectiveness, confidence in the drug should be engendered. The confidence the patient has in the dental hygienist can be conveyed to the analgesic drug suggested or prescribed.

One difficulty in evaluating an analgesic is related to the testing methods used. Reliable results are difficult to produce when measuring and comparing the analgesic potency of various agents, since the pain threshold is altered by many factors. Because experimentally induced pain does not produce reliable results, most modern studies on analgesics are done on "real" pain. The dental extraction presents an ideal pain model for testing analgesic efficacy.

CLASSIFICATION

The analgesic agents can be divided into two groups, the mild, nonnarcotic, nonopioid, peripheral antipyretic analgesics, and the strong, narcotic, opioid, central group.

An important difference between the nonopioid and the opioid analgesics is their site of action. Nonopioid analgesics act primarily at the peripheral nerve endings, although they also act centrally. Opioids act within the central nervous system (CNS).

Another difference between the narcotic and nonnarcotic analgesic agents is their mechanism of action. The action of the nonnarcotic analgesic agents is related to their ability to inhibit prostaglandin synthesis. The opioids affect pain perception by depressing the CNS. The side effect profiles of the two groups also differ.

The nonopioids can be divided into the aspirin and aspirin-like group and acetaminophen, or into the aspirin-like group, acetaminophen, and the nonsteroidal antiinflammatory agents. Aspirin, a member of the salicylates, is discussed first.

SALICYLATES

Since antiquity, extracts of willow bark containing salicin have been used to reduce fever. Since that time, many other salicylates have been synthesized, but aspirin is the most useful salicylate for analgesia. Since aspirin is the prototype salicylate, it will be discussed.

Chemistry

Acetylsalicylic acid is broken down into acetic acid and salicylic acid.

| Acetylsalicylic acid | Acetic acid | Salicylic acid |

Acetic acid imparts the characteristic vinegar odor to a bottle of aspirin. Therefore the degree of breakdown of aspirin can be roughly determined by smelling a bottle of aspirin tablets. Also, salicylic acid is a strong keratolytic agent and may cause additional adverse gastrointestinal effects if degraded aspirin is administered orally.

Mechanism of action

The mechanism of aspirin's analgesic, antipyretic, and antiinflammatory actions is related to its ability to inhibit prostaglandin synthesis. Aspirin inhibits the enzyme, prostaglandin synthetase (cyclooxygenase), by acetylating a serine resulting in an inhibition of the production of prostaglandins. Prostaglandins, lipids that are synthesized locally by inflammatory stimuli, can sensitize the pain receptors to substances such as bradykinin. Therefore a reduction in prostaglandins results in a reduction in painful perception. Because it blocks the synthesis of prostaglandins, aspirin's action is more effective if given before the painful stimuli is experienced. This explains why aspirin is not effective against "stabbing" pain (direct effect on nerve endings) and is effective against "throbbing" pain (caused by inflammation, and common in dentistry).

Pharmacologic effects

1. Analgesic effect. Although the analgesic potency of aspirin is weaker than that of the strongest opioids, its analgesic effect has been repeatedly demonstrated in clinical trials. In fact, it is often included as a treatment group when new analgesic drugs are tested. Aspirin typically relieves mild to moderate pain such as a headache or toothache. For more intense pain the opioids are required. Because of its easy accessibility and long history of use, aspirin's worth as an analgesic is not always recognized.

2. Antipyretic effect. The ability of aspirin to reduce fever results from its inhibition of prostaglandin synthesis in the hypothalamus. Hypothalamic prostaglandin synthesis is caused by elevated blood levels of leukocyte **pyrogens** induced by inflammation. Increased hypothalamic prostaglandin levels produce increased body temperature. Therefore the inhibition of hypothalamic prostaglandin synthesis results in a return to more normal body temperature. Aspirin reduces fever by inducing peripheral vasodilation and sweating. Although it reduces an elevated temperature, it has no effect on normal body temperature.

3. Antiinflammatory effect. Aspirin's antiin-

flammatory effect is derived from its ability to inhibit prostaglandin synthesis. The prostaglandins are potent vasodilating agents that also increase capillary permeability. Therefore aspirin causes decreased **erythema** and swelling of the inflamed area. Patients with arthritis are often given large doses of aspirin to provide symptomatic relief of pain and inflammation in the joints.

4. Uricosuric effect. Even though large doses (greater than 5 gm/day) of aspirin can produce a uricosuric effect, small doses (less than 1 gm/day) produce uric acid excretion. Aspirin can also counteract the uricosuric effect of probenecid (Benemid), used to treat gout. More effective uricosuric agents are available to treat gout.

5. Antithrombotic effect. Aspirin's antithrombotic effect has been shown to be effective in a selected male population. Since it can inhibit both prostacyclin (inhibits aggregation) and thromboxane A_2 (stimulates aggregation), depending on the dose, further studies are needed to determine aspirin's usefulness and dose in preventing clotting events.

Adverse reactions

In high enough doses, aspirin can produce a variety of undesirable effects. Some of aspirin's side effects can be minimized, but not eliminated.

Precautions and contraindications for the administration of aspirin are listed in Table 6-1.

1. Gastrointestinal effects. Aspirin's most frequent side effect is gastrointestinal. It may be simple dyspepsia or nausea, vomiting, or gastric bleeding. These adverse effects result from direct gastric irritation, as well as from inhibition of the cytoprotective mucus secondary to prostaglandin inhibition. In high doses, aspirin's stimulation of the chemoreceptor trigger zone in the CNS can also produce nausea and vomiting. Salicylate-induced gastric bleeding is painless and in most instances does not significantly affect a patient's health. However, salicylates may exacerbate preexisting ulcers, gastritis, or hiatal hernia.

2. Bleeding. At usual therapeutic doses, aspirin interferes with the clotting mechanism irreversibly by reducing platelet adhesiveness (stickiness or aggregation) caused by interfering with adenosine diphosphate (ADP) release. The bleeding time is prolonged and remains so until new platelets are formed (4 to 7 days). With repeated doses it also inhibits prothrombin synthesis resulting in hypoprothrombinemia. These bleeding effects can contribute to gastrointestinal bleeding.

3. Reye's (rīs) syndrome. In children and adolescents with either chickenpox or influenza the use of aspirin has been epidemiologically associ-

Table 6-1. Precautions and contraindications for the administration of aspirin

Disease or condition	Drug taken	Reason for precaution or contraindication
Peptic ulcer		Gastric irritant effect
Hemophilia		Gastric bleeding
Gout	Probenecid	Antagonizes uricosuric effect
Myocardial infarct	Warfarin	Displaces drug from protein-binding site, increasing its toxicity
Cancer, psoriasis	Methotrexate	
Asthma		High incidence of hypersensitivity reactions
Hypoprothrombinemia		Inhibition of platelet aggregation
Vitamin K deficiency		
Glucose-6-phosphate dehydrogenase deficiency		Hemolysis
Rheumatic fever		May be taking large quantities already
Pregnancy		Possible alteration of gestation period and labor

Adapted from Holroyd, S.V.: Clinical pharmacology in dental practice, ed. 2, St. Louis, 1978, The C.V. Mosby Co.

ated with Reye's syndrome. Acetaminophen is used in pediatrics for its antipyretic action. Hepatotoxicity and encephalopathy that can be fatal have been reported with Reye's syndrome.

4. Hepatic and renal effects. Rarely aspirin can produce hepatotoxicity. Renal papillary necrosis and interstitial nephritis associated with analgesic use may be caused by intake of aspirin concomitantly with the coal tar derivatives.

5. Pregnancy and nursing. Even though animal studies have shown that aspirin can produce birth defects, human studies have demonstrated only a slight positive correlation between chronic aspirin ingestion and congenital abnormalities. With aspirin abuse, increased risk of stillbirth or neonatal death, as well as decreased birthweight, have been shown to occur. With near-term, high-dose administration of aspirin, gestation can be prolonged, parturition delayed, and risk of hemorrhage increased in the newborn and mother. Although salicylates are excreted in the breast milk, usual occasional therapeutic doses of aspirin do not present a problem for the healthy nursing infant.

6. Allergy and hypersensitivity. The incidence of true aspirin allergy is about 0.2%. Many patients with an allergy to aspirin in their charts really, on questioning, have upset stomachs, rather than a true allergy. Allergic reactions can vary from rash, wheezing, urticaria, and angioneurotic edema, to anaphylactic shock. When a true aspirin allergy exists any aspirin-containing products should be avoided.

The aspirin hypersensitivity triad—aspirin hypersensitivity, asthma, and nasal polyps—often occur together. These patients exhibit cross-hypersensitivity between aspirin and other agents, including the nonsteroidal antiinflammatory agents.

Overdose toxicity

Symptoms. When the blood level of salicylates reaches a certain level a toxic reaction, referred to as *salicylism*, occurs. It is characterized by tinnitus, headache, nausea, vomiting, dizziness, and dimness of vision. Hyperthermia and electrolyte imbalance can also occur. With higher levels, stimulation of respiration leads to hyperventilation, producing respiratory alkalosis. Compensatory alkalosis results in renal loss of bicarbonate, sodium, and potassium. Both respiratory and metabolic acidosis ensues. The cause of death from aspirin poisoning is usually acidosis and electrolyte imbalance.

Prevention. Children are the primary accidental poisoning victims. The lethal adult dose of aspirin is between 10 and 30 gm. Education of the parents regarding the potential for poisoning and proper storage, as well as childproof containers for over-the-counter (OTC) aspirin have reduced accidental poisonings in children significantly.

Treatment. Treatment of aspirin poisoning includes removing excess drug in the stomach by inducing emesis or administering activated charcoal to adsorb the aspirin. Other symptoms are treated symptomatically. For example, acidosis is treated with sodium bicarbonate, hypokalemia with potassium, and hypoglycemia with glucose intravenously.

Drug interactions

The common drug interactions with aspirin are listed in Table 6-2. Some of the more notable are briefly discussed.

1. Warfarin. The drug interaction between aspirin and warfarin can result in bleeding. Warfarin, an oral anticoagulant, is highly protein bound to plasma protein binding sites. If aspirin is administered to a patient taking warfarin, it can displace the warfarin from its binding sites increasing its anticoagulant effect. Also, aspirin itself affects both platelets and the gastrointestinal tract.

2. Probenecid. Aspirin interferes with probenecid's uricosuric effect. Aspirin has been reported to have precipitated an acute attack of gout.

3. Methotrexate (MTX). MTX, an antineoplastic drug used to treat certain kinds of cancer and psoriasis, can also be displaced from protein binding sites. This results in an increase in side effects, such as bone marrow depression.

Table 6-2. Salicylate-drug interactions

Drug	Mechanism	Outcome
Ammonium chloride	Acidified urine increases reabsorption of salicylate	Increased plasma salicylate
Anticoagulants, oral	Reduced plasma prothrombin levels; displaced coumarin anticoagulants from plasma protein binding	Hemorrhage
Antidiabetic agents	Displaced agent from plasma protein binding site	Hypoglycemia
Ascorbic acid	Acidified urine reducing urinary excretion	Increased plasma salicylate
Corticosteroids	Increased filtration and decreased reabsorption of water	Decreased blood salicylate concentrations
Ethyl alcohol	Increased gastrointestinal bleeding produced by salicylates	Hemorrhage
Heparin	Inhibited platelet function impairing hemostasis	Hemorrhage
Methotrexate	Displaced methotrexate from plasma protein binding and blocked renal tubular secretion of methotrexate	Increased free methotrexate
Probenecid	Inhibited uricosuric activity; salicylates and probenecid may share common binding site on plasma albumin	Increased levels of uric acid precipitating acute attack of gout
Sulfinpyrazone	Inhibited uricosuric activity	Increased levels of uric acid precipitating acute attack of gout

Adapted from Hansten, P.D.: Drug interactions, ed. 3, Philadelphia, 1975, Lea & Febiger.

Pharmacokinetics

Aspirin is rapidly and almost completely absorbed from the stomach and small intestine producing a peak effect on an empty stomach in 30 minutes (90 minutes for salicylate). The buffered tablet reaches its peak in about 50 minutes (salicylate). Before a tablet of aspirin can be absorbed it must be dispersed and dissolve. Addition of a buffer to the tablet facilitates this process. This is borne out by the quicker peak of action and higher blood levels attained with the buffered aspirin preparations. The buffered aspirin has a higher proportion of the aspirin in the ionized form, which should make absorption slower, but this is offset by the dissolution process, which is facilitated. This difference in absorption has not been shown to translate into a quicker or more effective clinical effect.

Aspirin may be administered rectally when vomiting is present. Since this route is more erratic and unpredictable it should only be used when the oral route is not feasible. An aspirin tablet should never be applied topically to the oral mucosa to treat a toothache. A painful ulceration can occur. Any benefit from this practice would come from inadvertent swallowing of the aspirin or local damage to nerve endings.

Aspirin is widely distributed into most body tissues and fluids. It is poorly bound to plasma proteins. It is hydrolyzed to salicylate in the mucosa of the gastrointestinal tract and on first pass through the liver. Salicylate is conjugated with glycine and glucuronic acid by the liver microsomal enzymes. Salicylate is excreted by a capacity-limited process. For this reason, aspirin's half-life is dose dependent. With small doses the half-life is 2 to 3 hours; with higher doses a half-life of 15 to 30 hours can be attained. The half-life of unhydrolyzed aspirin is about 15 minutes. In a poisoning situation, the excretion of aspirin can be increased by alkalinization of the urine with sodium bicarbonate.

Uses

Aspirin's primary use is to provide analgesia for mild to moderate pain. Its antipyretic effect is useful in the control of fever. Its antiinflammatory action is employed in the treatment of inflammatory conditions such as rheumatic fever and arthritis.

Dosage and preparations

The usual adult dosage of aspirin for the treatment of pain or fever is 650 mg (two 5-grain tablets) every 4 hours. The dosage for children is 65 mg/kg/24 hours (maximum 3.6 gm/24 hours) divided into four to six doses. Dosage for children should never exceed 60 mg (1 grain) for each year of age, five times a day.

Many types of preparations containing aspirin are available by prescription and over the counter (Table 6-3). Some of these types are as follows:

1. Regular aspirin. A single-entity form of aspirin includes the commonly used 325 mg (5 grain) tablet and 75 mg (1¼ grain) flavored children's tablet. Many brand-name and generic products are available.

2. Enteric-coated aspirin. Aspirin can be formulated with an enteric coating that dissolves in the intestine rather than the stomach. These products can give erratic absorption and unreliable blood levels. The onset of action is too long to make them useful for acute dental pain. They have limited use in treatment of chronic arthritis because they have been shown to reduce gastric irritation.

3. Sustained-release aspirin. There is no justification at the present for these products.

4. Combinations

a. With buffer. Buffered tableted preparations, although claimed to produce fewer gastrointestinal side effects, have never been shown to do so. They do have a slightly quicker rate of absorption. The liquid buffered preparations do produce less gastrointestinal irritation, but contain sodium in the form of sodium bicarbonate. Sodium is relatively contraindicated in cardiovascular disease such as high blood pressure.

b. With another analgesic. Aspirin is often combined with acetaminophen or an opioid-like codeine. Most authors feel these combinations are additive. Mixing aspirin with acetaminophen may increase the chance of toxicity. Mixing aspirin with an opioid can reduce the amount of the opioid in the product, and therefore its side effects.

c. With sedatives. Adding a sedative to aspirin can make it more effective if anxiety is a substan-

Table 6-3.   Selected aspirin-containing products

Type of aspirin	Selected brand names	Amount of aspirin (mg)	Other ingredients	Approximate amount
Regular	Bayer	325	None	
	Empirin	325		
	St. Joseph	325		
Buffered tablets	Bufferin	324	Magnesium carbonate	100 mg
			Aluminum glycinate	50 mg
	Ascriptin	325	Magnesium-aluminum hydroxide	150 mg
Buffered solutions	Alka-Seltzer	324	Sodium bicarbonate	2 gm
			Citric acid	1 gm
Enteric	Ecotrin	325	None	
Sustained release	Measurin	650	None	
	Zorprin	· 800	None	
Combinations	Excedrin Tablets	250	Caffeine	65 mg
			Acetaminophen	250 mg
	Anacin	400	Caffeine	32 mg

tial component of the pain. Prescribing a separate antianxiety agent would give the prescriber more control and is preferred.

d. With caffeine. Caffeine may potentiate the analgesic effect of aspirin. Controlled studies are needed to verify this initial finding.

Other salicylates

Sodium, choline, and magnesium salicylate and salicylamide, and salsalate are other salicylates. These agents claim to have fewer gastrointestinal side effects, but this claim has little, if any documentation. Their efficacy as analgesic agents and the appropriate doses for analgesia need to be determined. Two advantages of these agents is that they have no platelet effects and no cross-hypersensitivity with aspirin. Magnesium is contraindicated in renal disease and sodium in cardiovascular disease.

Diflunisal

Diflunisal (Dolobid) is classified as a nonsteroidal antiinflammatory agent (NSAIA). Its peak of action occurs in 2 to 3 hours after ingestion and its half-life is 8 to 12 hours in the normal patient. It is as effective as the other NSAIAs in the treatment of pain. It can be administered before a dental procedure to delay the onset of pain postsurgically. Because of its long half-life, it is dosed only two or three times daily. The general comments relating to the NSAIAs also apply to diflunisal. Its antipyretic effect is not clinically useful.

NONSTEROIDAL ANTIINFLAMMATORY AGENTS (NSAIAs) OR DRUGS (NSAIDs)

The NSAIAs are a rapidly growing group of analgesics that have important application in dentistry. Their mechanism of action, and many of their pharmacologic effects and adverse reactions resemble those of aspirin. Many authors agree that the NSAIAs are the most useful drug group for the treatment of dental pain.

Mechanism of action

Like aspirin, NSAIAs inhibit the enzyme cyclooxygenase, resulting in a reduction in the formation of prostaglandin precursors and thromboxanes from arachidonic acid. Many of the actions, as well as the adverse reactions, of the NSAIAs result from their inhibition of prostaglandin synthesis.

Chemical classification

NSAIAs are divided into six chemical derivatives: the propionic acids, acetic acids, fenamic acids, pyrazolones, oxicams, and salicylates. Table 6-4 lists the NSAIAs by chemical classification and includes the pharmacokinetic parameters, analgesic dose, and dosing interval. Most members of the propionic acid derivative group, along with mefenamic acid and diflunisal, are approved for use for the management of pain.

Pharmacokinetics

Most NSAIAs peak in about 1 to 2 hours (see Table 6-4). The effect of food on absorption of the NSAIAs approved to treat pain is to reduce the rate but not the extent of absorption of ibuprofen, the naproxens, and diflunisal. There is no effect on absorption of the NSAIAs with oral antacids, except for diflunisal (antacids reduce absorption). They are metabolized in the liver and excreted by the kidney. The half-lives ($t_{1/2}$) of the individual agents are listed in Table 6-4. Biliary or fecal excretion occurs with the fenamic acids, piroxicam, sulindac, and tolmetin.

Pharmacologic effects

The analgesic, antipyretic, and antiinflammatory actions of the NSAIAs result from the same mechanism as aspirin—inhibition of prostaglandin synthesis by inhibiting cyclooxygenase. The antigout action of the NSAIAs is related to their analgesic and antiinflammatory action but is independent of their effect on serum uric acid. NSAIAs are useful for treating dysmenorrhea, or painful menstruation, because this condition is due to an excess in the uterine wall of prostaglandins producing painful contractions.

Adverse reactions

Gastrointestinal effects. Gastrointestinal irritation, pain, and bleeding problems leading to tarry stools can occur with all the NSAIAs. The

Table 6-4. Nonsteroidal antiinflammatory agents

Drug name	Peak (hr)	$t_{1/2}$ (hr)	Analgesic dose (mg)	Dosing interval (hr)	Comments
Propionic acid derivatives					
Ibuprofen (Motrin, Rufen)	1–2	1.8–2.5	400	4–6	a
Fenoprofen (Nalfon)	2	2–3	200	4–6	
Suprofen (Suprol)	0.5–2.0	2–4	200	4–6	b
Naproxen (Naprosyn)	2–4	12–15	500 stat; 250	6–8	
Naproxen sodium (Anaprox)	1–2	12–15	550 stat; 275	6–8	
Ketoprofen (Orudis)	0.5–2.0	2–4			c
Benoxaprofen (Oraflex)					b
Acetic acid derivatives					
Indomethacin (Indocin)	1–2	4.5–6.0	—	—	c
Sulindac (Clinoril)	1–2	7.8(16.4)	—	—	c,d
Tolmetin (Tolectin)	0.5–1.0	1.0–1.5	—	—	c
Zomepirac (Zomax)					b
Fenamic acid derivatives					
Meclofenemate (Meclomen)	0.5–2.0	2(3.3)	—	—	c,e
Mefenamic acid (Ponstel)	2–4	2–4	500 stat; 250	6	f
Pyrazolones					
Phenylbutazone (Butazolidin)	2.5	84	—	—	c,g
Oxyphenbutazone (Oxalid)	6	72	—	—	c,g
Oxicams					
Piroxicam (Feldene)	3–5	30–86	—	—	c,h
Salicylates					
Diflunisal (Dolobid)	2–3	8–12	1000 stat; 500	8–12	i

Modified from Holroyd, S.V., Wynn, R.L., and Requa-Clark, B.: Clinical pharmacology in dental practice, ed. 4, St. Louis, 1988, The C.V. Mosby Co.
a, Now available over the counter as Nuprin/Advil, Medipren/Haltran.
b, Not available in the United States (removed from the market).
c, Not approved for use as simple analgesic.
d, Half-life of active metabolite in parentheses.
e, Half-life with chronic use in parentheses.
f, Therapy not usually to exceed 1 week.
g, Rarely aplastic anemia and agranulocytosis.
h, qd dosing for arthritis.
i, A salicylate derivative.

prostaglandins stimulate the production of cytoprotective mucus and reduce gastric acid secretion. Prostaglandin inhibitors, like NSAIAs, can interfere with the normal protective mechanisms in the stomach, causing symptoms or even an ulceration or perforation.

Central nervous system effects. CNS side effects include sedation, dizziness, confusion, mental depression, headache, vertigo, and convulsions. Because of the CNS effects of the NSAIAs, patients taking them should be cautioned about driving an automobile. These agents are not addicting, tolerance does not develop and no withdrawal syndrome can be induced.

Blood clotting. The NSAIAs reversibly inhibit platelet aggregation because they inhibit TXA_2

production. In contrast to aspirin, their effect remains only as long as the drug is present in the blood.

Renal effects. Renal effects of the NSAIAs include renal failure, cystitis, and an increased incidence of urinary tract infections. The NSAIAs have little effect on the patient with normal kidney function; however, with disease, decreases in both renal blood flow and glomerular filtration rate can occur.

Other effects. Other adverse effects associated with the NSAIAs are muscle weakness, ringing ears, hepatitis, hematologic problems, and blurred vision. Peripheral edema with fluid retention has been noted. Oral manifestations reported include ulcerative stomatitis, gingival ulcerations, and dry mouth.

Hypersensitivity reactions. Like aspirin, the NSAIAs can induce a wide range of hypersensitivity reactions, including hives or itching, angioneurotic edema, chills and fever, Stevens-Johnson syndrome, exfoliative dermatitis, and epidermal necrolysis. Anaphylactoid reactions including bronchospasm (wheezing) have been reported. The pyrazolones are the only group that does not have cross-sensitivity with the other agents, and they are not approved for use in pain.

Zomepirac is an example of an NSAIA that was removed from the market in response to a few fatal hypersensitivity reactions reported. Some of the fatalities should never have been given zomepirac because of their positive history of aspirin hypersensitivity. The lesson that this product should teach us is that a new drug may have previously undiscovered adverse reactions and should not be used without a clear advantage over available drugs.

Pregnancy and nursing. Like aspirin, the NSAIAs given late in pregnancy can prolong gestation, delay parturition, and produce dystocia or premature closure of the ductus arteriosus. The uterine prostaglandins are responsible for parturition and closure of the ductus arteriosus. Fenoprofen, ibuprofen, naproxen, and tolmetin have not been shown to be teratogenic in animal studies (FDA pregnancy category B). Diflunisal and

mefenamic acid have been shown to be teratogenic in animals (FDA pregnancy category C).

Ibuprofen has not been detected in breast milk, whereas fenoprofen and mefenamic acid are present in very small quantities. Both naproxen (1% of serum) and diflunisal (5% of serum) are excreted in breast milk. Piroxicam has been shown to inhibit lactation in animals and is to be avoided in nursing mothers.

Drug interactions. The drug interactions of the NSAIAs are summarized in Table 6-5. Most of the interactions are still under investigation for

Table 6-5. Drug interactions of the nonsteroidal antiinflammatory agents (NSAIAs)

Specific NSAIA/ Interacting Drug	Potential outcome
All NSAIAs	
Warfarin (coumadin)	Increased anticoagulant action, possible GI bleeding
Propranolol (Inderal)	Decreased antihypertensive effect
Captopril (Capoten)	Decreased antihypertensive effect
Ibuprofen	
Phenytoin (Dilantin)	Increased phenytoin effect
Digoxin (Lanoxin)	Temporarily increased digoxin effect
Cimetidine (Tagamet)	Increased ibuprofen effect
Furosemide (Lasix)	Decreased diuretic effect
Naproxen	
Lithium (Lithobid)	Increased lithium effect
Methotrexate (MTX) (Mexate)	Impaired MTX elimination
Probenecid (Benemid)	Increased naproxen effect
Diflunisal	
Acetaminophen (Tylenol)	Increased acetaminophen effect and toxicity
Aluminum hydroxide (Amphojel)	Decreased diflunisal effect

their clinical significance and presence with each NSAIA. One interaction that is clinically significant but has only been demonstrated with indomethacin is the production of lithium toxicity in those patients taking lithium with bipolar affective disorders.

Contraindications and cautions

The contraindications and cautions for using an NSAIA are related to their adverse reactions. Patients with asthma, cardiovascular diseases with fluid retention, coagulopathies, peptic ulcer, and ulcerative colitis should be given NSAIAs cautiously, if at all.

Patients also at higher risk for adverse reactions include those with renal function impairment, a history of previous hypersensitivity to aspirin or other NSAIAs, and geriatric patients (more prone to adverse hepatic or renal adverse reactions).

Therapeutic uses
Medical

Depending on the specific NSAIA and the clinical trials that have been conducted, medical use of NSAIAs may include many conditions. Osteoarthritis, rheumatoid arthritis, gouty arthritis, fever, dysmenorrhea, and pain are indications for the NSAIAs. Accepted unlabeled indications for which NSAIAs are frequently prescribed include bursitis and tendonitis.

Dental

The NSAIAs are useful in the management of dental pain. Many studies that have compared the analgesic efficacy of the NSAIAs with that of the opioid analgesics find that they are equivalent in many clinical situations. For example, usual analgesic doses of the NSAIAs have been shown to be as effective as 650 mg of aspirin, 650 mg of aspirin or acetaminophen plus various amounts of codeine, and even as effective as the intermediate-strength opioid combinations (oxycodone plus aspirin or acetaminophen). In usual therapeutic doses, NSAIAs can be shown to be statistically significantly better than most doses of codeine alone, low doses of aspirin and acetaminophen,

and placebo. It is no wonder that the dental use of the NSAIAs has greatly increased.

Ibuprofen (Advil, Motrin, Rufen)

Ibuprofen, the oldest member of the NSAIAs, has the most clinical experience. It is rapidly absorbed orally, and food decreases its rate but not its extent of absorption; antacids have no effect. The half-life is about 2 hours. Its onset of action is about half an hour, and its duration of action is 4 to 6 hours. It undergoes hepatic metabolism and is excreted by the kidney. It is an effective analgesic and has been studied in many dental situations. Ibuprofen is the drug of choice for the treatment of dental pain when an NSAIA is indicated. Only in rare cases or if new information becomes available is there an indication for other NSAIAs. When a longer acting agent is desired for patient convenience, another relative of ibuprofen or diflunisal can be used.

Clinical trials in dental pain management testify to ibuprofen's effectiveness. Cooper[2] found that 400 mg of ibuprofen was more effective than 650 mg of aspirin, 600 mg of acetaminophen, and both aspirin and acetaminophen when combined with 60 mg of codeine. A shallow dose-response curve for ibuprofen has been demonstrated by various investigators with some finding no difference between the 200 and the 400 mg dose, while others finding no difference between the 400 and the 800 mg dose. Most studies can easily demonstrate that 400 mg of ibuprofen is better than any usual therapeutic doses of codeine.

The usual analgesic dose is 400 mg every 4 to 6 hours. It is available over the counter in 200 mg tablet. Patient instructions for the use of NSAIAs are:
1. Take with a full glass of water.
2. Take with food to minimize gastrointestinal irritation.
3. Do not use acetaminophen or aspirin concurrently.
4. Use caution with driving because of the possibility of drowsiness or dizziness.
5. If pain does not subside within a few days, call the dentist.

Naproxen (sodium) (Naproxyn, Anaprox)

These two propionic acid NSAIAs have slightly longer half-lives and can be dosed on an every-6-to-8-hour schedule. They should also be given with a loading dose (see Table 6-4). Their pharmacologic effects, adverse reactions, and efficacy are similar to those of ibuprofen. In addition to tablets, this product is available in suspension form.

ACETAMINOPHEN

Acetaminophen (paracetamol, N-acetyl para-aminophenol; Tylenol) is the only member of the para-aminophenols currently available for clinical use. Acetanilid, the parent compound, was introduced in 1886 and rapidly shown to be too toxic. Phenacetin, removed from the market in 1983, was more toxic than acetaminophen. It is used as an analgesic and antipyretic when aspirin is contraindicated. *NOT anti-inflammatory*

Administration, absorption, and metabolism

Acetaminophen is rapidly and completely absorbed from the gastrointestinal tract, achieving a peak plasma level in 1 to 3 hours. After therapeutic doses, it is excreted with a $t_{\frac{1}{2}}$ of 1 to 4 hours. Acetaminophen is metabolized by the liver microsomal enzymes to the glucuronide conjugate, the sulfuric acid conjugate, and cysteine. When large doses are ingested an intermediate metabolite is produced that is thought to be hepatotoxic and possibly nephrotoxic.

Pharmacologic effects

The analgesic and antipyretic effects of acetaminophen are approximately the same (milligram for milligram) as aspirin; however, acetaminophen does not possess any clinically significant antiinflammatory effect. Therefore, it is not useful in the treatment of arthritis. Differences in degree of prostaglandin synthesis inhibition at different sites may account for this difference in action.

Therapeutic doses of acetaminophen have no effect on the cardiovascular or respiratory system.

In contrast to aspirin, acetaminophen does not produce gastric bleeding, or affect platelet adhesiveness or uric acid excretion.

Adverse effects

The principal toxic effects of acetaminophen are hepatic necrosis and nephrotoxicity.

Hepatic effects. Hepatic necrosis may occur in adults after the ingestion of a single dose of 10 to 15 gm of acetaminophen; 25 gm or more is potentially fatal. Symptoms during the first 2 days after intoxication are minor. Nausea, vomiting, anorexia, and abdominal pain may occur. Liver injury becomes manifest on the second to third day, with alterations in plasma enzyme levels (elevated transaminase and lactic hydrogenase), elevated bilirubin levels, and prolongation of prothrombin time. Hepatotoxicity may progress to encephalopathy, coma, and death. If the patient recovers, no residual hepatic abnormalities persist. Patients with hepatic disease, such as alcoholics or patients with a history of hepatitis, should avoid acetaminophen.

Treatment. The treatment of overdose toxicity should begin with gastric lavage if a drug has recently been ingested. The administration of activated charcoal and magnesium or sodium sulfate solution should follow. The administration of sulfhydryl groups in the form of oral N-acetyl-cysteine reduces or even prevents liver damage if given soon enough after ingestion.

Nephrotoxicity. Nephrotoxicity has been associated with long-term consumption. The primary lesion appears to be a papillary necrosis with secondary interstitial nephritis. Although no single agent can be identified, prolonged consumption of analgesics can lead to kidney disease. Because analgesics are used in dental practice on a short-term basis, the possibility of nephrotoxicity does not present a significant problem in dental therapy. Concurrent chronic use of the combination of acetaminophen and aspirin or the NSAIA increases the risk of analgesic nephropathy, renal papillary necrosis, end-stage renal disease, and cancer of the kidney or urinary bladder.

Drug interactions

Acetaminophen is remarkably free of drug interactions at usual therapeutic doses.

Uses

Acetaminophen is employed as an analgesic and antipyretic. It is especially useful in patients who have aspirin hypersensitivity or in whom aspirin-induced gastric irritation would present a problem. In young children its use as an antipyretic has replaced aspirin because of aspirin's association with Reye's syndrome. It is not known to what degree the long-term use of therapeutic doses of acetaminophen might produce renal lesions. It has a greater propensity for producing hepatic necrosis when a large acute dose (overdose) is ingested.

Dosage and preparations

Acetaminophen is available in many combinations and elixirs (Datril, Tempra, Tylenol). The usual adult dose is one (325, 500 mg) or two tablets or capsules. Not more than 4 gm in 24 hours should be ingested by adults. Various elixirs, drops, and chewable tablets that are convenient for administration to children are available. The concentration of the elixir is 120 mg/5 ml (1 teaspoonful); the drops contain 60 mg/0.6 ml. Acetaminophen should not be administered to young children (less than 3 years old) or for more than 10 days except on a prescriber's advice. The dose for 1- to 3-year-old children is 120 mg; 4- to 5-year-olds, 200 mg; 6- to 8-year-olds, 240 mg; children over 9 years old can use the lowest adult dose.

SUMMARY

The drug of choice for mild to moderate pain is aspirin. Special caution must be exercised in regard to overdosage in children and in patients allergic to aspirin or susceptible to gastrointestinal distress. In cases in which aspirin is contraindicated or undesirable, acetaminophen is usually a good substitute. If aspirin or acetaminophen is inadequate for the relief of pain, an NSAIA may be used; its gastrointestinal and CNS effects must be

considered. If more severe pain is encountered, the opioid analgesic agents may be indicated although some authors state that the NSAIAs are equipotent in the treatment of dental pain to the opioid analgesic agents (see Chapter 7). Lastly, opioids can be combined with NSAIAs to provide additional pain relief than afforded by either alone.

DRUGS USED TO TREAT GOUT

Gout is an inherited disease occurring primarily in men with an onset that usually involves one joint, often the big toe or knee. Both hyperuricemia and urate crystals or tophi may be found in the joints or other tissues. The excess uric acid may be due to overproduction or underexcretion of uric acid. The disease responds to colchicine.

Both the NSAIAs and colchicine have been used to treat acute attacks of gout. Other agents, such as probenecid and allopurinol, are available to prevent gout. These are briefly mentioned here, although they are not analgesics per se.

Colchicine

Colchicine has only one indication—the treatment of an acute attack of gout. It is so specific in its action on gouty attacks that it is sometimes used to diagnose the disease. Colchicine is taken hourly at the onset of the attack or until symptoms are intolerable, which include nausea and vomiting. Its mechanism is complex, but it appears to inhibit the chemotactic property of the leukocytosis and interfere with the inflammatory response to urate crystals. Colchicine possesses many side effects, but gastrointestinal toxicity including nausea, vomiting, and diarrhea occur frequently (up to 80%). Bone marrow depression and hypersensitivity have also been reported.

Allopurinol (Zyloprim)

Allopurinol is a xanthine oxidase inhibitor that inhibits the synthesis of uric acid. It is used to prevent excessive uric acid from forming. It is also used in patients receiving either chemotherapy or irradiation for malignancy because the death of many cells causes a release of large amounts of uric acid precursors. The side effects associated with allopurinol include hepatotoxicity of a hypersensitivity type. If a pruritic rash should occur, the drug should be promptly discontinued because fatalities have been reported. This drug is not indicated for asymptomatic hyperuricemia.

Probenecid (Benemid)

The other approach to prevention of gout is to increase the excretion of uric acid by the administration of a uricosuric agent like probenecid. Probenecid, by blocking the tubular reabsorption of filtered urate, prevents new tophi and mobilizes those present. Increasing frequency or severity of acute gouty attacks is an indication for uricosuric administration. Gastrointestinal side effects and hypersensitivity may occur with probenecid use. Headaches and sore gums have also been reported. Concurrent administration of aspirin can interfere with the uricosuric action of probenecid. Diabetic tests using the copper sulfate urine test (Clinitest) may have false-positive results. Occasionally probenecid and colchicine are combined, with the colchicine preventing acute attacks while the probenecid enhances the excretion of uric acid. Probably a more rational approach is to administer each drug separately as needed. Maintenance of adequate urinary output (at least 2 L) is important to minimize the precipitation of uric acid in the urinary tract.

REVIEW QUESTIONS

1. Name the two components of pain, and state which one varies and which one is constant among patients.
2. List six factors that alter the patient's pain threshold.
3. Describe the placebo effect and discuss its place in treatment of dental pain.
4. Compare and contrast the nonopioid and opioid analgesics with respect to the following:
   a. Site of action
   b. Mechanism of action
   c. Efficacy
   d. Addiction and tolerance
   e. Toxicity
5. Explain the mechanism of action of aspirin.
6. State and describe three major effects and four other effects of aspirin.
7. Name and describe a toxic reaction to the salicylates.
8. Describe the nature and extent of the most serious drug interaction with aspirin.
9. Name the drug interactions and disease states contraindicating aspirin's use.
10. Explain the contrast between the uricosuric effect of aspirin and its interaction with probenecid.
11. Name the therapeutic uses of aspirin.
12. State the agents that are commonly combined with aspirin and describe their usefulness (or lack thereof).
13. List the various dosage forms of aspirin and their purported advantage, if any.
14. Compare and contrast the pharmacologic effects of aspirin and acetaminophen.
15. List an adverse effect of acetaminophen and describe its symptoms.
16. Explain two uses of acetaminophen.
17. Explain the role of acetaminophen in the treatment of dental pain.
18. Explain the role of the NSAIAs for the treatment of dental pain.
19. Name the major adverse reaction of the NSAIAs.
20. State three NSAIAs useful as analgesics. Describe one difference they possess.
21. State three contraindications to the use of the NSAIAs.

REFERENCES

1. Bennett, C.R.: Local anesthesia and pain control in dental practice, ed. 5, St. Louis, 1974, The C.V. Mosby Co.
2. Cooper, S.A.: Five studies on ibuprofen for postsurgical dental pain, Am. J. Med. **77**:70, 1984.

Chapter 7

Opioid analgesics and antagonists

9/8/93

The opioid analgesics are frequently used to manage dental pain that cannot be managed by the nonsteroidal antiinflammatory agents (NSAIAs). The dental hygienist should be aware of their properties and side effects.

HISTORY

Opium is the dried juice from the unripe seed capsules of the opium poppy. As early as 4000 BC, many cultures had recognized the euphoric effect of the poppy plant. In the early 1800s, morphine and codeine were isolated from opium. Until about 1920 patent medicines containing opium were promoted for numerous uses. When these agents, used orally, became unlawful, narcotic (opioid) abuse by injection began, and has continued until the present.

TERMINOLOGY

The terms used to describe this group of drugs, the opioids, is rapidly changing. The term *narcotic*, as a drug in this group was formerly referred to, is derived from the Greek word that means stupor and was used for agents that produced sleep. The term *opiate* was introduced to refer to drugs derived from opium. Since the development of synthetic opiate-like drugs the term *opioid* was coined. It is used to refer to all drugs with morphine-like action, as well as to drugs that antagonize morphine and also to the receptors involved.

CLASSIFICATION

The opioids useful clinically may be divided in several ways. The first is by mechanism of action at the receptor sites. The following are the three groups of opioids grouped by action at receptor sites:

1. Opioid agonists (e.g., morphine)
2. Mixed opioids including the agonist-antagonists (e.g., pentazocine) and the partial agonists (e.g., buprenorphine)
3. Antagonists (e.g., naloxone)

The opioids may also be classified either by their chemical structure (Table 7-1) or by their potency (Table 7-2). Structural classification is useful when a history of allergies is present. Potency classification assists in selection of the proper opioid based on the amount of pain relief needed.

MECHANISM OF ACTION

The opioids bind to receptors located in the central nervous system (CNS) producing an altered perception of and response to pain. Receptors that mediate specific pharmacologic effects and adverse reactions are stimulated to differing degrees by individual opioids. The discovery of three groups of endogenous substances with opioid-like action—the enkephalins, endorphins, and dynorphins—has helped explain the presence of these receptors. These naturally occurring peptides all possess analgesic action and have addiction potential. They probably function as neurotransmitters, but their exact function has not been elucidated. They may be involved in the analgesic action of a placebo and the enhancement of well-being that occurs with running (increase in β-endorphins).

Many opioid receptors, probably at least eight, exist in the body. Activity of three receptors, mu (μ), kappa (κ), and sigma (σ) has been defined. The μ-receptor is associated with respiratory depression, euphoria, physical dependence, and supraspinal analgesia. The κ-receptor mediates

59

Table 7-1. Opioid analgesic agents grouped by structure

NATURAL AND SEMISYNTHETIC OPIODS

Opium alkaloids (Pantopon)
Heroin (diacetylmorphine)
Morphine
Codeine (methylmorphine)
Semisynthetic derivatives of:

*Morphine

*Hydromorphone or dihydromorphinone
    (Dilaudid)
Oxymorphone (Numorphan)
Nalbuphine† (Nubain)

*Codeine

*Hydrocodone or dihydrocodeinone (Codone, in Vicodin,
    Tussend, Hycodan)
*Dihydrocodeine (in Synalgos-DC)
*Oxycodone (in Percodan, Percocet, Tylox)

SYNTHETIC OPIODS

Meperidine Group

*Meperidine (Demerol)
Ethoheptazine (Zactane)
*Alphaprodine (Nisentil)‡
Anileridine (Leritine)
Piminodine‡ (Alvodine)
Fentanyl (Sublimaze)
Diphenoxylate (in Lomotil)
Loperamide (Imodium)
Sufentanil (Sufenta)

Other

Buprenorphine (Buprenex)

Methadone Group

*Methadone (Dolophine)
*Propoxyphene (Darvon)

Morphinan Group

Levorphanol (Levo-Dromoran)
Methorphan‡
Butorphanol† (Stadol)

Benzomorphan Group

*Pentazocine† (in Talwin-NX)
Phenazocine‡ (Prinadol)

*More common opiods.
†Has antagonist properties.
‡Not marketed in the United States.

miosis, sedation, and spinal analgesia. Finally, the σ-receptor controls dysphoria, hallucinations, and respiratory and vasomotor stimulation. Differences in affinity for and action of opioids at these receptors, either agonist or antagonist action, may explain some of the differences among the effects and adverse reactions of the opioids. For example, the σ-receptor is responsible for dysphoria. Pentazocine, a σ-receptor agonist, produces dysphoria, while morphine has no effect on the σ-receptor and does not produce dysphoria.

PHARMACOKINETICS

1. Absorption. Most opioid analgesic agents are well absorbed taken orally; absorption occurs from the lungs and from the nasal and oral mucosa. A new dosage form for one opioid, a nasal spray, is being explored.

2. Distribution. After absorption, the opioids undergo first-pass metabolism in the liver or intestinal cell wall, which reduces their bioavailability. The oral/parenteral ratio determines the difference in bioavailability between the same opioid administered orally and parenterally. For example, the ratio is 0.2 to 0.3 for morphine, 0.25 to 0.7 for meperidine, and 0.4 to 0.7 for codeine. Therefore, about two thirds of codeine administered orally reaches the systemic circulation, while only about one fourth of morphine does. The opioids are bound to plasma proteins to vary-

Table 7-2. Selected opioid analgesics by strength, dosing interval, and usual doses

Drug name	Dosing interval (hr)	Usual dose (mg)*	Comments	Controlled Substances Schedule†
Strongest				
Morphine	4–6	IM: 10	Standard agent; prototype	II
Methadone	4–6‡	IM: 10 PO: 10?	Used PO for "methadone maintenance"	II
Meperidine (Demerol)	3–4	IM: 100 PO: 50	Abused by professionals	II
Hydromorphone (Dilaudid)	4–6	PO: 2	Most potent on a mg for mg basis	II
Intermediate				
Oxycodone (in Percodan, Percocet, Tylox)	4–6	PO: 5	Popular with addicts "shopping" for opioids	II
Pentazocine (in Talwin-NX)	4–6	PO: 50	Has antagonist properties	IV
Weakest				
Hydrocodone (in Vicodin)	4–6	PO: 5		III
Codeine (in Tylenol #3, Empirin #3)	4–6	PO: 30	#3 has 30 mg of codeine	III
Dihydrocodeine (in Synalgos-DC)	4–6	PO: 30	15 mg per dosage form	III
Propoxyphene (in Darvocet N-100)	4–6	PO: 65 or 100	65 mg of HCl salt equals 100 mg of napsylate	IV

*Average dose; PO, orally and IM, intramuscularly.
†Schedule for Controlled Substances (see Table 4-4).
‡Dosing interval in methadone maintenance is 24 hours.

ing degrees (morphine 35%, meperidine 60%). The opioids are also distributed to the fetus in pregnant women, accounting for the respiratory depression produced in the fetus when the mother is given opioids.

3. Metabolism. The major route of metabolism for the opioids is conjugation with glucuronic acid in the liver. The half-lives of the opioids are listed in Table 7-2. Given orally, the opioids have a similar duration of action for analgesia.

4. Excretion. Metabolized opioids are excreted by glomerular filtration as their metabolites. The metabolites as well as the unchanged drug are excreted in the urine.

The dosing interval and usual dose of some opioids are listed in Table 7-2. In general, their onset is within 1 hour and their duration necessitates dosing every 4 to 6 hours.

PHARMACOLOGIC EFFECTS

Although the pharmacologic effects and the adverse reactions of the opioids are closely related, they are discussed separately. A pharmacologic effect may also be an adverse reaction, depending on the clinical use of the agent. The degree of each of these effects is proportional to the agent's potency.

1. **Analgesia.** The opioid analgesics provide varying degrees of analgesia, depending on the strength of the agent. Table 7-2 lists the opioids from the strongest to the weakest. Morphine is the opioid against which other opioids are measured. The strongest opioids can reduce even the most severe pain; the weaker agents mixed with nonopioids are equivalent to the NSAIAs in their ability to relieve pain; the analgesic potency of the weakest agent (codeine) is difficult to demonstrate. Codeine raises the pain threshold and affects the cerebral cortex to depress the reaction to pain. Both μ- and κ-receptors are involved in producing analgesia. The opioids alter the patient's perception of painful stimuli, possibly by altering the release of certain central neurotransmitters.

2. **Sedation and euphoria.** In the usual therapeutic doses the opioid analgesics generally produce sedation by κ-receptor stimulation. This may potentiate their analgesic effect and relieve anxiety. This effect is additive with other agents that are CNS depressants, such as alcohol. With larger doses, or if the pain is suddenly removed, euphoria can result. This is due to stimulation of the μ-receptor. CNS excitation occurs rarely.

3. **Cough suppression.** The opioids exert their antitussive action by depressing the cough center, located in the medulla. The dose that produces the antitussive effect is much lower than that required for analgesia, so the least potent agents are effective (such as codeine). Related compounds, such as dextromethorphan, are often used as antitussives.

4. **Gastrointestinal effects.** The opioids increase the smooth muscle tone of the intestinal tract and markedly decrease its propulsive contractions and motility. This effect has made opioids useful in the symptomatic treatment of diarrhea. Opioid-like agents without analgesic properties, such as diphenoxylate, are used for this effect to treat diarrhea.

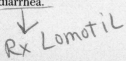

Rx Lomotil

ADVERSE REACTIONS

Unlike many drugs, the adverse reactions of the opioids are not related to a direct damaging effect on hepatic, renal, or hematologic tissues but rather are an extension of their pharmacologic effects. Like the pharmacologic effects, the adverse reactions of the opioid analgesics are proportional to their analgesic strength. Table 7-3 lists contraindications and cautions for the use of opioids.

1. **Respiratory depression.** The opioid analgesic agonists depress the respiratory center in a dose-related manner. This is usually the cause of death with an overdose. The depression is related to a decrease in sensitivity of the brainstem to carbon dioxide. Both the rate and depth of breathing are reduced. In elderly or debilitated patients, the usual therapeutic dose of morphine can produce a significant decrease in pulmonary ventilation. Reduced ventilation produces vasodilation, which results in an increase in intracranial pressure. For this reason, opioids should not be used in patients with head injuries. They may also mask the diagnostic symptoms. Patients with hyperthyroidism are more tolerant to the depression, whereas patients with myxedema are more sensitive.

2. **Nausea and emesis.** Analgesic doses of opioid analgesics often produce nausea and vomiting. This is due to their direct stimulation of the chemoreceptor trigger zone (CTZ), located in the medulla. This side effect is reduced by discouraging ambulation. Administration of repeated, regular doses of an opioid can prevent vomiting

Table 7-3. Contraindications and cautions to the use of opioids

Condition	Comment
Head injury	Can increase intracranial pressure
Chronic pain	Addiction potential limits duration
Respiratory disease	Respiratory depression can occur
Pregnancy	Respiratory depression near-term
Nursing	No problem; watch infant

by depressing the vomiting center, another area in the CNS distinct from the CTZ.

3. Constipation. The opioids produce constipation by producing a tonic contraction of the gastrointestinal tract. Small doses of even weak opioids frequently have this effect and its duration outlasts their analgesic effect. Even with continued administrations tolerance does not develop to this effect.

4. Miosis. The opioid analgesics cause miosis, an important sign (pinpoint pupils) in diagnosing an opioid overdose or identifying an addict. Tolerance does not develop to this effect.

5. Urinary retention. The opioids increase the smooth muscle tone in the urinary tract thereby causing urinary retention. They also produce an antidiuretic effect by stimulating the release of antidiuretic hormone (ADH) from the pituitary gland. This reaction may pose a problem in patients with prostatic hypertrophy.

6. CNS effects. Occasionally, opioids may produce CNS stimulation exhibited by anxiety, restlessness, or nervousness. Dysphoria can also occur from the opioids.

7. Cardiovascular effects. The opioids may depress the vasomotor center and stimulate the vagus nerve. With high doses postural hypotension, bradycardia, and even syncope may result.

8. Biliary tract constriction. In high doses, the opioids may constrict the biliary duct, resulting in biliary colic. This effect is important in patients with gallstones being treated with opioids.

9. Histamine release. Because the opioids can stimulate the release of histamine, itching and urticaria can result from their administration. This effect can occur at the site of intramuscular injection.

10. Pregnancy and nursing. Opioids have not been shown to be teratogenic although they may prolong labor or depress fetal respiration if given near-term. Infants born to mothers using high-dose opioids, as in an addict, can have marked depressed respiration and experience withdrawal symptoms. The amount of opioid excreted in the mother's milk when therapeutic doses are given to the mother would pose no problem to the nor-

mal infant. Morphine is Food and Drug Administration (FDA) pregnancy category C.

11. Addiction. All opioids are addicting—proportional to their analgesic strength. This fact limits the usefulness of the strongest of these agents. Because the duration of use in dentistry is usually short, this does not often pose a problem for the dentist. NSAIAs should be used to control dental pain in the addict. An addict will develop tolerance to the effects of the opioids, except for miosis and constipation. The rate of development of tolerance is related to the strength of the opioid and its frequency of use. After abruptly discontinuing the opioids a withdrawal syndrome occurs. The symptoms include lacrimation, perspiration, rhinorrhea, gooseflesh ("cold turkey"), irritability, nausea, vomiting, tachycardia and chills.

The dental hygienist should become suspicious if the patient:

1. Requests a certain drug and says it's better
2. Says he has many allergies and lots of pain medications don't work
3. Cancels dental appointments because he is going out of town on business
4. Experiences pain for days after scaling and root planing
5. Moves from dental office to dental office because others don't understand him
6. Says he has a low pain threshold

The major symptom of opioid overdose is respiratory depression. In addition to pinpoint pupils and coma, this symptom is pathognomonic for opioid overdose. Opioid overdose is treated with an antagonist, naloxone, discussed later in this chapter.

There are four general methods for treating opioid addiction. One method involves substituting the equivalent amount of an oral opioid (usually methadone) for the injectable form that the addict had been using (e.g., heroin) and then gradually withdrawing that oral form. Another method involves going "cold turkey" by abruptly withdrawing the opioid and using adjunctive medication to alleviate the symptoms of withdrawal, such as phenothiazines, clonidine, or benzodiazepines. A third method involves maintaining a patient on high doses of methadone, termed "methadone maintenance." With this method, the patient takes supervised large oral doses of methadone on a daily basis. Because the patient develops a tolerance for the effects of the opioids, a block is produced that prevents the "rush" resulting from injecting heroin-like agents. The last method involves administering an orally effective long-acting antagonist. This antagonist would block the action of small doses of opioid administered illicitly. No treatment for opioid addiction is successful in all patients.

Allergic reactions

The most common type of true allergic reactions to the opioids are dermatologic in nature, including skin rashes and urticaria. Reports of gastrointestinal side effects are frequently reported as allergies but are side effects of the opioids. Contact dermatitis can occur with topical exposure. These allergic reactions have to be differentiated from the symptoms related to the histamine-releasing properties of the opioids. If a patient gives a history of a **true** allergic reaction to an opioid, an opioid from a different chemical class should be chosen (see Table 7-1).

Drug Interactions

The respiratory depression produced by the opioids is additive with that produced by other CNS depressants. Alcohol or sedative-hypnotic agents can potentiate the opioids' respiratory depressant effect.

Meperidine, but not the other opioids, can interact with the monoamine oxidase inhibitors, a group of drugs rarely used to treat hypertension or depression. CNS excitation, hypertension, and hypotension have been reported to occur. The accumulation of a metabolite of meperidine, normeperidine, may be responsible for the increased effect of meperidine in the presence of the antipsychotic agents such as chlorpromazine.

SPECIFIC OPIOIDS
Agonist opioids

Morphine and meperidine (Demerol). Morphine is considered to be the prototype opioid

against which other opioids are measured. An equivalent number of milligrams of each opioid is compared to 10 mg of morphine. Both morphine and meperidine are used parenterally to control postoperative pain in hospitalized patients. These agents are also used orally, primarily in the treatment of terminal illnesses. The usual oral dosing interval and route of administration are listed in Table 7-2. Meperidine is the favorite drug of abuse of medical personnel. It requires 100 mg to equal about 10 mg of morphine. The drug interactions between meperidine and both the monoamine oxidase inhibitors and phenothiazines must be considered before using meperidine.

Fentanyl (Sublimaze), sufentanil (Sufenta), and alfentanil (Alfenta). These three short-acting parenterally administered agonist opioid analgesics are used perioperatively. They provide analgesia during and immediately following general anesthesia. They are also used with neuroleptic agents such as droperidol to induce or supplement general or regional anesthesia, and to produce general anesthesia. Postoperative ventilation and observation is needed when these agents are chosen.

Hydromorphone (Dilaudid). This orally effective opioid is reserved for the management of severe pain. It is more potent than morphine and better absorbed orally, but it tends to produce similar adverse reactions. Its use in dentistry should be limited to rare situations and carefully monitored. It is a favorite of the addict because of its strength.

Methadone. Methadone's primary use is in the treatment of opioid addicts. It is used either to gradually withdraw the patient or in "methadone maintenance." Its longer duration of action makes withdrawal from methadone easier than from heroin.

Oxycodone (in Percodan, Percocet, and Tylox). Oxycodone is combined with either aspirin or acetaminophen (see Table 7-4) to provide relief of moderate to severe pain. Combining an opioid with a nonopioid analgesic produces an additive analgesic effect with fewer adverse reactions. Oxycodone retains about two thirds of its action when given orally. It bridges the gap between codeine and hydromorphone in terms of strength of analgesic action.

Codeine, dihydrocodeine (in Synalgos-DC), and hydrocodone (in Vicodin). Codeine is the most commonly used opioid in dentistry. It is combined with aspirin (Empirin #3) or acetaminophen (Tylenol #3) for oral administration. Codeine, dihydrocodeine, and hydrocodone have weak analgesic action compared to morphine, hydromorphone, or even oxycodone. These weaker opioid analgesics produce fewer adverse reactions and have less addiction potential than the other stronger opioids. Some commonly used analgesic combinations are listed in Table 7-4.

The amount of codeine in a product containing codeine is designated by #1 (7.5 mg; ⅛ gr), #2 (15 mg; ¼ gr), #3 (30 mg; ½ gr) and #4 (60 mg; 1 gr). Generally doses above 30 mg of codeine are poorly tolerated by the patient. In pain studies it was difficult to show that 30 mg of codeine was any better than placebo; and 60 mg of codeine is about the same as 650 mg of aspirin or acetaminophen or 200 mg of ibuprofen. Because of codeine's lack of analgesic potency and presence of side effects, the use of NSAIAs has in-

Table 7-4. Constituents of common opioid analgesic combinations

Trade name	Opioid agent (mg)	Opioid potency (+ to + + + +)*	Other ingredients (mg)
Propoxyphene (Darvon) Compound-65	Propoxyphene HCl (65)	+	Aspirin (389) Caffeine (32.4)
Darvocet N-100	Propoxyphene napsylate (100)	+	Acetaminophen (650)
Synalgos-DC	Dihydrocodeine (16)	+ +	Aspirin (356.4) Caffeine (30)
Tylenol #1–4	Codeine #1 (7.5) #2 (15) #3 (30) #4 (60)	+ +	Acetaminophen (300)
Phenaphen #2–4	Codeine (15, 30, 60)	+ +	Acetaminophen (325)
Empirin #2–4	Codeine (15, 30, 60)	+ +	Aspirin (325)
Fiorinal #1–3	Codeine (7.5, 15, 30)	+ +	Aspirin (325) Butalbital (50) Caffeine (40)
Talwin-NX	Pentazocine (50)	+ + +	Naloxone (0.5)
Vicodin	Hydrocodone (5)	+ + +	Acetaminophen (500)
Percodan	Oxycodone (~5)	+ + +	Aspirin (325)
Percocet	Oxycodone (5)	+ + +	Acetaminophen (325)
Tylox	Oxycodone (~5)	+ + +	Acetaminophen (500)
Demerol	Meperidine (50,100)	+ + +	None
Demerol APAP	Meperidine (50)	+ + +	Acetaminophen (300)
Dilaudid	Hydromorphone (1,2,3,4)	+ + + +	None

*+ *to* + + + +, From least to most potent.

creased substantially for the management of dental pain. Whether codeine is merely additive or synergistic with aspirin or acetaminophen is debated.

Propoxyphene. This synthetic opioid is chemically similar to methadone. Its analgesic potency has been questioned. It is available combined with aspirin or acetaminophen. After reviewing the literature on propoxyphene Miller[1] concluded that "factors other than intrinsic therapeutic value are responsible for the commercial success of propoxyphene." Its adverse effects include nausea, vomiting, dizziness, and physical dependence. Hundreds of deaths have been associated with its overdose, often in combination with alcohol. With the availability of the NSAIAs, the use of propoxyphene is difficult to justify.

Mixed opioids

Mixed opioids include the agonist-antagonist opioid analgesics and the partial agonists. Only pentazocine is available for oral use in this mixed opioid group. This group is ripe for research to develop opioids with adequate analgesic potency and fewer side effects, such as respiratory depression and addiction potential, than the agonist opioids. Their place in dental therapeutics is at present unclear.

Agonist-antagonist opioids

Pentazocine (Talwin). This agonist-antagonist opioid, the first synthesized, is the only orally available agent in this group. It produces CNS effects not unlike the opioid agonists including analgesia, sedation, and respiratory depression. The type of analgesia it produces is somewhat different from that produced by the agonist opioids. This may be due to its agonist action at the κ-receptor.

The adverse reactions of pentazocine include sedation, dizziness, nausea, vomiting, and headache. Opioid-like effects on the gastrointestinal tract occur with pentazocine. Psychomimetic effects including nightmares and hallucinations, as well as dysphoria, have been reported. With high doses, respiratory depression can occur. Unlike the agonist opioids, increasing the dose of penta-

zocine does not result in a commensurate increase in respiratory depression, that is, respiratory depression is nonlinear. Unlike the opioid agonists, pentazocine can increase both the blood pressure and heart rate. This may be related to its catecholamine-releasing properties.

The drug of choice to treat pentazocine overdose is naloxone. With abuse, repeated injections in the same location can result in severe sclerosis, fibrosis, and ulceration. Because pentazocine was initially thought to be absent of abuse potential, many pentazocine abusers have been produced. A popular mixture termed "Ts and Blues" is a combination of pentazocine (Talwin) and pyribenzamine (blue-colored tablet). Because of its weak antagonist property, it can precipitate withdrawal in the addict.

Pentazocine is available as tablets containing 50 mg of pentazocine and 0.5 mg of naloxone, a pure opioid antagonist (Talwin NX). If used by injection, the naloxone will counteract the agonist action of pentazocine. Since naloxone is rapidly inactivated if taken orally, it will not affect analgesic potency if taken by the intended route, oral. This combination makes the tablets of pentazocine plus naloxone more difficult to abuse and their street value is reduced.

Nalbuphine (Nubain) and butorphanol (Stadol). These members of the agonist-antagonist group are only available parenterally. They have agonist action at the κ-receptor and antagonist action at the μ-receptor. Their analgesic strength is comparable to morphine at usual therapeutic doses. Like pentazocine, these agents demonstrate nonlinear respiratory depression. Sedation, nausea, vomiting, xerostomia, and headache are side effects of these drugs. These agents produce fewer psychomimetic effects than pentazocine, but more than the agonists. Their addiction potential seems to be less than the agonists.

Partial agonists

Buprenorphine (Buprenex) is the first and only available partial agonist. It is a partial μ-receptor agonist, but has no σ-receptor action. In abstinent morphine-dependent patients, buprenorphine suppresses withdrawal; while in stabilized opioid-dependent patients it precipitates withdrawal. It is currently available only for parenteral use, but alternative dosage forms such as sublingual or nasal spray are being investigated.

Opioid antagonists

Naloxone (Narcan). This is an essentially pure opioid antagonist. It antagonizes the μ-, κ-, and σ-receptors. When given alone, it produces no pharmacologic effects. Naloxone is the drug of choice for treating agonist or mixed-opioid overdoses. It will reverse opioid-induced respiratory depression. If another agent, for example a barbiturate, is responsible for the depression, naloxone does not add to the respiratory depression. If administered to an addict who has taken an overdose of an opioid, small doses must be carefully titrated or withdrawal may be produced. This drug is being investigated for a wide range of problems. It also serves as a useful tool to determine the role of the opioid receptors in the mechanisms of action of hypnosis, acupuncture, and the placebo effect. Naloxone is given in a 0.4 to 2 mg dose intravenously. Effects should occur within 1 to 2 minutes. Doses may be repeated at 2- to 3-minute intervals. If no response occurs after 10 mg is administered, the diagnosis of opioid overdose must be questioned. Dental office emergency kits should contain naloxone if any opioid is used in the dental office.

Naltrexone (Trexan). Naltrexone is a long-acting, orally effective opioid antagonist. It is indicated for the maintenance of the opioid-free state in detoxified, formerly opioid-dependent patients. It should not be administered until the patient has remained opioid free for at least 1 week and has had a negative naloxone challenge. It is administered daily or in some instances three times weekly. Patients on naltrexone should not be given opioid analgesic agents for management of dental pain.

DENTAL USE OF OPIOIDS

The advent of the nonsteroidal antiinflammatory agents has produced a dramatic decrease in the use of the opioids in dental practice. Most dental pain can be better managed by the use of NSAIAs. In the patient in whom NSAIAs are contraindicated, the dentist has a wide range of opioids to choose from. Beginning with codeine or hydrocodone combinations and progressing to oxycodone combinations almost all dental pain can be managed. Only in rare cases, and for very short periods of time (1 to 2 days) should hydromorphone or meperidine be prescribed for outpatient dental pain. Patients with chronic pain should be managed with nonopioid therapies and referred to appropriate specialists depending on the nature of their chronic pain. New patients with a complaint of pain should be seen in the dental office and definitive treatment rendered. Opioid prescriptions should be given only for small amounts, without refills, and only if the patient has dental treatment performed. If dental pain persists the patient should be seen in the dental office for evaluation and local treatment.

REVIEW QUESTIONS

1. Name the two ways in which opioid analgesic agents may be classified, and state an advantage of each system.
2. How are the pharmacologic effects and adverse reactions of the opioids related in contrast to the pharmacologic effects and adverse reactions of other groups of drugs?
3. Name four pharmacologic effects of the opioids.
4. Describe the two adverse reactions of the opioids to which tolerance does not develop.
5. Describe the two most common adverse reactions associated with the opioids.
6. Define the following terms:
   a. Physical dependence
   b. Withdrawal
   c. Tolerance
7. Discuss three conditions in which opioids would be contraindicated or in which they should be used with caution.
8. Explain the additive respiratory depression with the opioid analgesic agents and state the other drug with which they are additive.
9. Describe the four major therapeutic uses of the opioids.
10. State the ways in which the opioids differ from one another.
11. Describe what is meant by "morphine is the prototype."
12. State the most potent orally effective opioid.

13. Describe the major use of methadone at the present time.
14. Explain the place for the use of meperidine in dentistry.
15. Describe two major disadvantages to the use of pentazocine.
16. Explain the agonist and antagonist properties of pentazocine, and describe how this can produce a problem in an opioid addict.
17. Explain why pentazocine is combined with naloxone in Talwin-NX.
18. Describe the use of the most frequently employed opioid in dental practice.
19. Explain the use of propoxyphene in dentistry, and state the degree of its proven clinical effectiveness.
20. Explain the use of naloxone for any emergency situation. State what situation in which it would be indicated. Contraindicated.
21. Discuss the disease states in which a particular analgesic drug should be avoided, and select an alternative choice.
22. Discuss the partial agonists in dentistry.

REFERENCES

1. Miller, R.R., Reingold, A., and Paxinos, J.: Propoxyphene hydrochloride: a critical review, J.A.M.A. **213:**996, 1970.

Chapter 8

Antiinfective agents

The antiinfective agents play an important role in dentistry because infection, after pain, is the most important dental problem manageable with drugs. As knowledge of the etiology of dental diseases increases, dental professionals understand the involvement of microorganisms. There are at least three types of infective dental processes:

1. Caries. Caries, produced by *Streptococcus mutans,* is the first important dental problem that the young patient faces. At present, traditional antiinfective agents have not been useful for this problem for the general population. The treatment of choice is local physical removal on a regular basis (good oral hygiene).

2. Periodontal disease. Since dental hygienists are intimately involved in the treatment of periodontal disease, knowledge about a variety of antiinfective agents will guide them in their understanding of new treatments for this disease that are being researched. Since we now know that microorganisms such as *Actinobacillus actinomycetemcomitans,* black-pigmented bacteroides, motile rods, and spirochetes are involved in periodontal disease, the development of a more rational approach to treatment of periodontal disease may be possible. Also, treatments using localized methods of drug delivery hold promise for the future.

3. Localized or systemic dental infection. Although antiinfective agents are often not indicated in localized dental infections, when systemic infection is involved the use of the correct antiinfective agent may be critical.

The following are two other situations in which the hygienist will see the use of antiinfective agents:

1. Prophylactic use. In certain at-risk patients, antiinfective agents are indicated before dental procedures to prevent an infection. An example is the patient with rheumatic heart disease who is premedicated with penicillin before a dental procedure.

2. Physician-generated prescriptions. Dental patients may be receiving antimicrobial agents from their physician for systemic infections. The effect of these agents on the patient's oral health and how that patient's treatment plan may need to be altered must be considered.

HISTORY

In 1932, Gerhard Domagk of Germany observed that Prontosil protected mice against infection by streptococcal bacteria. This milestone in medical history led to the development of the sulfonamides and marked the beginning of systemic antimicrobial therapy.

In 1940, Chain and Florey (England) made the observation that interest had been focused on the sulfonamides and that other possibilities, notably those connected with naturally occurring substances, should be considered. Fleming (England) in 1928 had observed that a mold, *Penicillium notatum,* produced a naturally occurring substance that inhibited the growth of certain bacteria. He had named this substance "penicillin" and suggested that it might be useful for application to infected wounds. In their classic paper Chain and co-workers reported the low toxicity and systemic antibacterial effectiveness of penicillin. The excitement, begun with the sulfonamides, was transferred to the antibiotics. Today, as each new antibiotic is marketed, this excitement is again transferred.

DEFINITIONS

A discussion of the individual antimicrobial agents should be preceded by the definition of certain terms.

antiinfective agents Substances that act against or tend to destroy infections

antimicrobial agents Substances that kill or suppress the growth or multiplication or prevent the action of microorganisms.

antibacterial agents Substances that destroy or suppress the growth or multiplication of bacteria

antibiotic agents Chemical substances produced by microorganisms that have the capacity, in dilute solutions, to destroy or suppress the growth or multiplication of organisms or prevent their action. The difference between the terms *antibiotic* and *synthetic antibacterial agents* is that antibiotics are produced by microorganisms and antibacterial agents are made in a laboratory. Often the above four terms are used interchangably without regard for their exact definition.

antiviral agents Substances that destroy or suppress the growth or multiplication of viruses.

antifungal agents Substances that destroy or suppress the growth or multiplication of fungi.

The following are definitions of terms commonly used to compare and contrast various antimicrobial agents:

spectrum Range of activity of a drug. An antibacterial agent may have either a narrow or broad spectrum. A narrow-spectrum agent acts primarily against either gram-positive or gram-negative organisms, whereas a broad-spectrum agent is effective against a wide variety of organisms, including both gram-positive and gram-negative bacteria, as well as some viruses.

resistance Microorganisms unaffected by an antimicrobial agent. *Natural* resistance occurs when an organism has always been resistant to the antimicrobial agent. *Acquired* resistance occurs when an organism that was previously sensitive to an antimicrobial agent develops resistance. This can occur by natural selection of a spontaneous mutation or by transfer of genetic material from one organism to another. The second strain thus becomes resistant to the same antibiotics as the first strain

without ever having been exposed to the antibiotic.

bactericidal The ability to kill bacteria. This effect is irreversible; that is, if the bacteria are removed from the drug, they do not live.

bacteriostatic The ability to inhibit or retard the multiplication or growth of bacteria. This is a reversible process because the bacteria are able to grow and multiply when removed from the agent.

Whether an antibacterial agent is labeled "bactericidal" or "bacteriostatic" depends on variables such as the dose used or the organism being treated. Table 8-1 lists the most common antimicrobial agents and classifies them as bacteriostatic or bactericidal.

blood level Concentration of antiinfective agent present in the blood or serum. This level is an important index to drug dosage, since a certain concentration of the drug is required in the body fluids to inhibit or kill the microorganisms.

minimum inhibitory concentration (MIC) Lowest concentration needed to inhibit visible growth of an organism on media after 18 to 24 hours of incubation. This in vitro test is more reliable and quantitative than the disc tests.

synergism Combination of two antibiotics more rapidly bactericidal than either drug used alone. Combinations of antibiotics that are bactericidal (Table 8-1) generally are synergistic. Combina-

Table 8-1. Classification of antiinfective agents—bactericidal or bacteriostatic

Bactericidal	Bacteriostatic
Penicillins	Erythromycin*
Cephalosporins	Tetracyclines
Metronidazole	Clindamycin*
Aminoglycosides	Chloramphenicol
Bacitracin	Spectinomycin
Vancomycin	Sulfonamides
Polymyxin	
Ciprofloxacin	
Rifampin	

*Erythromycin and clindamycin may be bactericidal against some organisms at higher blood levels.

tions of those that are bacteriostatic are merely additive.

antagonism Bactericidal rate for the combination of two drugs less than for either drug used alone. This is often exhibited when bacteriostatic and bactericidal agents are used in combination (Table 8-1).

superinfection, suprainfection Infection caused by the proliferation of microorganisms different from those causing the original infection. When antiinfectives disturb the normal flora of the body, the emergence of organisms unaffected by or resistant to the antibiotic used can occur. Superinfection is often caused by broad-spectrum antibiotics such as tetracycline. In this case a reduction in the number of gram-positive and gram-negative bacteria allows the overgrowth of the fungus *Candida albicans*.

The pathogenic organisms emerging in a superinfection generally are more difficult to eradicate than the original organism. The fact that the practitioner can *cause* as well as *eliminate* infections emphasizes the importance of determining a definite need before these drugs are used.

Infection is not only an invasion of the body by pathogenic microorganisms but also a reaction of the tissues to their presence. The presence of a pathogen does not constitute "invasion." The oral cavity is inhabited by many microorganisms, some of which are potentially pathogenic. The factors that determine the likelihood of a microorganism causing an infection are (1) virulence of the microorganism, (2) number of organisms present, and (3) resistance of the host. Host resistance should be considered as having both local and systemic components. Systemically, both drugs and diseases may reduce a patient's immunity (Table 8-2).

CULTURE AND SENSITIVITY

Ideally, all infections requiring antimicrobial therapy should be cultured and sensitivity tests performed. This is the only way to be sure that a drug will kill or inhibit the growth of the infecting microorganisms in a specific infection. In practice this is often difficult. In cases of a serious infection, an infection in a compromised patient, or an

Table 8-2. Diseases and drugs that decrease resistance to infection

Diseases	Drugs
Addison's disease	Immunosuppressive drugs
ARC	Antineoplastic agents
AIDS	Cytotoxic drugs
Alcoholism	Adrenal corticosteroids
Blood dyscrasias	
Diabetes mellitus	
Immunoglobulin deficiency	
Leukemia	
Malnutrition	

Modified from Holroyd, S.V., Wynn, R.L., and Requa-Clark, B.: Clinical pharmacology in dental practice, ed. 4, St. Louis, 1988, The C.V. Mosby Co.

infection that is not responding to treatment, it is imperative that a culture be taken.

Culture

When a culture is taken dental personnel need to communicate to the laboratory the organisms to consider. The laboratory personnel should perform a Gram stain so that they may report all of the bacteria present in high numbers. Proper collection materials (tubes or vials with the correct media) and methods must be used to obtain reliable results. Both obligate and facultative anaerobes should be preserved. Depending on the site, the collection method varies. With an abscess, aspiration with a needle, with a draining lesion, a swab from an anaerobic pack, and with endodontic treatment, absorbent points can be used if they are handled properly to keep the anaerobes alive.

Sensitivity

After the organism is identified, it is grown on culture media, to test the effect of different antimicrobial agents on the organism. One to two days are required before the results of this test are available. Although therapy is begun before this time, it may be changed after the results are available. If clinical response has been adequate often the original antibiotic is continued despite sensitivity results.

INDICATIONS FOR ANTIMICROBIAL AGENTS

There is considerable controversy regarding the need for antimicrobial agents in various situations. There are two categories of indications, prophylactic and therapeutic, that will be discussed briefly.

Therapeutic indications

Although there is no simple rule to determine whether antimicrobial therapy is needed in dentistry, many infections do not require it. Before a decision is made, the following factors must be considered:

1. The patient. The best defense against a pathogen is the host response. A properly functioning defense mechanism is of primary importance. When this defense is lacking, the need for antimicrobial agents is more pressing.

2. The infection. The virulence and invasiveness of the microorganism are important in deciding the acuteness, severity, and spreading tendency of the infection. An acute, severe, rapidly spreading infection should generally be treated with antimicrobial agents, whereas a mild, localized infection in which drainage can be established need not be so treated.

Prophylactic indications

There are few situations when a definite indication for prophylactic antibiotic coverage exists. One clear-cut indication is a history of rheumatic or congenital heart disease or the presence of a heart prosthesis. Since dental procedures may precipitate bacteremia, prophylactic antibiotics must be given to prevent bacterial endocarditis. Other prophylactic uses of antimicrobial agents in dental practice are less clear. Some clinicians suggest antibiotic prophylaxis for patients with total hip replacement. In cases of compound mandibular fracture, the use of prophylactic antimicrobial agents has reduced the rate of infection.[1] Situations in which the need for prophylaxis is uncertain include coronary bypass operations, Teflon implants, and surgical procedures. Although dental studies concerning the value of prophylactic antibiotics are lacking, the failure of prophylactic antibiotic coverage to prevent postsurgical infections is well documented in the medical literature. The following analysis concerns periodontal patients:

Most patients who undergo periodontal surgery are not going to develop a postoperative infection. Infections that do evolve might have been prevented by prophylactic antibiotics if the invading organism was susceptible to the particular drug selected. Some individuals who would not have developed a postoperative infection may do so if prophylactic antibiotics are used. Thus, one must balance the infections caused against those prevented. The gains and losses in using antibiotics to prevent postsurgical infection are approximately equal.[2]

Dental treatment

When antimicrobial agents are to be used in the treatment of dental infections the organisms likely to be producing the infection and their susceptibility to antimicrobial agents must be considered. Table 8-3 lists the antimicrobials of choice for various dental situations and alternatives if the drugs of choice cannot be used. For example, if antibiotics are used for a soft tissue dental infection, penicillin V is the choice, while in an adult periodontal case unresponsive to standard treatment, tetracycline is used.

GENERAL ADVERSE REACTIONS ASSOCIATED WITH ANTIINFECTIVES
Suprainfection (superinfection)

All antiinfective agents can produce an overgrowth of organisms that are different from the original infection and resistant to the agent being used. The wider the spectrum of the antiinfective agent and the longer the agent is administered, the greater the chance of superinfection occurring. This side effect can be minimized by using the most specific antiinfective agent, the shortest course of therapy effective, and adequate doses.

Table 8-3. Antimicrobial use in dentistry

Infection*/situation	Drug of choice	Alternative drug(s)
Periodontal disease		
ANUG† (Vincent)	Penicillin V	Metronidazole Tetracycline
Abscess (perio)	Penicillin V	Erythromycin Tetracycline
Periodontitis		
Juvenile	Tetracycline	—
Adult‡	Tetracycline	Metronidazole Clindamycin
Oral infections		
Soft tissue (abscess, cellulitis, postsurgical pericornitis)	Penicillin V	Erythromycin Cephalosporin Clindamycin Tetracycline
Osteomyelitis	Penicillin V	Cephalosporin Clindamycin Erythromycin
Penicillinase-producing staphylococci	Cloxacillin Dicloxacillin	Cephalosporin Clindamycin
Mixed infections insensitive to penicillin		
Aerobes	Amoxicillin	Cephalosporin Sulfonamides Tetracycline
Anaerobes	Clindamycin	Cephalosporin Metronidazole Erythromycin Tetracycline
Prophylactic for infective endocarditis	**No penicillin allergy**	**Penicillin allergy**
Rheumatic heart disease	Penicillin V	Erythromycin

Prosthetic heart valve	Ampicillin +
	  gentamicin, then
	  penicillin
		Vancomycin

From Holroyd, S.V., Wynn, R.L., and Requa-Clark, B.: Clinical pharmacology in dental practice, ed. 4, St. Louis, 1988, The C.V. Mosby Co.)
*Only if antibiotic indicated.
†Local debridement alone preferred.
‡Not responsive to standard treatment.

Allergic reactions

All antiinfective agents can produce a variety of allergic reactions, ranging from a mild rash to fatal anaphylaxis. Some antiinfective agents, such as the penicillins, are more allergenic than other agents.

Drug interactions

Antiinfective agents can interact with oral antico-agulants and contraceptives. The antibiotics can also interact with each other. Although extremely rare, most of the antiinfective agents have been implicated in a drug interaction with the oral contraceptives. Antiinfective agents lower the blood levels of the estrogenic component in the combination estrogen-progestin birth control pills. This interaction has been documented by several reported pregnancies that were conceived while the patient was taking oral contraceptives and given antibiotics. This rare drug interaction should be discussed with the patient whenever a patient using oral contraceptive agents receives a prescription for an antibiotic. Of those antibiotics used in dentistry, the ampicillins and tetracyclines are the most implicated groups. The effect of oral antico-agulants may be potentiated by antibiotics that destroy gastrointestinal flora that produce vitamin K.

Gastrointestinal complaints

All antiinfective drugs can produce a variety of gastrointestinal complaints. The incidence varies greatly, depending on the particular agent employed, the dose of that agent, and whether the patient takes the drug "with food." More serious gastrointestinal complaints, like pseudomembranous colitis (PMC), which has been historically linked with clindamycin, is now known to occur not only in the absence of antimicrobial agents but also with a wide variety of antiinfective agents.

Pregnancy

During pregnancy the choice of antimicrobial agents to treat infections is difficult. Although the risk-to-benefit ratio must be considered whenever pregnant women are given any medication, penicillins and erythromycin have not been associated with teratogenicity and are frequently used. The tetracyclines are contraindicated during pregnancy because of their effect on developing teeth. Sulfonamides are contraindicated near-term because of their association with hyperbilirubinemia.

ANTIINFECTIVE AGENTS USED IN DENTISTRY
Penicillins

The penicillins can be divided into three major groups (Table 8-4). The first group contains penicillins G and V, the second group is composed of the penicillinase-resistant penicillins, and the third group includes the extended-spectrum penicillins. Because the penicillins have many properties in common, their similarities are discussed first.

Source and chemistry

The mold *Penicillium notatum* and related species produce the naturally occurring penicillins. The semisynthetic penicillins are produced by chemically altering the naturally produced penicillins. All penicillins contain the nucleus 6-aminopenicillanic acid, which by itself has little antibacterial activity.

The addition of organic groups at the R position confers antibacterial activity to the compounds formed from 6-aminopenicillanic acid. These R groups create the various penicillins. The penicillins can be inactivated by any reaction that removes the R group or, in the case of penicillinase, breaks the β-lactam ring *(B)*. Salts of the penicillins are made by reactions at the thiazolidine *(T)* carboxyl (—COOH) group.

Although many naturally occurring penicillins have been produced, only penicillin G (benzyl penicillin) is of use today. The various semisynthetic penicillins are formed by substituting other groups at the R position.

Table 8-4. Penicillins

Drug name	Routes	Penicillinase-resistant	Acid stable	Absorbed orally (%)	Protein bound (%)
Penicillin G/V					
Penicillin G (Pentids)	PO, IM, IV	No	No	20–30	60
Penicillin G procaine (Cysticillin)	IM	No	No		60
Penicillin G benzathine (Bicillin L-A)	IM	No	No		60
Penicillin V (Pen Vee K, V-Cillin K)	PO	No	Yes	75	75–80
Penicillinase-resistant					
Methicillin (Staphcillin)	IM, IV	Yes	No	0	30–45
Nafcillin (Unipen, Nafcil)	PO, IM, IV	Yes	Yes	10–15	90
Oxacillin (Prostaphlin, Bactocil)	PO, IM, IV	Yes	Yes	20–30	95
Cloxacillin (Tegopen, Cloxapen)	PO	Yes	Yes	40–60	95
Dicloxacillin (Dycill)	PO	Yes	Yes	40–60	98
Extended spectrum					
Ampicillin-like					
Ampicillin (Polycillin, Omnipen)	PO, IM, IV	No	Yes	30–40	20
Bacampicillin (Spectrobid)	PO	No	Yes	80	20
Amoxicillin (Amoxil, Larotid)	PO	No	Yes	80	20
Cyclacillin (Cyclapen-W)	PO	No	Yes	80	20
Carbenicillin-like					
Carbenicillin indanyl (Geocillin)	PO	No	Yes	80	50
Carbenicillin (Geopen, Pyopen)	IM, IV	No	No		50
Ticarcillin (Ticar)	IM, IV	No	No		45
Mezlocillin (Mezlin)	IM, IV	No	No		16–42
Piperacillin (Pipracil)	IM, IV	No	No		16
Azlocillin (Azlin)	IV	No	No		25–45
Amdinopenicillins					
Amdinocillin (Coactin)	IM, IV	Yes	No		5–10

From Holroyd, S.V., Wynn, R.L., and Requa-Clark, B.: Clinical pharmacology in dental practice, ed. 4, St. Louis, 1988, The C.V. Mosby Co.

Pharmacokinetics

Penicillin can be administered either orally or parenterally but should not be applied topically because of its great allergenicity. When penicillin is administered orally, the amount absorbed depends on the type of penicillin given. The percentage can vary from 0% to 80% (Table 8-4). When the percentage absorbed is too low, as with methicillin, the penicillin is available only for injection. Note that penicillin V is better absorbed orally than penicillin G. The oral route provides the advantages of convenience and less likelihood of a life-threatening allergic reaction. The disadvantages of using the oral rather than the parenteral route are that the blood levels rise slower and are less predictable owing to variable absorption or lack of patient compliance and gastric acid degrades some penicillins. Highest blood levels are obtained if the patient takes the penicillin orally at least 1 hour before, or 2 hours after meals. Penicillin V and amoxicillin can be taken without regard to meals.

After absorption, penicillin is distributed throughout the body, with the exception of cerebrospinal fluid (CSF), bone, and abscesses. This includes the tissue, saliva, and kidneys. Penicillin crosses the placenta and appears in breast milk.

Penicillin is metabolized, mainly in the liver, and undergoes tubular secretion in the kidney. The elimination half-life for both penicillin G and penicillin V is about 0.5 hour. In five half-lives, about 2.5 hours, these penicillins are virtually eliminated from the body. Probenecid, a uricosuric agent, interferes with penicillin's excretion and therefore prolongs its action. This may be used to therapeutic benefit when higher blood levels are desired.

Spectrum

Penicillin is a very potent bactericidal agent that acts by interfering with the synthesis of the bacterial cell wall (Table 8-5). It affects rapidly multiplying bacteria by inhibiting the formation of cross-linkages in the cell wall and some enzymatic activity. Its narrow spectrum of activity includes cocci (streptococci, staphylococci, pneumococci), spirochetes, *Actinomyces*, and certain gram-negative cocci such as *Neisseria gonorrhoeae* and *N. meningitidis*. Bacterial resistance to penicillin can develop.

The antibacterial activity of penicillin is standardized in international units. One unit has the activity of 0.6 μg of sodium penicillin G, so 1 mg of sodium penicillin G = 1667 units. About 400,000 units of penicillin V is equivalent to approximately 250 mg. Penicillin G is usually measured in units, whereas other penicillins are expressed in milligrams.

Resistance

Resistance to penicillin usually develops in a slow, stepwise fashion. Staphylococci became resistant by producing penicillinases. These inactivate the penicillin moiety by cleaving the β-lactam ring. In hospital environments, over 95% of the population of staphylococci are penicillinase producing. Although most oral strains of *Streptococcus viridans* are sensitive to penicillin, an increasing number of strains that are currently sensitive to penicillins G and V are growing resistant.

Adverse reactions

The untoward reactions to the penicillins can be divided into toxic reactions and allergic or hypersensitivity-type reactions. Penicillin is the most common cause of drug allergies.

Toxicity. Because penicillin's toxicity is almost nonexistent, large doses have been tolerated without adverse effects. For this reason there is a large margin of safety when penicillin is administered. With massive intravenous doses, direct central nervous system (CNS) irritation can result in convulsions. Large doses of penicillin G have been associated with renal damage manifested as fever, eosinophilia, rashes, albuminuria, and a rise in blood urea nitrogen (BUN). Hemolytic

Table 8-5. Antiinfective mechanisms of action

| Inhibits bacterial cell wall synthesis | Affects cell membrane | Inhibits bacterial protein synthesis | | Inhibits nucleic acid synthesis | Antimetabolites |
		50S subunit	30S subunit		
Penicillins	Polymycin	Chloramphenicol	Aminoglycosides	Rifampin	Trimethoprim
Cephalosporins	Colistimethate	Erythromycin	Tetracyclines	Quinolones	Sulfonamides
Cycloserine		Clindamycin		Metronidazole	
Vancomycin					
Bacitracin					

From Holroyd, S.V., Wynn, R.L., and Requa-Clark, B.: Clinical pharmacology in dental practice, ed. 4, St. Louis, 1988, The C.V. Mosby Co.

anemia and bone marrow depression have also been induced by penicillin. The penicillinase-resistant penicillins are significantly more toxic than penicillin G. Gastrointestinal irritation can manifest itself as nausea with or without vomiting. The irritation caused by injection of penicillin can produce sterile abscesses if given intramuscularly or thrombophlebitis if given intravenously.

Allergy and hypersensitivity. An allergic reaction to penicillin represents the greatest danger with therapy. These reactions include all types of hypersensitivity reactions, type I through type IV (see Chapter 3). The following are types of allergic reactions associated with the penicillins:

1. Anaphylactic reactions. Anaphylactic shock, an acute allergic reaction, occurs within ½ hour after the administration of penicillin. It presents the most serious danger to patients. It is characterized by smooth muscle contraction (e.g., bronchoconstriction), capillary dilation (shock), and urticaria caused by the release of histamine and bradykinin. If treatment does not begin immediately, death can result. The treatment of anaphylaxis is the immediate administration of parenteral epinephrine.

2. Rash. All types of skin rashes have been reported in association with the administration of penicillin. This type of reaction accounts for 80% to 90% of allergic reactions to the penicillins. They are usually mild and self-limiting but can occasionally be severe. Even contact dermatitis has occurred as a result of topical exposure, for example, while preparing an injectable solution (type IV).

3. Delayed serum sickness. Serum sickness is manifested as fever, skin rash, and eosinophilia or severely as arthritis, purpura, lymphadenopathy, splenomegaly, mental changes, abnormal electrocardiogram, and edema. It usually takes at least 6 days to develop and can occur during treatment or up to 2 weeks after treatment has ceased.

4. Oral lesions. Delayed reactions to penicillin can exhibit themselves in the oral cavity. These include severe stomatitis, furred tongue, black tongue, acute glossitis, and cheilosis. These oral lesions can occur most commonly with topical application but have been reported from other routes.

5. Other. Interstitial nephritis, hemolytic anemia, and eosinophilia occasionally reported during penicillin therapy are types of allergic reactions.

The extent and severity of an allergic reaction to penicillin are enormous. Some studies indicate that between 5% and 10% of patients receiving penicillin will have a reaction. Allergic reactions to oral penicillin are less common than with parenteral penicillin. Anaphylactic reactions are more frequent in patients pretreated with β-blockers and subsequently given oral penicillin. These anaphylactic reactions have been reported to be difficult to treat.

When reactions to penicillin occur, the consequences are often serious. It is estimated that an anaphylactic reaction occurs in up to 0.05% of penicillin-treated patients, with a mortality of 5 to 10%. If statistics from other studies[3,4] are projected, they indicate that 100 to 300 deaths caused by an allergic reaction to penicillin occur annually in the United States. Although the chance of a serious allergic reaction to penicillin is greater after parenteral administration, anaphylactic shock and death after oral use have also been reported. Patients who have a history of any allergy are more likely to be allergic to penicillin.

Allergic reactions of any nature may be followed by more serious allergic reactions on subsequent exposure. Any history of an allergic reaction to penicillin contraindicates the use of this substance, and another antibiotic should be substituted for penicillin. However, a negative history does not guarantee the lack of a penicillin allergy. When penicillin must be given to a penicillin-allergic patient and other antibiotics are not available, desensitization, that is, giving a small dose and increasing the dose gradually, may be instituted. Because anaphylaxis can be precipitated, this procedure is not useful for any outpatient situation.

Testing. In certain clinical cases when the use

of penicillin is critical, testing for penicillin allergy can be done. Because the testing itself may precipitate an anaphylactic reaction, it should only be undertaken in a situation where life support equipment, drugs, and personnel are immediately available. It should never be done in an outpatient dental office.

Penicillin itself does not act as a haptene, but is metabolized to a haptene. Allergic reactions from penicillin can be in response to the major determinant, resulting in a skin reaction, or to the minor determinant, producing anaphylaxis. The major determinant, termed major because of the frequency rather than the severity of the reaction, is produced by a reaction to penicilloyl acid. The minor determinant, termed so because it happens less often, is produced by either penicilloic acid or penicillin itself. Penicilloyl-polylysine (PPL, Pre-Pen), the major determinant, and the minor determinant mixture (MDM) or aqueous penicillin itself both must be used to test for allergy to penicillin. Both false-positive and false-negative reactions may occur, but when both of these determinants are negative giving penicillin is probably safe. These tests only are sensitive to type I allergic reactions.

Uses

Penicillin is an important antibiotic in medical and dental practice. Its use in dentistry results from its bactericidal potency, lack of toxicity, and spectrum of action, which includes many oral flora. It is often employed for the treatment of dental infections. Table 8-3 demonstrates the number of dental infections for which penicillin is the drug of choice if patients are not allergic to it. Penicillin is also used for specific prophylactic indications. It is the agent of choice for the prophylaxis of infective endocarditis in nonallergic patients who have a history of rheumatic heart disease or valve damage (see the discussion on antibiotic prophylaxis of infective endocarditis at the end of this chapter). Its effectiveness in the treatment of oropharyngeal strains of *Bacteroides* species explains its effectiveness in many anaerobic dental infections.

Specific Penicillins

Penicillin G. Penicillin G, the prototype penicillin, is available as the sodium, potassium, procaine, or benzathine salts. These salts differ in their onset and duration of action and the plasma levels attained. Fig. 8-1 compares the blood levels attained by the intravenous (IV) administration of the potassium salt and the intramuscular (IM) administration of the potassium, procaine, and benzathine salts. Note that the potassium salt given IV produces the most rapid and highest blood level, whereas the benzathine salt given IM produces a much lower and more sustained level. The potassium salt and the procaine salt given intramuscularly produce intermediate blood levels.

The sodium salts of penicillin should be avoided in patients with a limited sodium intake such as cardiovascular patients. Renal patients should not be given potassium salts, which can result in hyperkalemia. Patients may be allergic to the procaine moiety in procaine penicillin G. Both procaine and benzathine penicillins are suspensions, given IM, from which the penicillin is slowly released. The benzathine form is given once monthly to patients with a history of rheumatic heart disease for prophylaxis.

Penicillin V. Penicillin V has a spectrum of action very similar to that of penicillin G. Given orally, penicillin V produces higher blood levels than an equivalent amount of penicillin G. Penicillin V has never been proved to be of greater therapeutic value than penicillin G given in higher doses. Because of the higher blood levels, penicillin V is used almost exclusively in the treatment and prevention of dental infections. The potassium salt of penicillin V (K penicillin V or penicillin VK) is more soluble than the free acid and therefore is better absorbed when taken orally. Table 8-3 lists some situations in which penicillin is the drug of first choice if the patient is not allergic to penicillin. The usual dose is 500 mg qid for treatment of an infection. For infective endocarditis prophylaxis, 2 gm is given 1 hour before the procedure followed by 1 gm in 6 hours.

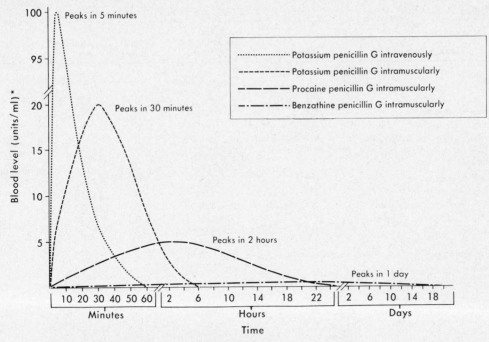

Fig. 8-1. Comparative blood levels of penicillin G salts.

Penicillinase-resistant penicillins. Table 8-6 lists the penicillinase-resistant penicillins. These drugs should be reserved for use only against penicillinase-producing staphylococci. Compared to penicillin G, the penicillinase-resistant penicillins are less effective against penicillin G–sensitive organisms. They also produce more side effects such as gastrointestinal discomfort, bone marrow depression, and abnormal renal and hepatic function. Patients allergic to penicillin are also allergic to the penicillinase-resistant penicillins.

Since cloxacillin and dicloxacillin are better absorbed than the others, they are the penicillinase-resistant penicillins of choice.

Extended-spectrum penicillins

Ampicillin and amoxicillin. These agents are frequently used in medicine. These penicillinase-susceptible penicillins have a spectrum of action that includes gram-positive cocci, some *Haemophilus influenzae*, and some enterococci such as *Escherichia coli*, *Proteus mirabilis*, *Salmonella*, and *Shigella*. Ampicillin is usually used to treat gonococcal infections, either alone or with probenecid as a single oral dose (3.5 gm). Ampicillin is also used in combination with gentamicin for infective endocarditis prophylaxis for prosthetic heart valves (Table 8-7). Amoxicillin, a relative of ampicillin, is preferred for most other indications because it produces higher blood levels, is better absorbed, requires less frequent dosing (tid versus qid for ampicillin), and its absorption is not impaired by food. Amoxicillin is used to treat upper respiratory tract infections (*H. influenzae*), urinary tract infection (*E. coli*), and meningitis (*H. influenzae*). Otitis media in children is often treated with amoxicillin. Amoxicillin is also available mixed with clavulanic acid, a β-lactamase inhibitor (Augmentin). Since clavulanic acid can in-

Table 8-6. Penicillins

Drug name	Routes	Penicillinase-resistant	Acid stable	Absorbed orally (%)	Protein bound (%)
Penicillin G/V					
Penicillin G (Pentids)	PO, IM, IV	No	No	20–30	60
Penicillin G procaine (Cysticillin)	IM	No	No		60
Penicillin G benzathine (Bicillin L-A)	IM	No	No		60
Penicillin V (Pen Vee K, V-Cillin K)	PO	No	Yes	75	75–80
Penicillinase-resistant					
Methicillin (Staphcillin)	IM, IV	Yes	No	0	30–45
Nafcillin (Unipen, Nafcil)	PO, IM, IV	Yes	Yes	10–15	90
Oxacillin (Prostaphlin, Bactocil)	PO, IM, IV	Yes	Yes	20–30	95
Cloxacillin (Tegopen, Cloxapen)	PO	Yes	Yes	40–60	95
Dicloxacillin (Dycill)	PO	Yes	Yes	40–60	98
Extended spectrum					
Ampicillin-like					
Ampicillin (Polycillin, Omnipen)	PO, IM, IV	No	Yes	30–40	20
Bacampicillin (Spectrobid)	PO	No	Yes	80	20
Amoxicillin (Amoxil, Larotid)	PO	No	Yes	80	20
Cyclacillin (Cyclapen-W)	PO	No	Yes	80	20
Carbenicillin-like					
Carbenicillin indanyl (Geocillin)	PO	No	Yes	80	50
Carbenicillin (Geopen, Pyopen)	IM, IV	No	No		50
Ticarcillin (Ticar)	IM, IV	No	No		45
Mezlocillin (Mezlin)	IM, IV	No	No		16–42
Piperacillin (Pipracil)	IM, IV	No	No		16
Azlocillin (Azlin)	IV	No	No		25–45
Amdinopenicillins					
Amdinocillin (Coactin)	IM, IV	Yes	No		5–10

hibit the β-lactamases produced by bacteria, this combination offers an advantage if amoxicillin has not been successful in treating a variety of infections.

Ampicillin has the propensity to produce rashes more often than other penicillins. Some suggest that this rash, more common in patients with mononucleosis or those taking allopurinol, is not of an allergic nature. Allergy is still an adverse reaction that can occur with these agents. Cross-allergenicity between other penicillins and the ampicillins is complete.

Carbenicillins. Carbenicillin has a wider spec-trum of action than does penicillin G, with special activity against *Pseudomonas aeruginosa* and some strains of *Proteus*. It is not penicillinase re-sistant and is available parenterally to treat sys-temic infections. Carbenicillin indanyl is used or-ally only for the treatment of urinary tract infec-tions. This is because even though it produces high levels in the urine, it does not produce high tissue levels when given orally. Ticarcillin and azlocillin are similar to carbenicillin but they are more active against *P. aeruginosa*. Mezlocillin and piperacillin have greater activity against *Kleb-siella* than carbenicillin. The carbenicillins are

Table 8-7. Antibiotic regimens suggested for prophylaxis before dental procedures

Parenteral prophylaxis

a. No penicillin allergy—give ½ hr before

    (1) Adult
        Ampicillin 1 to 2 gm IM or IV **plus**
        Gentamicin 1.5 mg/kg IM or IV
        Repeat above in 8 hrs *or* give:
        Penicillin VK 1 gm in 6 hr PO

    (2) Child*
        Ampicillin 50 mg/kg IM or IV **plus**
        Gentamicin 2.0 mg/kg IM or IV
        Repeat above in 8 hr *or* give:
        Penicillin VK in 6 hours:
           >60 lb: 1 gm PO
           <60 lb: 500 mg PO

b. Penicillin allergy

    (1) Adult
        Vancomycin 1 gm IV by infusion over course of
        1 hr beginning 1 hr before procedure

    (2) Child*
        Vancomycin 20 mg/kg IV by infusion over course of
        1 hr beginning 1 hr before procedure

Oral prophylaxis

a. No penicillin allergy

    (1) Adult
        Penicillin VK 2 gm 1 hr before procedure, then
        1 gm in 6 hr
        Unable to take orally: 2 million units aqueous
        penicillin G IV or IM (½ to 1 hr) before procedure;
        then 1 million units in 6 hr

    (2) Child*
        (a) >60 lb: see adult dose
        (b) <60 lb: one half the adult dose:
           Penicillin VK 1 gm 1 hr before procedure, then
           500 mg in 6 hr
        (c) Unable to take orally:
           >60 lb: adult dose
           <60 lb: 50,000 U/kg penicillin G IV or IM 30
           minutes before procedure; then 25,000 U/kg in
           6 hr

b. Penicillin allergy

    (1) Adult
        Erythromycin 1 gm 1 hr before procedure, then
        500 mg in 6 hr

    (2) Child*
        Erythromycin 20 mg/kg 1 hr before procedure,
        then 10 mg/kg in 6 hr

Adapted from Prevention of bacterial endocarditis: a statement prepared by the Committee on Prevention of Rheumatic Fever and Bacterial Endocarditis of the American Heart Association, J.A.D.A. 110:98-100, Jan. 1985.
*The child's dose should never exceed the adult dose.

used to treat hospitalized patients with serious infections produced by gram-negative bacteria They are often combined with an aminoglycoside and are very expensive.

    Amdinocillin. This agent has poor action against gram-positive organisms and *Pseudomonas,* but good action against Enterobacteriaceae organisms. Because it binds to different proteins than do the other penicillins, it tends to be synergistic with other β-lactam antibiotics.

Erythromycin

Erythromycin is a macrolide antibiotic whose spectrum against gram-positive organisms is similar to penicillin V. It is ineffective against the typ-

ical anaerobes producing dental infections such as *Bacteroides.* It was isolated from the bacterial strain *Streptomyces erythraeus* in 1952. Erythromycin is a high molecular weight organic base called a macrolide.

Pharmacokinetics

Erythromycin is administered orally as tablets, capsules, or oral suspensions, and in IV and IM forms. Because erythromycin is broken down in the gastric fluid, it is formulated as an enteric-coated tablet, capsule, or insoluble ester to reduce degradation by the stomach acid. It should be administered 2 hours before meals or several hours after meals. The peak blood level is usually

Table 8-8. Erythromycins

Drug	Route of administration
Erythromycin base (E-mycin ERYC, PCE)	Oral
Erythromycin stearate (Erythrocin stearate, Erypar)	Oral
Erythromycin ethylsuccinate (E.E.S. 400, Pediamycin)	Oral, IM
Erythromycin estolate (Ilosone)	Oral
Erythromycin lactobionate (Erythrocin piggyback)	IV
Erythromycin glucceptate (Ilotycin glucceptate)	IV

attained in 1 to 4 hours after ingestion. Although food reduces the absorption of erythromycin, it may be necessary to administer it with food to minimize its adverse gastrointestinal effects. Its $t_{1/2}$ is 2 hours. No therapeutic difference has been demonstrated among the different erythromycin products (Table 8-8). Erythromycin is distributed to most body tissues, excreted in the bile, and partially reabsorbed through enterohepatic circulation. It is excreted in the urine and feces.

Activity and spectrum

Erythromycin is usually bacteriostatic and interferes with protein synthesis by inhibiting the enzyme peptidyl transferase at the 50S subunit of the 70S ribosome. Its spectrum of action closely resembles that of penicillin against gram-positive bacteria. It is also the drug of choice for whooping cough (*Bordetella*), diphtheria, *Legionella* (Legionnaires' disease), some *Chlamydia* infections, *Actinomyces,* and *Mycoplasma pneumoniae*. It is also indicated for streptococcal and staphylococcal infections, syphilis, and gonorrhea. Bacterial resistance can occur as a result of demethylation of an adenine residue in the 23S ribosomal ribonucleic acid. Cross-resistance has been reported between erythromycin and clindamycin. About one half of hospital staphylococcal infections are resistant to erythromycin.

Because erythromycin is not effective against many infections caused by obligate anaerobes involved in some dental infections, it is a poor second choice to penicillin to treat dental infections. If the infection is serious, erythromycin should not be used unless culture and sensitivity tests are available. If the causative agent is a gram-positive agent, erythromycin may be effective. The therapeutic effectiveness of erythromycin to treat dental infections may be the result of local intervention measures such as debridement and drainage.

Adverse reactions

With usual therapeutic doses of erythromycin, side effects other than gastrointestinal are usually minimal. Allergic reactions to erythromycin are uncommon.

Gastrointestinal effects. The side effects most often associated with erythromycin administration are gastrointestinal and include stomatitis, abdominal cramps, nausea, vomiting, and diarrhea. These effects occur more frequently in qid versus bid dosing and with higher (2 gm/day) versus lower doses (1 gm/day). Requa-Clark found that the incidence of at least one gastrointestinal side effect occurring averaged about 46% with about 16% discontinuing their medication because of side effects.[4a]

Cholestatic jaundice. Cholestatic jaundice has been reported with erythromycin estolate as well as erythromycin ethylsuccinate. Erythromycin base has not been associated with this reaction. Symptoms include nausea, vomiting, and abdominal cramps followed by jaundice and elevated liver enzyme levels. The mechanism of this adverse effect is believed to be a hypersensitivity reaction.

Drug interactions

Erythromycin may interact with theophylline, digoxin, triazolam, warfarin, carbamazepine, and cyclosporine. Erythromycin can increase the effects of these drugs, possibly producing toxicity. The mechanism by which erythromycin produces these drug interactions is not known, but may involve interference with metabolism.

Uses

Because erythromycin is active against essentially the same aerobic microorganisms as penicillin, it is the drug of first choice against these infections in patients penicillin-allergic. Erythromycin is not effective against the anaerobic *Bacteroides* species implicated in many dental infections. It is indicated in certain situations for the prophylaxis of rheumatic heart disease (see Table 8-7). A major difference is that erythromycin is bacteriostatic rather than bactericidal, as is penicillin. This may be a factor in treating a compromised patient (Table 8-2). The various preparations of erythromycin are shown in Table 8-8.

The base form is the drug of choice for erythromycin. No clinical advantages have been demonstrated for other forms of erythromycin. The usual dose is 250 or 500 mg qid. For infective endocarditis the dose is 1 gm 1 hour before the procedure and 500 mg in 6 hours.

Tetracyclines

The tetracyclines are broad-spectrum antibiotics affecting a wide range of microorganisms. Their adverse effects on the developing teeth are well-known.

The first tetracycline was isolated from a *Streptomyces* strain in 1948. Since then, other tetracyclines have been derived from different species of *Streptomyces*, and the rest have been produced semisynthetically. The tetracyclines (see Table 8-9) are closely related chemically.

Pharmacokinetics

The tetracyclines are most commonly given by mouth. Absorption following oral administration varies but is fairly rapid. There is wide tissue distribution, and tetracyclines are secreted in the saliva and in the milk of lactating mothers (one-half plasma concentration). Tetracyclines are concentrated by the liver and excreted into the intestines by the bile. Enterohepatic circulation prolongs the action of the tetracyclines after they have been discontinued. The tetracyclines are also stored in the dentine and enamel of unerupted teeth and are concentrated in the gingival crevicular fluid. The long-acting agents are concentrated to at least four times serum levels.

The various tetracyclines differ clinically in their duration of action, in the percent absorbed when taken orally, half-lives, and mechanism of elimination. Doxycycline is excreted in the feces, whereas tetracycline is eliminated by glomerular filtration essentially unchanged and minocycline is metabolized in the liver and excreted in the urine. Both doxycycline and minocycline may be given safely to patients with renal dysfunction. They all cross the placenta and enter the fetal circulation.

The concomitant administration of foods with a high calcium content, such as dairy products, oral iron supplements, or antacids containing aluminum, calcium, or magnesium decreases the oral absorption of some tetracyclines. Unlike tetracycline itself, concomitant administration of food or

Table 8-9. The Tetracyclines

Drug name	Serum protein binding (%)	Normal serum $t_{1/2}$ (hr)	Usual oral adult dosage	Lipid solubility	Comments
Tetracycline (Achromycin V, Sumycin)	20–65	6–10	250–500 mg q.6h.	Intermediate	
Doxycycline (Vibramycin, Doxychel)	60–90	14–25	50 mg q.12h. or 100 mg q.24h.	High	*
Minocycline (Minocin)	55–75	11–20	100 mg q.12h.	High	*,†

Modified from Holroyd, S.V., Wynn, R.L., and Requa-Clark, B.: Clinical pharmacology in dental practice, ed. 4, St. Louis, 1988, The C.V. Mosby Co.
*May be taken with food or milk.
†Vestibular side effects.

dairy products with doxycycline or minocycline does not appear to inhibit absorption significantly. The decrease in absorption with tetracycline itself is about 50%, whereas the decrease in absorption with the long-acting agents is only about 20%. The mechanism involves tetracycline chelating the divalent (calcium, magnesium, iron) or trivalent (aluminum) cations. Sodium bicarbonate also reduces the absorption of the tetracyclines.

Spectrum

The tetracyclines are bacteriostatic and interfere with the synthesis of bacterial protein by binding at the 30S subunit of bacterial ribosomes. As broad-spectrum antibiotics, they are effective against a wide variety of gram-positive and gram-negative bacteria (both aerobes and anaerobes), *Rickettsia*, spirochetes (*Treponema pallidum*), some protozoa (*Entamoeba histolytica*), *Chlamydia*, and *Mycoplasma*.

Bacterial resistance develops slowly to the tetracyclines in a stepwise fashion. Cross-resistance is probably complete. This resistance is caused by a decreased uptake of the tetracycline by the organism. In the study of sensitivity of organisms isolated from dental infections, one fifth to three fifths of *Streptococcus viridans* and one fifth to two fifths of *S. aureus* were found to be resistant to tetracycline. The advantage of penicillin over tetracycline in these aerobic gram-positive infections is clear.

Adverse reactions

Although most adverse reactions to the tetracyclines occur infrequently, gastrointestinal distress is not uncommon.

1. Gastrointestinal effects. The gastrointestinal adverse effects include anorexia, nausea, vomiting, diarrhea, gastroenteritis, glossitis, stomatitis, xerostomia, and superinfection (moniliasis). The side effects are largely related to local irritation from alteration of the oral, gastric, and enteric flora.

If diarrhea occurs in a patient receiving tetracycline, the possibility of infectious enteritis such as staphylococcal enterocolitis, intestinal candidiasis, and pseudomembranous colitis (PMC) (secondary to *Clostridium difficile* overgrowth) must be ruled out. Patients taking tetracyclines have developed a yellowish brown discoloration of the tongue. This can occur with either topical or systemic administration. Patients with ill-fitting dentures are likely to have candidosis (moniliasis) associated with the areas of oral mucosa tissue breakdown caused by superinfection.

2. Effects on teeth and bones. Tetracyclines are incorporated in calcifying structures. If they are used during the period of enamel calcification, they can produce permanent discoloration of the teeth and enamel hypoplasia. Consequently, they should not be used during the last half of pregnancy or in children up to 9 years of age. Tetracycline will affect the primary teeth if given to the mother during the last half of pregnancy or to the infant during the first 4 to 6 months of life. If tetracycline is administered between 2 months and 7 or 8 years of age, the permanent teeth will be affected. The mechanism involves the deposition of tetracycline in the enamel of the forming teeth. These stains are permanent and darken with age and exposure to light. They begin as a yellow fluorescence and progress with time to a brown color. This process is accelerated by exposure to light. The permanent discoloration ranges from light gray to yellow to tan. With large doses of tetracyclines, a decrease in the growth rate of bones has been demonstrated in the fetus and in infants.

The treatment of tetracycline-stained teeth is now done almost exclusively with veneers. In the past, heat plus 30% hydrogen peroxide (Superoxol) was applied to the affected teeth to bleach the stain. This process was often not as satisfactory because the stain sometimes returned, and the bleaching process did not completely remove the existing stain.

3. Hepatoxicity. The incidence of liver damage increases with the intravenous use of tetracyclines. Deaths have occurred, especially in pregnant women. Renal impairment leads to accumulation of tetracyclines and an increase in the likelihood of hepatic damage.

4. Nephrotoxicity. Toxic renal effects producing the **Fanconi syndrome**[5] have been reported after

the use of old (degraded) tetracycline. Old or outdated tetracycline should be discarded to prevent future use. Since the nephrotoxic effect of the tetracyclines is additive with that of other drugs, tetracyclines should not be used concomitantly with other nephrotoxic drugs.

5. Hematologic effects. Although hematologic changes are uncommon, hemolytic anemia, leukocytosis, and thrombocytopenic purpura have been reported after tetracycline therapy.

6. Superinfection. With superinfection, resistant organisms multiply and may cause disease. One common situation, especially prevalent in the compromised host (Table 8-2), is an overgrowth of *C. albicans*. This can result in vaginal candidal infections in women treated with tetracyclines.

7. Photosensitivity. Patients taking tetracyclines who are exposed to the sunlight sometimes react with an exaggerated sunburn. Although the incidence seems to vary with the different tetracyclines, patients receiving a prescription for a tetracycline should be told to use a sunscreen before exposure to the sun.

8. Other effects. Minocycline has been associated with CNS side effects, including lightheadedness, dizziness, or vertigo. Patients who will be driving a car should be warned about this reaction. Another side effect associated with minocycline is a blue-black discoloration of the oral cavity. Whether the color arises from discoloration of the underlying teeth and whether minocycline can discolor permanent teeth is being debated.

9. Allergy. Anaphylactic and various dermatologic reactions to the tetracyclines have occasionally occurred, but the overall allergenicity of these drugs is low. Glossitis and cheilosis have also been attributed to a hypersensitivity reaction to tetracycline. A patient who is allergic to one tetracycline is almost certain to be allergic to all tetracyclines.

Drug interactions

1. Cations. Divalent (Ca^{++}, Mg^{++}, Fe^{++}) and trivalent (Al^{+++}) cations decrease the intestinal absorption of tetracycline by chelating with it. Dairy products containing calcium, antacids

(Ca^{++}, Mg^{++}, Al^{+++}), and mineral supplements (iron, calcium, fortified foods) should not be taken within 2 hours of ingesting tetracycline itself. Reasonable quantities of dairy products can be taken with doxycycline and minocycline because there is less interference with absorption.

2. Enhanced effect of other drugs. Tetracycline enhances the effect of the oral sulfonylureas potentially resulting in hypoglycemia. The effects of digoxin, lithium, and theophylline may also be enhanced leading to toxicity from these agents with narrow therapeutic indices. Furosemide's toxicity may also be increased by tetracycline.

3. Reduced tetracycline effect. The barbiturates and phenytoin could reduce the action of the tetracyclines, most notably doxycycline. The mechanism is stimulation of hepatic microsomal enzymes so that doxycycline is metabolized more rapidly.

4. General antibiotic interactions. Like all the antibiotics, the tetracyclines may reduce the effectiveness of oral contraceptives or increase the effectiveness of oral anticoagulants. Also, in most instances, mixing tetracyclines with another antibiotic results in antagonism, especially if the other antibiotic is bactericidal.

Uses

Medical. Although active against a wide variety of microorganisms, the tetracyclines are rarely the drug of choice for a specific infection. Occasionally, they are alternative drugs to treat chlamydial and rickettsial infections. They are used to treat acne (topically and systemically), pulmonary infections in patients with chronic obstructive pulmonary disease (COPD) and traveler's diarrhea. Tetracyclines should not be used for prophylaxis against infective endocarditis except in one unusual situation in dentistry discussed below.

Dental. The tetracyclines are not indicated as either the drug of choice or the alternative drug of choice for dental infections unrelated to periodontal disease. Although controversial, they show some promise for certain periodontal conditions. Conventional treatment with local mea-

chelates = binds

sures should have been undertaken and failed before tetracycline therapy is initiated. A potential advantage of the tetracyclines in the treatment of certain periodontal situations may relate to their concentrating in the gingival crevicular fluid. Because the long-acting tetracyclines are most concentrated in the gingival fluid and they require once-a-day dosing, they may have some limited advantage over tetracycline itself. The ideal tetracycline therapy would be delivered directly to the gingival crevice, thereby reducing the systemic dose greatly. A variety of plastic tubes or collars to deliver the tetracycline directly to the site are currently being evaluated.

Although tetracycline is not a drug of choice for prophylaxis of infective endocarditis before dental appointments, it has a role. Penicillin-resistant *A. actinomycetemcomitans* has been shown to produce endocarditis. It is also present in about one half of adult and almost all juvenile periodontitis patients. Therefore to prevent endocarditis infection from *A. actinomycetemcomitans* after dental treatment in patients at risk, Genco[5] recommends that a full course of tetracycline be administered several weeks before dental treatment is begun. The American Heart Association guidelines for using penicillin (or erythromycin) 1 hour before treatment and 6 hours after treatment should also be followed.

Graykowski and Kingman[6] advocated a mixture of equal parts of tetracycline syrup and lidocaine viscous for the management of recurrent aphthous stomatitis. Acute necrotizing ulcerative gingivitis (ANUG) may also be treated with tetracycline, although local measures are preferred.

Clindamycin

Clindamycin is a bacteriostatic antibiotic effective primarily against gram-positive organisms and the anaerobic *Bacteroides* species. Clindamycin (Cleocin) is produced by adding a Cl group to lincomycin, that is elaborated by *Streptomyces lincolnensis*, found in a soil sample taken near Lincoln, Nebraska. Clindamycin is structurally unrelated to any other antimicrobial agent other than lincomycin, which is not used.

Pharmacokinetics

Clindamycin may be administered orally, topically, intramuscularly, or intravenously. Oral clindamycin is well absorbed, and food does not interfere with its absorption. It reaches its peak concentration in 45 minutes, with a $t_{1/2}$ of about 2.5 hours. Clindamycin is distributed throughout most body tissues, including bone, but not to the cerebrospinal fluid. Concentration in the bone can approximate that of the plasma. It crosses the placental barrier. It is more than 90% bound to plasma proteins. Only about 10% of the active drug is eliminated in the urine. The majority of clindamycin is excreted as inactive metabolites in the urine and feces by the bile.

Spectrum

The antibacterial spectrum of clindamycin includes many gram-positive organisms and some gram-negative organisms. The antibacterial action results from interference with bacterial protein synthesis. Clindamycin is bacteriostatic in most cases, although occasionally it can be bactericidal at higher blood levels.

Clindamycin's activity, similar to erythromycin's, includes *Streptococcus pyogenes* and *S. viridans*, pneumococci, and *S. aureus*. In contrast to erythromycin, it is very active against several anaerobes, including *Bacteroides fragilis* and *Bacteroides melaninogenicus*, *Fusobacterium* species, *Peptostreptococcus* (anaerobic streptococci) and *Peptococcus* species, and *Actinomyces israelii*.

Bacterial resistance to clindamycin develops in a slow, stepwise manner. It occurs by mutations in the bacterial ribosomes that result in a decrease in affinity and binding capacity of these drugs. Cross-resistance between clindamycin and erythromycin is frequently noted. An antagonistic relationship has been observed between clindamycin and erythromycin because of competition for the same binding site (50S subunit) on the bacteria.

Adverse reactions

1. Gastrointestinal effects. The most commonly observed side effects of clindamycin are gastroin-

testinal, including diarrhea, nausea, vomiting, enterocolitis, and abdominal cramps. Glossitis and stomatitis have also been reported with these agents. The incidence of diarrhea has been reported to be between 5% and 20%, with one study reporting an incidence of 7% for clindamycin.[7]

A more serious consequence associated with these agents has been the development of pseudomembranous colitis characterized by severe, persistent diarrhea and the passage of blood and mucus. This colitis, which can be fatal, is due to a toxin produced by the bacterium *C. difficile*. It is associated not only with clindamycin but also with other antibiotics such as tetracycline and ampicillin. The treatment of colitis includes discontinuation of the drug, vancomycin or cholestyramine administered orally, and fluid and electrolyte replacement. Systemically administered corticosteroids have sometimes proved helpful. Opioid-like agents such as diphenoxylate and atropine (Lomotil) may exacerbate the condition and should not be used. Pseudomembranous colitis may occur during treatment or as long as several weeks after the cessation of antibiotic therapy.

2. Superinfection. As with other antibiotics, superinfection by *C. albicans* is sometimes associated with the use of clindamycin.

3. Other effects. Adverse reactions affecting the formed elements in the blood include neutropenia, thrombocytopenia, and agranulocytosis. Abnormal liver function tests and renal dysfunction have been noted.

4. Allergy. Morbilliform skin rashes occur in about 10% of patients given clindamycin. Oral allergic manifestations include glossitis and stomatitis. More severe allergic reactions include urticaria, angioneurotic edema, erythema multiforme, serum sickness, and anaphylaxis.

Uses

Although clindamycin is effective against many gram-positive organisms, other agents are available that are at least as effective as clindamycin and do not usually cause PMC. The indications for treatment with clindamycin are limited to a small number of infections caused by anaerobic organisms, especially *Bacteroides* species and some staphylococcal infections, when the patient is allergic to penicillin.

Many oral infections have been shown to contain a predominance of anaerobic organisms. Many of these anaerobes, such as *Bacteroides oralis*, *Peptostreptococcus*, *Fusobacterium*, and *Veillonella* species, as well as clostridia, are sensitive to 2 gm of oral penicillin G daily.[8] Only for *B. fragilis* infections (see Table 8-3) is clindamycin the drug of choice.

As the importance of the anaerobes in both oral infections and a wide variety of periodontal conditions become documented in the literature, the use of clindamycin will increase. Also mixed gram-positive and gram-negative anaerobic infections may be treated with clindamycin. The use of clindamycin when anaerobic osteomyelitis is suspected is indicated if the organism is susceptible. It is important to emphasize that clindamycin should be used only when specifically indicated, not ever indiscriminately, and the patient should be informed of the potential for and appraised of the symptoms of PMC. The dose of clindamycin is 75 to 150 mg q6h (qid).

Metronidazole

Metronidazole (Flagy 1) is a synthetic nitroimidazole with trichomonocidal (*Trichomonas vaginalis*), ambicidal (*E. histolytica*), and bactericidal action. It has exceptional action against obligate anaerobes such as the *Bacteroides* species.

Pharmacokinetics

Taken orally, metronidazole is well absorbed, with a peak level occurring between 1 and 2 hours after administration. Between 60% and 80% of a dose is excreted in the urine. Metabolites account for about 20% of the dose. Its half-life is 8 hours. It is less than 20% protein bound. Metronidazole is distributed into the cerebrospinal fluid, saliva, and breast milk in levels approximating that of the serum.

Spectrum

Metronidazole is bactericidal and penetrates all bacterial cells. It reacts with deoxyribonucleic acid (DNA), producing inhibition of replication and fragmentation of existing DNA. The spectrum of action of metronidazole includes *T. vaginalis* and *E. histolytica*. Metronidazole is active against obligate anaerobic bacteria such as *Bacteroides*, *Fusobacterium*, *Veillonella*, *Treponema*, *Clostridium*, *Peptococcus*, *Campylobacter*, and *Peptostreptococcus*. Few cases of resistance have been documented.

Adverse reactions

1. Gastrointestinal effects. The most common adverse effect involving the GIT occurs in 12% of patients taking metronidazole. It includes nausea, anorexia, diarrhea, and vomiting. Epigastric distress and abdominal cramping have also been reported.

a. Oral effects. An unpleasant metallic taste has frequently been reported. Altered taste of alcohol has been noted. Glossitis, stomatitis, and a black furred tongue are side effects the dental practitioner should note. These side effects may be related to monilial overgrowth. Dryness of the mouth has also been reported.

2. CNS effects. Headache, dizziness, vertigo, and ataxia have been reported. Confusion, depression, weakness, insomnia, and serious convulsive seizures are associated with metronidazole use.

3. Renal toxicity. Cystitis, polyuria, dysuria, and incontinence can occur with metronidazole. Rarely, darkening of the urine as a result of a metabolite has been reported.

4. Other effects. Transient neutropenia in humans and carcinogenicity and mutagenicity or tumorigenicity in lower life-forms have been seen. Metronidazole is in FDA pregnancy category B because intraperitoneal administration to pregnant mice caused toxicity to the fetus. Administration during the first trimester is contraindicated. Nursing mothers should not be given metronidazole.

Drug interactions

When alcohol is ingested with metronidazole, a disulfiram-like reaction can occur. Symptoms include nausea, abdominal cramps, flushing, vomiting, or headache. Alcohol should be avoided during metronidazole administration and for 1 day after therapy has stopped. Mouthwashes or elixirs containing alcohol should not be used during this period. Metronidazole can potentiate the oral anticoagulants. Drugs that stimulate liver microsomal enzymes can reduce the plasma levels of metronidazole.

Uses

Medical. The medical uses of metronidazole include treatment of trichomoniasis, giardiasis, amebiasis, and susceptible anaerobic bacterial infections. It is effective against serious anaerobic infections of the abdomen, skeleton, and female genital tract. Endocarditis and lower respiratory tract infections caused by *Bacteroides* species are treated with metronidazole.

Dental. Metronidazole is not the drug of choice for any dental infections. It may have some usefulness in the treatment of anaerobic infections when clindamycin is contraindicated or ineffective. Rood and Murgatroyd[9] demonstrated metronidazole's effectiveness in reducing the incidence of "dry socket." Loesche[10] found that a 1-week course of metronidazole produced clinical improvement that persisted for 6 months in periodontal patients. The appropriate clinical place for metronidazole still awaits double-blind controlled clinical trials with adequate patient numbers.

Cephalosporins

The cephalosporin group of antibiotics are chemically related to the penicillins. They are active against a wide variety of both gram-positive and gram-negative organisms. The oral products listed in Table 8-10 are first generation. Second- and third-generation cephalosporins are available for parenteral use.

The source of the original cephalosporins was

Cephalosporium acremonium, isolated near a sewer outlet near Sardinia. These compounds are relatively acid stable and highly resistant to penicillinase, but they are destroyed by cephalosporinase, an enzyme elaborated by some microorganisms.

Spectrum

The cephalosporins are bactericidal agents that are active against most gram-positive cocci and penicillinase-producing staphylococci and some gram-negative bacteria. The cephalosporins inhibit most *Salmonella* and *Klebsiella,* some paracolon strains, *E. coli,* and *H. influenzae. Enterobacter* species, indole-positive *Proteus, Serratia,* methicillin-resistant staphylococci, and most *Pseudomonas* strains are unaffected. The generation of the cephalosporin (first, second, or third) designates the breadth of antimicrobial action, with the first generation being narrower than the second, and the third generation possessing the broadest spectrum of action.

Mechanism of action

The mechanism of action of the cephalosporins is similar to that of the penicillins—inhibition of cell wall synthesis.

Pharmacokinetics

The cephalosporins can be administered orally, intramuscularly, or intravenously. The agents that cannot be used orally are too poorly absorbed to provide adequate blood levels. After absorption they are widely distributed throughout the tissues. The degree of protein binding for the oral agents is between 5% and 20%. The oral cephalosporins are excreted in the urine, with a $t_{1/2}$ that varies between 30 and 150 minutes.

Adverse reactions

In general, the cephalosporins have a low incidence of adverse reactions and are well tolerated. The following reactions may occur.

1. Gastrointestinal effects. The most common adverse reaction associated with the cephalosporins is gastrointestinal, including diarrhea, nausea, vomiting, abdominal pain, anorexia, dyspepsia, and stomatitis.

2. Nephrotoxicity. Evidence suggests that the cephalosporins may produce nephrotoxic effects under certain conditions. Although some have suggested that this is a toxic reaction, it may be an allergic reaction.

3. Superinfection. As with all antibiotics, especially those with a broader spectrum of action, superinfection has been reported. Gram-negative organisms are often the culprits.

4. Local reaction. As with penicillin, the irritating nature of the cephalosporins can produce localized pain, induration, and swelling when given intramuscularly and abscess and thrombophlebitis when given intravenously.

5. Hemostasis and disulfiram-like reaction. Certain parenteral cephalosporins can impair hemostasis or produce a disulfiram-like reaction. The tetrazolethiomethyl side chain appears responsible.

6. Allergy. Various types of hypersensitivity reactions have been reported in approximately 5% of patients receiving cephalosporins. These reactions include fever, eosinophilia, serum sickness, rashes, and anaphylaxis. Large doses frequently produce a direct positive Coombs reaction. This can lead to a significant degree of hemolysis.

Theoretically, because the cephalosporins and penicillin have a similar structure, cross-sensitivity could be expected. Clinically, the incidence of hypersensitivity reactions to the cephalosporins is higher in patients who have a history of penicillin allergy. The degree of cross-sensitivity reported is about 10%. Clinically cephalosporins are frequently given to patients with a history of penicillin allergy.

Uses

The cephalosporins are indicated for infections that are sensitive to these agents but resistant to penicillin. They are especially useful in certain infections caused by gram-negative organisms such as *Klebsiella.* They are used parenterally in hos-

Table 8-10.   Oral cephalosporins

Drug name	t½ (min)	Usual daily adult dose (gm)*	Dosing interval (hr)
First generation			
Cephalexin (Keflex)	30–70	1–4	6
Cephradine (Velosef, Anspor)	45–120	1–4	6
Cefaclor (Ceclor)	36–54	1–4	8
Cefadroxil (Duricef, Ultracef)	70–80	1–2	12–24
Second generation			
Cefuroxime (Ceftin)	60–114	0.75–1.5	8

Modified from Holroyd, S.V., Wynn, R.L., and Requa-Clark, B.: Clinical pharmacology in dental practice, ed. 4, St. Louis, 1988, The C.V. Mosby Co.
*Varies in renal failure and with type of infection.

pitalized patients with a variety of infections. Their dental use is limited to the treatment of infections with sensitive organisms when other agents are ineffective or cannot be used. Their dose is listed in Table 8-10. They are not substitutes for penicillin V or erythromycin if these agents are effective. They may be used before dental treatment to prevent bacterial endocarditis in patients with a history of rheumatic heart disease when other agents cannot be used. Orthopedic surgeons frequently request that the cephalosporins be used as prophylaxis before a dental procedure in patients with an artificial hip prosthesis.

OTHER ANTIMICROBIAL AGENTS
Vancomycin

Vancomycin (Vancocin) is a glycopeptide antibiotic elaborated by *Streptomyces orientalis*, an actinomycete with a complex structure found in soil samples from India and Indonesia. It is unrelated to any other antibiotic currently marketed. Because it has minimal gastrointestinal absorption and causes irritation when used intramuscularly, it is administered only intravenously for a systemic effect.

Spectrum

Vancomycin is bactericidal and has a narrow spectrum of action against many gram-positive cocci, including both staphylococci and streptococci. It acts by inhibition of bacterial cell wall synthesis. Resistance does not seem to develop readily, and cross-resistance with other antibiotics is not believed to occur.

Adverse reactions

Except when vancomycin is given in large doses, significant toxic reactions are infrequent. With large doses or prolonged therapy, some degree of ototoxicity and nephrotoxicity may occur. Permanent deafness and fatal uremia have resulted. Anaphylaxis and superinfection may occur rarely. Prolonged, repeated use can cause thrombophlebitis. The "red-neck syndrome," including chills, fever, and shock, can occur during IV administration. Occasionally, there may be rash, urticaria, chills, fever, and nausea.

Dental uses

Vancomycin is useful in the prophylaxis of infective endocarditis for patients with prosthetic heart valves who are allergic to penicillin (see Table 8-

7). It must be given by IV infusion over 1 hour. It is also used orally to treat PMC through its local action inside the gastrointestinal tract.

Aminoglycosides

As the name implies, the aminoglycoside antibiotics are made up of amino sugars in glycosidic linkage. In 1943, a strain of *Streptomyces griseus* was isolated that elaborated streptomycin. Further strains of *Streptomyces* furnished neomycin, kanamycin, tobramycin, amikacin, and *Micromonospora* produced gentamicin and netilmicin. Note the use of the ending -*micin* rather than -*mycin* for these derivatives. The aminoglycosides are listed below:

Neomycin (Mycifradin)
Streptomycin
Kanamycin (Kantrex)
Gentamicin (Garamycin)
Tobramycin (Nebcin)
Amikacin (Amikin)
Netilmicin (Netromycin)

They appear to inhibit protein synthesis and to act directly on the 30S subunit of the ribosome.

Pharmacokinetics

These agents are poorly absorbed after oral administration and so must be administered by IM or IV injection for a systemic effect. After injection they are rapidly excreted by the normal kidney, with half-lives between 1 and 3 hours. With renal failure, these half-lives may be increased from 10 to 40 times. Therefore in renal failure, the dose of aminoglycosides must be reduced or the interval between doses prolonged considerably.

Spectrum

The aminoglycosides are bactericidal and have a broad antibacterial spectrum. Their use is primarily in the treatment of aerobic gram-negative infections when other agents are ineffective. They have little action against gram-positive anaerobic or facultative bacteria.

Resistance to the aminoglycosides can occur rapidly with a single mutation. Another mechanism of resistance is the metabolism of the agents by the bacterial membrane-bound enzymes. Because the carrier-mediated uptake by bacteria requires oxygen to function, anaerobic and facultative organisms are resistant to these agents. Resistance is also mediated by R factor transfer so that bacteria that have never been exposed to the aminoglycosides are already resistant.

Adverse reactions

The adverse reactions of the aminoglycoside antibiotics seriously limit their use in clinical practice. Their major adverse effects include the following:

1. Ototoxicity. The aminoglycosides are toxic to the eighth cranial nerve, which can lead to auditory and vestibular disturbances. Patients may have difficulty in maintaining equilibrium and can develop vertigo. Hearing impairment and deafness, which can be permanent, have resulted from the administration of these agents. This side effect is more common in patients with renal failure because the drug accumulates in the body. The elderly are also more susceptible.

2. Nephrotoxicity. The aminoglycosides can cause kidney damage by concentrating in the renal cortex. The blood levels and total amount of drug given correlate with the incidence of nephrotoxicity.

3. Neuromuscular blockade. The aminoglycosides act as weak neuromuscular blocking agents, potentially producing apnea. This is a problem if aminoglycosides are given in combination with general anesthetics or skeletal muscle relaxants, agents that are frequently used during surgical procedures.

Uses

The aminoglycosides are indicated for the treatment of hospitalized patients with serious gram-negative infections. Gentamicin, combined with ampicillin, is used in dentistry for the prophylaxis of patients with prosthetic heart valves.

Chloramphenicol

Chloramphenicol (Chloromycetin), a broad-spectrum, bacteriostatic antibiotic, inhibits bacterial protein synthesis by acting primarily on the 50S ribosomal unit. It is active against a large number of gram-positive and gram-negative organisms, rickettsiae, and some chlamydiae. It is particularly active against *Salmonella typhi.*

Chloramphenicol has fallen into disuse primarily because of its serious adverse effects that include fatal blood dyscrasias such as aplastic anemia, agranulocytosis, hypoplastic anemia, and thrombocytopenia. Chloramphenicol can produce bone marrow suppression with pancytopenia. Although its incidence is low (1:40,000), this condition is often fatal. Gray baby syndrome occurs when infants given chloramphenicol cannot conjugate it, causing accumulation and toxicity. Only in the treatment of life-threatening *H. influenzae* and *S. typhi* (typhoid fever) infections is chloramphenicol still the antibiotic of first choice. It is unlikely that any use for chloramphenicol in dentistry is justified.

Sulfonamides

The sulfonamides currently on the market cannot strictly speaking be classified as antibiotics because they are not produced by living organisms.

The introduction of many newer antibiotics limited the use of the sulfonamides until the introduction of trimethoprim-sulfamethoxazole.

Mechanism of action

The sulfonamides' structural similarity to *para-aminobenzoic acid (PABA)* is the basis for most of their antibacterial activity. Because many bacteria are unable to use preformed folic acid, an essential component of several enzyme systems, they must synthesize folic acid from PABA. Because of their structural similarity to PABA, the sulfonamides competitively inhibit the bacterial enzyme dihydropterate synthetase that incorporates PABA into dihydrofolic acid, a precursor of folic acid (Fig. 8-2). Thus by competitive inhibition, adequate folic acid cannot be synthesized by the bacteria. Drugs that are metabolized to PABA, for example, the ester local anesthetics, could theoretically interfere with the action of the sulfonamides.

Spectrum

The sulfonamides are bacteriostatic against many gram-positive and some gram-negative bacteria. They are ineffective against *S. viridans* but are active against some *Chlamydia.*

The amount of the sulfonamide absorbed varies with its solubility. The readily absorbed sulfonamides are used for their systemic effects. Some sulfonamides that produce relatively low systemic blood levels but high urine concentrations are used for the treatment of urinary tract infections. Other relatively insoluble sulfonamides are used in the treatment of ulcerative colitis or before surgical procedures on the bowel. Because these sulfonamides are poorly absorbed, they have only a local effect on the gastrointestinal tract.

After absorption, the sulfonamides are distributed throughout the body, including the cerebrospinal fluid. They are metabolized by acetylation or conjugation to the glucuronide in the liver.

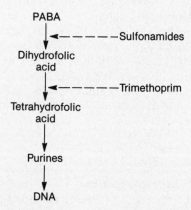

Fig. 8-2. Location of action of sulfonamides and trimethoprim. (Modified from Holroyd, S.V., Wynn, R.L., and Requa-Clark, B.: Clinical pharmacology in dental practice, ed. 4, St. Louis, 1988, The C.V. Mosby Co.)

Metabolites, some of which are less soluble, and some free drugs are excreted in urine.

Adverse reactions

The most common adverse effects of the sulfonamides are allergic reactions. These may be manifested as rash, urticaria, pruritus, fever, a fatal exfoliative dermatitis, or periarteritis nodosa. Other cutaneous allergic reactions include erythema nodosum, erythema multiforme, Stevens-Johnson syndrome, and epidermal necrolysis. These eruptions usually occur after 1 week of therapy. Cross-hypersensitivity can, but does not always, occur.

Other relatively common side effects include nausea, vomiting, abdominal discomfort, headache, and dizziness. Liver damage, depressed renal function, blood dyscrasias (agranulocytosis, thrombocytopenia, aplastic and hemolytic anemia), and precipitation of lupus erythematosus are seen less frequently.

The possibility of renal crystallization must always be kept in mind with the sulfonamides. The earlier sulfonamides had low solubility in the urine, and the danger of crystallization in the kidney was high. The new sulfonamides are more soluble and therefore less likely to precipitate in the kidney. Forcing fluids is generally advisable.

Dental uses

Even though sulfonamides have been reported to be effective in some dental infections, almost without exception antibiotics are more effective and generally safer. Because of their high allergenicity, they should **not** be used topically on oral lesions. Patients with a history of rheumatic heart disease may be taking a sulfonamide for long-term prophylaxis of bacterial endocarditis (sulfisoxazole 1 gm orally bid for a minimum of 5 years).

Trimethoprim-sulfamethoxazole (TMP-SMX)

No less than five products that contain trimethoprim, an antibacterial and antimalarial agent, and sulfamethoxazole, a sulfonamide, are listed in the top 200 drugs (see Appendix). Because sulfamethoxazole inhibits the incorporation of PABA into folic acid and trimethoprim inhibits the reduction of dihydrofolate to tetrahydrofolate (Fig. 8-2), this combination inhibits two separate steps in the essential metabolic pathway of the bacteria, thus leading to a synergistic effect.

Trimethoprim-sulfamethoxazole (Bactrim, Septra), like the sulfonamides, is bacteriostatic against a wide variety of gram-positive bacteria and some gram-negative bacteria. Its adverse effects are similar to those of the sulfonamides. About 75% of the adverse reactions associated with this combination involve the skin. The trimethoprim portion produces adverse effects of antifolate agents such as the hematologic reactions of megaloblastosis, thrombocytopenia, and leukopenia, as well as anemia, granulocytopenia, agranulocytosis, and coagulation disorders. Jaundice and renal damage can occasionally occur.

TMP-SMX is indicated in the treatment of selected urinary tract infections, certain cases of acute gonococcal urethritis, and selected respiratory and gastrointestinal infections. It is used extensively to treat acute otitis media in children often caused by *H. influenzae*. A combination of erythromycin and sulfisoxazole (Pediazole) is also used for otitis media in children. It is the drug of choice for *Pneumocystis carinii* pneumonia (AIDS [acquired immunodeficiency syndrome] patients), *Serratia* sepsis, systemic *Salmonella* (ampicillin-resistant), and *Shigella* infections.

Nitrofurantoin

Nitrofurantoin (Macrodantin) possesses a wide antibacterial spectrum including both gram-positive and gram-negative bacteria. It is bacteriostatic against many common urinary tract pathogens, including *E. coli*. Many strains of *Klebsiella* and *Enterobacter* and all strains of *P. aeruginosa* are resistant. It is rapidly absorbed from the gastrointestinal tract, but plasma antibacterial concentrations are not reached because the drug is rapidly excreted with a $t_{1/2}$ of less than 1 hour.

The most common adverse reactions are nausea, vomiting, and diarrhea, but taking the drug with food decreases these effects. Hypersensitivity reactions include chills, fever, leukopenia, granulocytopenia, hemolytic anemia, cholestatic jaundice, chronic active hepatitis, allergic pneumonitis and interstitial pulmonary fibrosis. Neurologic disorders observed include headache and a polyneuropathy with denervation and muscle atrophy. Nitrofurantoin is used in the treatment of certain urinary tract infections.

Quinolones (ciprofloxacin)

The quinolones are orally effective antibacterial agents chemically related to nalidixic acid (NegGram). Nalidixic acid is considered a first-generation quinolone, whereas the fluoroquinolones are third-generation quinolones. They are bactericidal against most gram-negative organisms and many gram-positive organisms. They are the first orally active agents against certain *Pseudomonas* species. There is no cross-resistance with other antimicrobial agents. The currently available members of the fluoroquinolones are norfloxacin (Noroxin) and ciprofloxacin (Cipro). The discussion will concentrate on ciprofloxacin, the most promising agent.

The mechanism of action of the quinolones involves antagonism of the A subunit of DNA gyrase; the enzyme is involved in DNA synthesis. Interference of DNA gyrase results in cell death. Because DNA gyrase is found only in microorganisms, human cells are unaffected by the quinolones' action. Resistance is not transferred from one resistant bacteria to an unexposed bacteria because plasmid and chromosomal DNA are destroyed.

Pharmacokinetics

Ciprofloxacin is well absorbed but antacids interfere with its absorption. It is eliminated with a half-life of 4 hours. Probenecid interferes with its absorption and increases its serum concentration by about 50%. Patients should be well hydrated to prevent any possibility of crystalluria.

Spectrum

Ciprofloxacin is bactericidal against a wide range of gram-negative organisms including *E. coli,*

Klebsiella species, *Enterobacter* species, *P. aeruginosa* and gram-positive organisms such as *S. aureus*. Unlike other antiinfective agents, an additive action may result when ciprofloxacin is combined with other antimicrobial agents.

Adverse reactions

1. Gastrointestinal tract. Nausea, diarrhea, vomiting, painful oral mucosa, bad taste, and oral candidiasis have been reported.

2. CNS effects. CNS adverse reactions include headache, restlessness, lightheadedness, and insomnia.

3. Hypersensitivity. Rash, pruritus, urticaria, cutaneous candidiasis, hyperpigmentation, photosensitivity, and edema of the lips have been noted.

4. Other effects. Disturbed vision, joint pain, renal problems, and palpitations have rarely been reported.

5. Pregnancy and nursing. Ciprofloxacin is contraindicated in the pregnant woman or nursing mother.

Uses

Ciprofloxacin is indicated for lower respiratory tract, skin, bone and joint, and urinary tract infections caused by susceptible organisms. Dental patients taking this agent may have candidal overgrowth or an altered oral flora.

In summary, the new quinolones have an advantage over other antimicrobial agents by having a unique mechanism of action, making the development and transfer of resistance more difficult. Their unique gram-negative spectrum coupled with their oral efficacy and bactericidal action makes these agents a welcome addition to the antimicrobial armamentarium. Many more members of this group of agents currently await in the wings.

Antituberculosis agents

The treatment of tuberculosis, a disease caused by the acid-fast bacterium *Mycobacterium tuberculosis,* is difficult for several reasons. First, patients with tuberculosis often have inadequate defense mechanisms. Second, tubercle bacilli develop resistant strains easily and possess unusual metabolic characteristics, including long periods of inactivity. Finally, most of the drugs available are not bactericidal and because of their toxicity often cannot be used in sufficient doses.

The treatment of tuberculosis relies almost entirely on chemotherapy. Because of the problem of resistance, at least two drugs are administered concurrently in all active cases. Isoniazid, rifampin, and pyrazinamide are combined for the treatment of pulmonary tuberculosis. With susceptible organisms, a patient, if compliant, usually becomes noninfective within 2 to 3 weeks.

The Centers for Disease Control (CDC) recommend that the following patients receive INH because they are at risk of developing tuberculosis: close contacts of recently diagnosed patients, patients with a positive skin test and radiographic findings consistent with nonprogressive tuberculosis, patients whose skin test has become positive (converted), and immunosuppressed patients (see Table 8-2).

Isoniazid

Isoniazid (INH) is bactericidal only against actively growing tubercle bacilli. "Resting" bacilli exposed to the drug are able to resume normal growth when the drug is removed. Within a few weeks after beginning therapy, resistant strains develop.

Pharmacokinetics. INH is readily absorbed from the gastrointestinal tract and is distributed throughout the body. Its metabolism varies by race. Most Eskimos and Japanese are fast acetylators, whereas North American whites are slow acetylators; in the United States the fast and slow acetylators are split 50-50. The ability to acetylate rapidly is inherited as an autosomal dominant trait. Whether this ability to metabolize INH rapidly is related to the chance of developing INH-induced hepatitis is unknown. The half-life for fast acetylators is 1½ hours; for the slow, 3 hours.

Adverse reactions. The incidence of all adverse reactions to INH is approximately 5%. The most common adverse reaction, occurring in about 20% of patients, involves the nervous system. Peripheral and optic neuritis, muscle twitching, toxic encephalopathy, insomnia, restlessness, sedation, incoordination, convulsions, and even psychoses have been reported. These neurotoxic symptoms can be prevented by coadministration of pyridoxine (vitamin B_6).

The other type of adverse effect associated with INH is hepatotoxicity. About 1% of patients taking INH exhibit clinical hepatitis, and up to 10% develop abnormal laboratory values. Some cases of hepatitis have been fatal. The risk for development of this adverse effect is age related; that is, it rarely occurs in patients less than 20 years old, whereas 2.5% of patients older than 50 exhibit hepatitis.

Other side effects include hematologic effects, gastrointestinal effects, dryness of the mouth, and a lupuslike reaction or rheumatic syndrome with arthralgia. Urinary retention and gynecomastia have been noted in males. Hypersensitivity reactions, including rashes, hepatitis, lymphadenopathy, and fever, are occasionally reported.

Uses. INH is used alone in the parameters discussed above and in combination, first with rifampin and pyrazinamide in the treatment of tuberculosis. The dose is 300 mg daily.

Rifampin (Rifadin, Rimactane)

Rifampin is a semisynthetic derivative of rifamycin, an antibiotic produced by *Streptomyces mediterranei*. Its mechanism of action involves inhibition of DNA-dependent ribonucleic acid (RNA) polymerase, which then suppresses the initiation of chain formation. It is active against *M. tuberculosis* and many gram-positive and some gram-negative bacteria. Rifampin's spectrum also includes *S. aureus*, *N. meningitidis*, *H. influenzae*, and *Legionella* species. In tuberculosis, resistance quickly develops to rifampin administered alone in a one-step process as a result of a change of the β subunit of RNA polymerase. Administering ri-

may be in "triple antibiotic ointments" *avoid*

fampin with another antituberculosis agent reduces the development of resistance.

Pharmacokinetics. Rifampin is absorbed from the gastrointestinal tract and eliminated in the bile, where enterohepatic circulation occurs. Its $t_{1/2}$, 1.5 to 5 hours, is increased in hepatic disease, but unaltered by renal disease. The half-life is reduced by INH coadministration because of enzyme induction. By blocking the hepatic uptake of rifampin, probenecid increases the concentration of rifampin in the serum.

Adverse reactions. The most common adverse reactions are gastrointestinal, including anorexia, stomach distress, nausea, vomiting, abdominal cramps, and diarrhea. Occasionally rashes, thrombocytopenia, nephritis, and impairment of liver function are seen. A "flulike" reaction can occur with infrequent administration. Rifampin gives a red-orange color to body fluids including tears (which affects contact lenses), urine, feces, saliva, and sweat.

Uses. Rifampin is used in combination with INH and pyrazinamide for treatment of tuberculosis. The adult dose is 600 mg daily. It is also used alone to treat meningococcal carriers and children exposed to *H. influenzae* meningitis.

Pyrazinamide (PZA)

Pyrazinamide (PZA) is a relative of nicotinamide that is well absorbed and widely distributed throughout the body. It is hepatotoxic and can produce rash, hyperuricemia, and gastrointestinal disturbances. Now recommended by the CDC to be used for the first 2 months with INH and rifampin to treat tuberculosis, pyrazinamide now plays a more important role than formerly.

Ethambutol

Ethambutol (Myambutol) is a synthetic tuberculostatic agent effective against *M. tuberculosis*. Resistance among tubercle bacilli develops very rapidly when used alone.

The most important side effect is optic neuritis, resulting in a decrease in visual acuity and loss of ability to perceive red and green colors. Periodic ophthalmologic examinations are recommended.

Other side effects include rash, joint pain, gastrointestinal upset, malaise, headache, and dizziness. This drug is used when other antituberculosis agents cannot be used or resistance is encountered.

Topical antibiotics

In general, the use of antibiotics topically is discouraged. Systemic administration is superior in most cases. If an agent is used topically, it should be one that cannot be used systemically. One old and one new product are mentioned briefly.

Neomycin, polymyxin, bacitracin. This combination, available in ointment form (Neosporin), contains an aminoglycoside (neomycin) and two polypeptide antibiotics (polymyxin and bacitracin). Although used clinically, the literature contains little evidence of its success.

Mupirocin (Bactroban). Mupirocin is a new topical antibiotic indicated for the treatment of impetigo. Local itching and stinging have been reported. It may be as effective as the usual systemic treatments, but further clinical trials are needed. *Not use in dental, cuts, abrasions skin*

ANTIFUNGAL AGENTS

Although fungal infections are not frequently encountered in dental practice, when they are, they are difficult to treat because immunocompromised patients are often involved. Fungal infections can be divided into those that affect primarily the skin or mucosa (mucocutaneous), and those affecting the whole body (systemic). Infections affecting the skin produce athlete's foot, "jock itch," and ringworm. Over-the-counter (OTC) products (Table 8-11) often manage these conditions. Dental practitioners manage the mucocutaneous fungal infections, primarily caused by *C. albicans* using nystatin, clotrimazole, or ketoconazole (Table 8-12). Systemic mycoses can be produced by many fungi such as aspergillosis, blastomycosis, coccidioidomycosis, cryptococcosis, histoplasmosis, mucormycosis, and paracoccidioidomycosis. Chromomycosis, mycetoma, and sporotrichosis may produce deep mycotic infections. These serious infections are medical management situations be-

Table 8-11. Topical over-the-counter antifungal agents

Drug name	Route
Undecylenic acid (Desenex, Cruex)	Powder, ointment, cream, liquid, foam, soap
Miconazole (Micatin)	Cream, powder, spray
Triacetin (Enzactin, Fungacetin)	Cream, ointment
Tolnaftate (Tinactin, Aftate)	Cream, powder, liquid, solution, gel
Haloprogin (Halotex)	Cream, solution

Modified from Holroyd, S.V., Wynn, R.L., and Requa-Clark, B.: Clinical pharmacology in dental practice, ed. 4, St. Louis, 1988, The C.V. Mosby Co.

yond the scope of this chapter. Amphotericin B and miconazole administered IV may be used to treat these serious infections.

Nystatin

Nystatin (Hycostatin) is a polyene macrolide antibiotic produced by *Streptomyces noursei*. Its mechanism of action involves binding to sterols in the fungal cell membrane. This produces a change in membrane permeability and allows the loss of potassium and other essential cellular constituents. Because bacteria do not contain sterols in their cell membranes, nystatin is not active against these organisms.

Nystatin is not absorbed from the mucous membranes and is essentially unabsorbed from the gastrointestinal tract. In the usual therapeutic doses, blood levels are not detectable. When administered orally, it is excreted unchanged in the feces. Nystatin is fungicidal and fungistatic against a variety of yeasts and fungi. In vitro, nystatin inhibits *C. albicans* and some other species of *Candida*.

The adverse reactions associated with nystatin are minor and infrequent. When higher doses have been used, nausea, vomiting, and diarrhea have occasionally occurred. Rarely, hypersensitivity reactions have been reported.

Nystatin is used for both the treatment and prevention of oral candidiasis in susceptible cases. Although *C. albicans* is a frequent inhabitant of the oral cavity, only under unusual conditions does it produce disease. Frequently, patients affected are immunocompromised (see Table 8-2).

Table 8-12. Dentally useful antifungal agents

Drug name	Dosage forms	Indication	Comments	Dose		Sucrose/ dose (gm)
Nystatin (Mycostatin, Nilstat, others)	Aqueous suspension, vaginal tablets, cream, ointment, powder, oral tablets, pastilles	Oral candidosis (monilia, thrush)	Side effects uncommon	Susp: Vag tab: Pastilles:	5 ml q.i.d. 1 q.i.d. 1–2 4–5 x/d	2.5 0.8 1.0*
Clotrimazole (Mycelex)	Troches (lozenges)	Candidiasis; tinea pedis, cruris, corpus, versicolor	Nausea	Troche:	1 5 x/d	0.9
Ketoconazole (Nizoral)	Oral tablets, cream	Systemic fungal infections, oral candidosis	Hepatotoxic, anaphylaxis, teratogenic, drug interactions	Tablet: Cream	1 daily	

Modified from Holroyd, S.V., Wynn, R.L., and Requa-Clark, B.: Clinical pharmacology in dental practice, ed. 4, St. Louis, 1988, The C.V. Mosby Co.
*Dextrose.

For the treatment of oral candidiasis, nystatin is available in the form of an aqueous suspension (100,000 units/ml) containing 50% sucrose. The dose is listed in Table 8-12. (Note: diabetics, 2.5 gm of sucrose per dose.) The pastilles are licorice-flavored and contain 0.8 gm of sucrose plus 1 gm of dextrose per dosage form.

A form of nystatin used vaginally are tablets containing 100,000 units each. The tablet is dissolved in the mouth qid. The lozenge allows the drug to be in contact with the infected oral mucosa longer than the aqueous suspension, but it is not flavored.

Patients should be instructed to use the nystatin product for at least 2 weeks or for 48 hours after the symptoms have subsided and cultures have returned negative. Some patients require prophylactic doses to control candidiasis.

Imidazoles

Two members of the imidazoles are useful in dentistry: clotrimazole and ketoconazole.

Clotrimazole

Clotrimazole (Mycelex) is a synthetic antifungal agent available in the form of a slowly dissolving lozenge for oral use. It is also available in forms for topical and vaginal use.

Clotrimazole's mechanism of action involves alteration of cell membrane permeability. It binds with the phospholipids in the cell membrane of the fungus. As a result of the alteration in permeability, the cell membrane loses its function, and the cellular constituents are lost.

The oral lozenge dissolves in approximately 15 to 30 minutes. Patients with xerostomia may have difficulty dissolving this product. Saliva concentrations that are sufficient to inhibit most *Candida* species are maintained in the mouth for about 3 hours. The drug is bound to the oral mucosa and slowly released from it. The amount of clotrimazole absorbed systemically by this route is unknown. Each lozenge also contains 0.9 gm of dextrose. The spectrum of action of clotrimazole includes *Tinea* species and *Candida*.

The most common adverse reactions associated with clotrimazole involve the gastrointestinal tract, including abdominal pain, diarrhea, and nausea. Clotrimazole has been reported to produce an elevated aspartate aminotransferase level in approximately 15% of patients. Other changes in laboratory tests have also been reported.

Clotrimazole has been assigned to FDA pregnancy category C. Very high doses have been embryotoxic in rats and mice. High doses have caused impairment of mating and a decrease in both the number and survival of the young. No teratogenic effects have been found in several other species tested. No carcinogenicity has been demonstrated in rats.

Clotrimazole is indicated for the local treatment of oropharyngeal candidiasis. Patients should be instructed to dissolve the lozenge in the mouth slowly, like a "cough drop," to minimize gastrointestinal discomfort. They should also be told to take the medication "until gone" to minimize relapse. The usual adult dosage is one lozenge (10 mg) five times daily for at least 14 days (or longer for immunosuppressed patients). Some clinicians advocate dissolving one 100 mg clotrimazole (Mycelex) vaginal tablet daily in the oral cavity, like a lozenge or troche.

Ketoconazole (Nizoral)   *oral thrush*

Ketoconazole, the other imidazole used in dentistry, alters cellular membranes and interferes with intracellular enzymes. By interfering with the synthesis of ergosterol, a cellular component of fungi, membrane permeability is altered and purine transport inhibited. The imidazoles inhibit the C-14 demethylation of lanosterol, an ergosterol precursor. It also inhibits sex steroid biosynthesis, including testosterone, perhaps by blocking several P-450 enzyme steps.

Pharmacokinetics

To be adequately absorbed systemically, ketoconazole requires an acidic environment. Patients taking medications that interfere with the normal production of stomach acid, such as histamine (H_2) blockers, or those with achlorhydria may absorb less ketoconazole. With the exception of the cerebrospinal fluid, it is well distributed in humans. It crosses the placenta and is excreted in breast milk. The peak serum concentration occurs between 1 and 4 hours.

Ketoconazole is metabolized in the liver, and approximately 13% is excreted by the kidney, with a half-life between 2 and 8 hours. Because of the small contribution of the kidney to the excretion of ketoconazole, patients with renal impairment do not generally require a reduction in their dose. The primary route of excretion for ketoconazole is biliary. Patients with hepatic impairment may require a lower dose.

Spectrum

Ketoconazole is effective against a wide variety of fungal infections. It is indicated in many systemic fungal infections, including blastomycosis, candidiasis, coccidioidomycosis, and histoplasmosis. It is not the drug of choice for the tinea fungi unless traditional agents have failed.

Adverse reactions

1. Gastrointestinal. The most frequent adverse reactions (3% to 10%) associated with ketoconazole are nausea and vomiting. These adverse effects can be minimized by taking with food.

2. Hepatotoxicity. The most serious adverse reaction associated with ketoconazole is hepatotoxicity. Its incidence is approximately 1:10,000. It is usually reversible on discontinuation of the drug but has occasionally been fatal. Patients taking other hepatotoxic agents, those with liver disease (e.g., alcoholic hepatitis), or those on prolonged therapy should be watched closely because they may be more susceptible to this hepatotoxicity.

3. Endocrine effects. Rarely, male patients have reported gynecomastia that is usually reversible and a decrease in sexual ability, including impotence. This may be the result of ketoconazole's effect on testosterone levels or its effect on adrenal steroid production.

4. Other effects. Other adverse reactions reported include headache, dizziness, drowsiness, photophobia, skin rash or pruritus, and insomnia.

Fever, chills, dyspnea, tinnitus, arthralgias, and thrombocytopenia have occurred in a few patients. When applied topically, irritation, pruritus, and stinging are the most commonly reported side effects.

5. Pregnancy and nursing. Animal studies have shown that ketoconazole can produce syndactyly, oligodactyly, dystocia, and embryotoxicity. The FDA pregnancy category for ketoconazole is C. Because ketoconazole is excreted in breast milk, the risk-to-benefit ratio must be considered before it is used in the nursing mother.

Drug interactions

Many drug interactions with ketoconazole have been reported in the literature. Because an acidic environment is required for dissolution and absorption of ketoconazole, agents that alter the amount of stomach acid could theoretically reduce the absorption of ketoconazole (H_2 blockers, anticholinergic agents, antacids). There should be at least 2 hours between the ingestion of these agents and ketoconazole's administration.

Ketoconazole may interact with warfarin and cyclosporin to increase their effects; it alters blood levels of rifampin, INH, and phenytoin. It may have a disulfiram-like reaction or enhanced hepatotoxicity with alcohol.

Dental uses

Ketoconazole is indicated in the treatment and management of mucocutaneous and oropharyngeal candidiasis (oral thrush). It is also effective in other susceptible fungal infections. Because of its adverse reaction profile, ketoconazole should be used only after other topical antifungal agents have been ineffective or there is reason to believe that they will be ineffective.

Dose

The usual adult dose of ketoconazole for the treatment of *Candida* is 200 to 400 mg daily. It should be used for at least 2 weeks, and 6 to 12 months may be required for chronic mucocutaneous candidiasis. Maintenance therapy may be necessary for certain patients. Ketoconazole is now available in a 2% aqueous vehicle (cream) for local administration in tinea infections. It is applied once or twice daily for at least 2 weeks.

Other antifungal agents

Because amphotericin B is still the mainstay of treatment for most serious systemic fungal infections, it is discussed briefly.

Amphotericin B (Fungizone)

Amphotericin B is an amphoteric polyene macrolide antibiotic produced by *Streptomyces nodosus*. It binds to the sterols in the fungus cell membrane, altering membrane permeability and allowing the loss of potassium and small molecules from the cells. This binding to sterols accounts for some adverse effects of amphotericin B. Because kidney cells and erythrocytes contain sterols, they can be adversely affected.

Amphotericin B is widely distributed, except to the cerebrospinal fluid. Because it is poorly absorbed from the intestinal tract, it must be administered parenterally to treat systemic fungal infections. Its metabolic fate is undetermined, and its elimination is complex.

The spectrum of amphotericin includes many fungi, such as certain strains of *Aspergillus*, *Paracoccidioides*, *Coccidioides*, *Cryptococcus*, *Histoplasma*, *Mucor*, and *Candida*. It is also effective against the protozoa *Leishmania*.

The adverse reactions associated with amphotericin are wide-ranging and potentially serious, but it is often the only effective treatment for certain serious systemic fungal infections. Most patients experience hypokalemia, headache, chills (50%), fever, malaise, muscle and joint pain, gastric complaints and some nephrotoxicity (80%). Amphotericin has many potentially serious drug interactions.

With topical administration, amphotericin has produced burning, itching, and in rare cases an allergic contact dermatitis. It is available in the form of a 3% cream or ointment.

Griseofulvin

Griseofulvin (Fulvicin P/G, Grisactin Ultra, Gris-PEG) is an antibiotic produced by *Penicillium gri-*

seofulvum. Its antifungal action is produced by disrupting the cell's mitotic spindle structure and arresting cell division in metaphase. Taken orally, the ultramicrosize griseofulvin is almost completely absorbed. Unlike many drugs, griseofulvin's absorption is enhanced by taking it with a fatty meal. It is tightly bound and preferentially deposited in diseased keratin percursors (hair, nails, skin). Its spectrum includes tineas (e.g., ringworm), *Trichophyton*, *Microsporum*, or *Epidermophyton* but does not include *Candida*.

The adverse reactions of griseofulvin include headache, gastrointestinal complaints, and overgrowth of *Candida* in the oral cavity (thrush). Hypersensitivity reactions include urticaria, photosensitivity, and lupuslike reactions. The possibility of some cross-sensitivity with penicillins should be considered. Depression of hematopoietic functions and carcinogenicity in animals have been demonstrated. It can also produce a disulfiram-like (Antabuse) reaction.

Griseofulvin is indicated in the treatment of susceptible infections of the skin, hair, and nails. Because the drug is deposited only in the growing tissues, the duration of treatment depends on the time it takes for the affected area to grow out completely; this may be from 2 weeks to 8 months. Although there is no known use in dentistry, the side effects of griseofulvin must be considered when a dental patient is taking this drug.

ANTIVIRAL AGENTS

The search for drugs useful in the treatment of viral infections has posed the greatest problem of all infectious organisms. This is probably because by their very nature viruses are obligate intracellular organisms that require cooperation from their host's cells. Therefore to kill the virus, often the host's cell must also be harmed. The herpesvirus, because of the location of the lesions around the oral cavity and, in some cases, on the dentist's finger, has been of the most interest to the dentist. Now, with the symptoms of AIDS being seen clinically in the mouth, the treatment of this virus takes on more importance. Table 8-13 lists some antiviral agents along with their routes of administration and indications.

Table 8-13. Antiviral agents

Drug name	Route(s)	Indication(s)	Comments
Acyclovir (Zovirax)	Oral, topical, IV	Primary and recurrent herpes, in non- and immunocompromised patients	Local: burning Oral: nausea, CNS effects
Vidarabine (Ara-A, Vira-A)	IV, ophth. oint.	Herpes encephalitis, keratoconjunctivitis, recurrent epithelial keratitis	
Ribavirin (Virazole)	Aerosol	Infants with severe respiratory syncytial virus	Very costly, difficult to administer, requires special machine
Amantadine (Symmetrel)	Oral	Prophylaxis of influenza A virus	Also used to treat parkinsonism
Idoxuridine (IDU, Herplex, Stoxil)	Ophth. oint., solution	Herpes simplex keratitis	Irritation, pruritus, edema, inflammation
Interferon (Intron A, Roferon-A)	IM, subcutaneous	Hairy cell leukemia	Many investigations underway currently

Acyclovir *reduce symptoms*

Acyclovir (zovirax) is a purine nucleoside that is first converted to acyclovir monophosphate by the herpes simplex virus–coded thymidine kinase. Cellular enzymes convert the monophosphate to the diphosphate, and then to the triphosphate. The triphosphate exerts its antiviral action on herpesviruses by interfering with DNA polymerase and inhibiting DNA replication. It is much less toxic to normal uninfected cells because it is preferentially taken up by infected cells. In the host's cells acyclovir is only minimally phosphorylated. This explains its excellent adverse reaction profile.

Pharmacokinetics

When acyclovir is taken orally, between 15% and 30% is absorbed. Peak concentrations occur within about 2 hours. Food does not affect the drug's absorption. Acyclovir is distributed widely throughout the body. In animals, acyclovir crosses the placenta but its presence in the human placenta or milk is unknown. The half-life of acyclovir in the initial phase is 0.3 hour and in the terminal phase is 2.1 to 3.5 hours. As the patient's creatinine clearance rises, the half-life of the drug

is prolonged. Approximately 10% of the dose of acyclovir is metabolized in the liver. It is excreted primarily unchanged in the urine by glomerular filtration and tubular secretion.

Spectrum

The antiviral action of acyclovir includes various herpesviruses, including herpes simplex types 1 and 2 (HSV-1 and HSV-2), varicella-zoster, Epstein-Barr, Herpesvirus simiae (B virus), and cytomegalovirus. Several mechanisms of resistance to acyclovir have been found.

Adverse reactions

The type and extent of the adverse reactions experienced depend on the route of administration of acyclovir.

1. Topical. When administered topically, acyclovir produces burning, stinging, or mild pain in about one third of patients. Itching and skin rash have also been reported.

2. Oral. One of the most common adverse effects associated with oral acyclovir is headache (13%). Other CNS effects include vertigo, dizziness, fatigue, insomnia, irritability, and mental depression. Oral acyclovir also commonly pro-

duces gastrointestinal adverse reactions, including nausea, vomiting, and diarrhea. Anorexia and a funny taste in the mouth have also been rarely reported. Other side effects associated with oral acyclovir include acne, accelerated hair loss, arthralgia, fever, menstrual abnormalities, pars planitis, sore throat, lymphadenopathy, thrombophlebitis, edema, muscle cramps, leg pain, and palpitation.

3. Parenteral. With parenteral administration, local reactions at the injection site are the most common side effects reported; these include irritation, erythema, pain, and phlebitis. Because acyclovir can precipitate in the renal tubules, it can occasionally affect the BUN or serum creatine levels. Encephalopathic effects, including lethargy, obtundation, tremors, confusion, hallucination, agitation, seizures, and coma, have been reported in about 1% of patients given parenteral acyclovir.

Uses

1. Topical. The indications for topical acyclovir include **initial** herpes genitalis and limited non–life-threatening initial and recurrent mucocutaneous herpes simplex (HSV-1 and HSV-2) in **immunocompromised** patients. Topical treatment has not been effective in the treatment of recurrent herpes genitalis or herpes labialis infections in nonimmunocompromised patients. It does produce a limited shortening in the duration of viral shedding in males by 1 day. It does not prevent the transmission of infection, nor does it prevent recurrence. The available literature does not support the use of topical acyclovir for management of herpes labialis in dentistry.

2. Oral. The oral form of acyclovir is indicated in the treatment of initial and management of recurrent herpes genitalis infections in both immunocompromised and nonimmunocompromised patients. It is effective in the prophylaxis of recurrent genitalis infections in both patient groups. It is not indicated to suppress recurrent herpes genitalis in patients with mild infections. In the treatment of herpes labialis, oral acyclovir's place has yet to be established.

3. Injectable. The parenteral form of acyclovir is used for severe initial herpes genitalis infections in the nonimmunocompromised patient. It is also indicated for the treatment of initial and recurrent mucocutaneous herpes simplex infections in the immunocompromised patient. Other uses include herpes zoster and varicella treatment.

Dose

The usual oral adult dosage of acyclovir for the treatment of initial genital herpes or intermittently for the treatment of recurrent episodes is 200 mg every 4 hours while the patient is awake 5 times daily for 5 days. Treatment should be started as soon as the prodromal stage is noticed. The prophylactic dosage for recurrent episodes is 200 mg 2 to 3 times daily not to exceed 6 months. Some patients may need up to 200 mg 5 times daily.

Other antiviral agents

Table 8-13 lists some other antiviral agents.

Amantadine (Symmetrel). Amantadine inhibits the penetration of the adsorbed virus into the host's cells or inhibits the uncoating of the influenza A viruses. It can be used prophylactically to prevent or for treatment to reduce the symptoms of an influenza A viral infection. It is used for institutional patients to prevent the spread of infection during outbreaks. It also has antiparkinson action.

Nucleic acid synthesis inhibitors. Vidarabine and idoxuridine are inhibitors of nucleic acid synthesis, like acyclovir. They are used topically to treat ophthalmologic infections caused by the herpesvirus.

Interferon. Interferons are a large group of proteins that have antiviral, cytotoxic, and immunomodulating action. Recombinant DNA technology now produces interferon. So far, the FDA has approved two interferons (alfa-2b [Intron A] and alfa-2a [Roferon-A]) for treatment of hairy cell leukemia. Interferon therapy is being studied for many other types of cancers, as well as herpes and hepatitis.

document in chart when using tetracycline, followups, ✓, call, ✓ again, call again.

Table 8-14. Determining antibiotic prophylaxis for dental procedures

Prophylaxis indicated:

Antibiotic prophylaxis must be considered for all patients potentially at risk when an anticipated dental procedure is likely to produce bacteremia. Procedures that produce bacteremia can be defined as any manipulation of tooth or periodontal structures that produce gingival, mucosal, or pulpal bleeding and any procedure that disturbs an area of infection. The following is a list of procedures believed to produce transient bacteremias but it is not to be construed as all-inclusive. These procedures include:

1. Periodontal probing
2. Intraoral examination, in which an explorer or other sharp instruments are used
3. Local anesthetic injection
4. Dental prophylaxis and oral hygiene procedures
5. Scaling and root planing
6. Any surgical procedure
7. Endodontic procedures
8. Operative procedures to include: cavity preparation, packing gingival tissues, taking impressions, placement of restorative materials and placement of matrix bands (either celluloid or metal), and polishing amalgams
9. Crown and bridge procedures including: Crown and bridge preparations, packing retraction cord, taking impressions, removing temporaries, and placing or removing temporaries
10. Dental insertions (complete and removable temporaries)
11. Pericoronitis treatments
12. Dressing changes
13. Suture removal
14. Postoperative treatments

Prophylaxis not indicated:

Antibiotic coverage is usually **not** indicated when performing the following procedures. However, sound clinical judgment should be exercised in the presence of inflammation or when trauma is anticipated. Under such circumstances, antibiotic coverage should be considered.
1. Edentulous impressions unless lacerations or ulcerations occur before or during treatment
2. Taking jaw relationships for complete dentures
3. Removable denture try-ins
4. Intraoral soft tissue exam when sharp instruments are not used
5. Adjustment of orthodontic appliances
6. Taking of intraoral radiographs*
7. Alginate impressions*

*There is controversy on whether or not the taking of intraoral radiographs and alginate impressions produce bacteremias. It is believed that in these procedures, as well as many of the procedures listed above, the production of bacteremias is altered by the cleanliness of the mouth, and the operator's ability.

UMKC Clinic Handbook 1987.

ANTIBIOTIC PROPHYLAXIS USED IN DENTISTRY
Prevention of bacterial endocarditis

In 1984 the Committee on Prevention of Rheumatic Fever and Bacterial Endocarditis of the American Heart Association provided dental professionals with guidelines for antibiotic prophylaxis before dental procedures.[11] Even periodontal probing or wax chewing can induce a transient bacteremia. If damaged or abnormal heart valves are present, bacteria can lodge on these valves and produce serious damage. For this reason, antibiotics are recommended for certain dental patients undergoing certain dental procedures.

Determining which patients should receive

prophylactic antibiotics is not always easy. Many situations are unclear. When the patient's history and the dental treatment indicate it, then the dental professional should administer prophylactic antibiotics. Past recommendations (e.g., in 1974) suggested other regimens, but only the current regimen should be used. Checking the literature for the newest regimen is the responsibility of all dental care professionals. In addition to patient protection, the dental professional must also consider the legal ramifications of withholding appropriate prophylactic antibiotics.

The recommendations of the Committee cannot possibly cover every potential clinical situation. The practitioner must exercise clinical judgment when situations exist that do not fall within these guidelines. Even with antibiotic coverage, infective endocarditis may occur. Also, patients at risk may not be identified by a health history. Clinical trials of these prophylactic measures have never been conducted. The recommendations are based on the serious deliberations and considerations of available data.

Dental procedures

Many dental procedures produce bacteremia. For these procedures, in patients at risk, prophylactic antibiotics should be administered. Table 8-14 lists some dental procedures that may produce bacteremia and therefore require prophylactic antibiotic coverage for susceptible patients. Situations when prophylaxis is not indicated are also listed. For intraoral radiographs and alginate impressions differences to consider if bacteremia may be produced may be related to the cleanliness of the mouth. Clinical judgment may suggest the need either for or against antibiotic coverage.

Medical conditions

Patients can be divided into three groups based on their medical conditions for discussing antibiotic prophylaxis before dental procedures (Table 8-15). The first group contains the patients at highest risk for developing bacterial endocarditis, in whom parenteral antibiotics are usually required. This group includes the patient with a prosthetic heart valve or a history of bacterial endocarditis. The second group poses a high risk, and oral antibiotics may be used. Many clinical conditions fall within this group including those with a history of rheumatic heart disease. The last group are those conditions that most clinicians feel do not require prophylactic antibiotic coverage, such as coronary bypass surgery after 6 months.

Patients with other medical conditions that also require antibiotic coverage before dental proce-

Table 8-15. Cardiac conditions indicating antibiotic prophylaxis

---

Endocarditis prophylaxis recommended:
Parenteral antibiotics (highest risk patients):
a. Previous episode of infective endocarditis
b. Heart valve prosthesis
c. Coarctation of aorta
d. Indwelling vascular catheter

Oral antibiotics (high-risk patients):
a. Rheumatic heart disease
b. Congenital heart disease
  (1) Ventricular septal defect
  (2) Patent ductus arteriosus
  (3) Tetralogy of Fallot
  (4) Aortic stenosis
  (5) Complex cyanotic heart disease
  (6) Systemic–pulmonary artery shunt
c. Mitral valve prolapse **with** insufficiency
d. Heart valve disease
e. Ventriculoatrial shunts for hydrocephalus
f. Tricuspid valve disease
g. Asymmetric hypertrophy
h. Vascular grafts
i. Intravenous drug addicts

Endocarditis prophylaxis not recommended:
a. Isolated secundum atrial septal defect
b. Six months or longer after surgery for:
  (1) Ligated ductus arteriosus
  (2) Vascular grafts (autogenous)
  (3) Surgically closed atrial or septal defects without Dacron patches
  (4) Coronary bypass surgery
c. Mitral valve prolapse **without** insufficiency

UMKC Clinic Handbook 1987.

High risk		Highest risk	
No PCN allergy	PCN allergy	No PCN allergy	PCN allergy
PCN,PO	ERY,PO	AMP + GM,IM	VANC,IV

PCN, penicillin; PO, orally; ERY, erythromycin; AMP, ampicillin; GM, gentamicin; IM, intramuscular; VANC, vancomycin; IV, intravenous.

dures include those with artificial joints (questionable), indwelling transvenous pacemakers, shunts for renal dialysis, or hydrocephaly. Much debate exists for some conditions—whether to premedicate or not.

Antibiotic regimens for dental procedures

Table 8-7 lists the antibiotic regimens for dental procedures. Note that there are four situations as diagrammed above. (Study Table 8-7 for further clarification.)

In unusual situations, whether antibiotics are indicated should be determined by those involved most closely with the patient's condition. For example, when a patient with a prosthetic hip replacement is seeking dental treatment the dental professional should contact the patient's orthopedic surgeon. Documentation in the chart should be complete and a follow-up letter summarizing the conversation sent and a copy retained. Antibiotics that have been suggested when the official recommendations were not appropriate include the cephalosporins and clindamycin. Tetracycline is not indicated just before dental procedures likely to produce bacteremia.

REVIEW QUESTIONS

1. Explain the rationale for the use of agents effective mainly against gram-positive organisms in the treatment of most dental infections.
2. Describe the proper use of prophylactic antibiotics in dentistry (other than for infective endocarditis).
3. Define the following terms:
   a. Spectrum
   b. Bacteriostatic
   c. Bactericidal
   d. Blood level
   e. Synergism
   f. Antagonism
   g. Resistance
4. List the three groups of penicillins and explain the differences among these groups.
5. State the most serious adverse reaction associated with the penicillins.
6. Explain the use of erythromycin in dentistry.
7. Name the major adverse reaction associated with all erythromycins, and state the one adverse reaction associated primarily with the estolate ester.
8. Explain the major adverse reaction associated with the clindamycin group of antibiotics.
9. Describe two major therapeutic uses for the clindamycin antibiotics. Explain its special interest (renewed) to dentistry.
10. Name two oral cephalosporins useful in the treatment of systemic infection.
11. State one similarity and two differences between the cephalosporins and penicillin G.
12. List three aminoglycoside antibiotics and state two major adverse reactions associated with their use.
13. State one major adverse reaction associated with the tetracyclines that is seen in the dental office.
14. Name two special instructions that a patient given tetracycline should be told.
15. Name two differences between tetracycline and doxycycline.
16. Describe metronidazole's special spectrum of interest in dentistry. Name an activity to avoid while ingesting it.
17. State the adverse reaction associated with chloramphenicol that precludes its use in dentistry.
18. Name the most common antifungal agent useful in the treatment of oral candidosis. State the three dosage forms useful in dentistry.
19. State two other agents (not no. 18 answer) useful for oral candidiasis. State one problem with each agent.
20. Describe the reason for difficulty associated with the

treatment of herpes labialis with antiviral agents. Describe its oral use.

21. State three agents commonly used together in the treatment of tuberculosis.

22. Describe the drug regimen for the prophylaxis of bacterial endocarditis in patients with a history of rheumatic heart disease, without any allergy to penicillin and with an allergy to penicillin. Separate both very high and high risk groups.

REFERENCES

1. Zallen, R.D., and Curry, J.T.: A study of antibiotic usage in compound mandibular fractures, J. Oral Surg. **33**:431, 1975.

2. Holroyd, S.V.: Antibiotics in the practice of periodontics, J. Periodontol. **42**:584, 1971.

3. Feinberg, S.M., and Feinberg, A.R.: Allergy to penicillin, J.A.M.A. **160**:778, 1956.

4. Welch, H., Lewis, C.N. and Putnam, L.E.: Acute anaphylactoid reactions attributable to penicillin, Antibiot. Chemother. **3**:891, 1953.

5. Genco, R.J.: Antibiotics in the treatment of human periodontal diseases, J. Periodontol. **52**:545, 1981.

6. Graykowski, E.A., and Kingman, A.: Double-blind trial of tetracycline in recurrent aphthous ulceration, J. Oral Path. **7**:376, 1978.

7. Swartzberg, K.E., Maresca, R.M.; and Bennington, J.S.: Gastrointestinal side effects associated with clindamycin: 1000 consecutive patients, Arch. Intern. Med. **136**:876, 1976.

8. Olsen, R.E., Morello, J.A., and Kieff, E.D.: Antibiotic treatment of oral anaerobic infections, J. Oral Surg. **33**:619, 1976.

9. Rood, J.P., and Murgatroyd, J.: Metronidazole in the prevention of dry socket, Brit. J. Oral Surg. **17**:62, 1979-1980.

10. Loesche, W.J., et al.: Treatment of periodontal infections due to anaerobic bacteria with short-term treatment with metronidazole, J. Clin. Periodontol. **8**:29, 1981.

11. Prevention of bacterial endocarditis: a statement prepared by the Committee on Prevention of Rheumatic Fever and Bacterial Endocarditis of the American Heart Association, J.A.D.A. **110**:98-100, Jan. 1985.

Chapter 9

Local anesthetics

No drugs are employed in the dental office more often than the local anesthetic agents. Because their use can become routine, it is easy to forget that these agents have a potential for systemic effects as well as the local effects desired. In some states the dental hygienist is responsible for the administration of local anesthetic agents in certain situations. With this duty comes the need for an in-depth knowledge of the local anesthetic agents.

HISTORY

The advent of "painless" dentistry through the use of local anesthetic agents is relatively recent. It began with the observation that the natives of the South American Andes chewed certain leaves that made them feel better. Their active ingredient was cocaine, isolated by Niemann in 1860. He noted that tasting this substance produced the loss not only of taste but also the sensation of pain. In 1884 Koller noted that cocaine instilled in the eye produced complete anesthesia. Its use in eye surgery was immediately adopted. During this time Sigmund Freud was also experimenting with cocaine and its effects on the central nervous system (CNS). CNS stimulation, toxicity, and the potential for abuse were quickly recognized as major problems with the widespread use of cocaine as a local anesthetic.

The search for a more acceptable local anesthetic for dentistry continued. Einhorn synthesized procaine in 1905, but it was not until many years later that its use in dentistry became common. In 1952 the amide lidocaine (Xylocaine) was released, and mepivacaine (Carbocaine) was released in 1960. Most recently, bupivacaine (Marcaine) was made

available for dental use. The search for the perfect local anesthetic agent continues.

IDEAL LOCAL ANESTHETIC

Although local anesthesia can be produced by several different agents, many are not clinically acceptable. The ideal local anesthetic should possess the following properties:

1. Potent local anesthesia
2. Reversible local anesthesia
3. Absence of local reactions
4. Absence of systemic reactions
5. Absence of allergic reactions
6. Rapid onset
7. Satisfactory duration   *& safety*
8. Adequate tissue penetration
9. Low cost
10. Stability in solution (long shelf-life)
11. Sterilization by autoclave
12. Ease of metabolism and excretion

No local anesthetic agent in use today meets all of these requirements, although many acceptable agents are available.

CHEMISTRY

The injectable local anesthetic agents are divided chemically into two major groups: the esters and the amides (Table 9-1). The clinical importance of this division is associated with allergic reactions.

The structure of the local anesthetics is composed of the following parts:

1. Aromatic nucleus (R_1)
2. Linkage (This may be either an ester or an amide, followed by an aliphatic chain, R_2.)
3. Amino group

107

Aromatic nucleus	Linkage	Amino group
	Ester	
R_1-	$\overset{O}{\overset{\|}{-C-O-R_2-}}$	$-N\overset{R_3}{\underset{R_4}{\diagdown}}$
	or	
	Amide	
R_1-	$\overset{H}{\overset{\|}{-N}}\overset{O}{\overset{\|}{-C-R_2-}}$	$-N\overset{R_3}{\underset{R_4}{\diagdown}}$

The aromatic nucleus (R_1) is lipophilic (lipid soluble), and the amino group $\left(-N\overset{R_3}{\underset{R_4}{\diagdown}}\right)$ is hydrophilic (water soluble). The esters are largely metabolized in the plasma, and the amides in the liver.

MECHANISM OF ACTION
Action on nerve fibers

A resting nerve fiber has a large number of positive ions (cations) on the outside (electropositive) and a large number of negative ions (anions) on the inside (electronegative). The nerve action potential results in the opening of the sodium channels and an inward flux of sodium resulting in a change from the -90 mV potential to $+40$ mV. The outward flow of potassium ions repolarizes the membrane and closes the sodium channels. Many theories have been postulated to explain the action of all the local anesthetics. The most popular one says that local anesthetics attach themselves to specific receptors in the nerve membrane. After combining with the receptor, the permeability of the nerve membrane to sodium ions is reduced. Because there is a close re-

Table 9-1. Chemical classification of local anesthetics

	Esters	
Of benzoic acid	**Of meta-aminobenzoic acid**	**Of para-aminobenzoic acid (PABA)**
Ethyl aminobenzoate* (Benzocaine)	Cyclomethycaine (Surfacaine)	Procaine (Novocain)
Cocaine*		Propoxycaine (in Ravocaine)
Butacaine* (Butyn)		Chloroprocaine (Nesacaine)
Hexylcaine (Cyclaine)		Proparacaine (Ophthaine)
Tetracaine (Pontocaine)		

	Amides		
Xylidine derivatives	**Toluidine derivatives**	**Other**	**Other local anesthetics**
Lidocaine (Xylocaine)	Prilocaine (Citanest)	Dibucaine (Nupercaine)	Chlorobutanol* Dyclonine*
Mepivacaine (Carbocaine)			
Bupivacaine (Marcaine)			
Etidocaine (Duranest)			

*Used only topically.

lationship between the sodium and calcium ions in the nerve membrane, an increase in sodium permeability may release bound calcium. Local anesthetics may then compete with calcium and prevent the onset of nerve conduction.

Ionization factors

Local anesthetics are weak bases that occur equilibrated between their two forms: the fat-soluble (lipophilic) free base and the water-soluble (hydrophilic) hydrochloride salt (Fig. 9-1). The proportion of drug in each form is determined by the

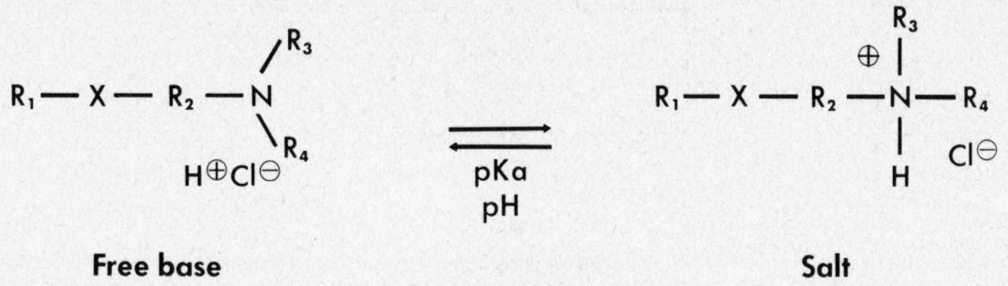

Fig. 9-1. Properties of base and salt forms of local anesthetics. X, ester or amide.

Free base	Salt
1. Viscid liquids or amorphous solids	1. Crystalline solids
2. Fat soluble (lipophilic)	2. Water soluble (hydrophilic)
3. Unstable	3. Stable
4. Alkaline	4. Acidic
5. Uncharged, nonionized	5. Charged, cation (ionized)
6. Penetrates nerve tissue	6. Active form at site of action
7. Form present in tissue (pH 7.4)	7. Form present in dental cartridge (pH 4.5-6.0)

pK_a of the local anesthetic and the pH of the environment. In the acidic environment of the dental cartridge, the proportion of the drug in the ionized form increases, thereby increasing solubility. Once injected into the tissues (pH 7.4), more local anesthetic is in the free-base form. This provides for greater tissue penetrations (Fig. 9-2). In the presence of an acid environment such as infection or inflammation, the amount of free base is reduced. This is one reason that dental anesthesia with a local anesthetic is more difficult when infection is present. Although the free base is needed to penetrate the nerve membrane, the cationic form is the form that exerts its blocking actions by binding to the specific receptor site.

PHARMACOKINETICS

1. Absorption. The absorption of a local anesthetic depends on its route. When injected into the tissues the rate of absorption depends on the vascularity of the tissues. This is a function of the degree of inflammation present, the vasodilating properties of the local anesthetic agent, the presence of heat, or the use of massage. For topical application, if the surface is denuded, absorption can approximate that produced by intravenous injection. Absorption is also determined by the proportion of the agent present in the free-base form (nonionized).

When used for dentistry, it is desirable to decrease the systemic absorption of a local anesthetic agent. This can be accomplished by adding a vasoconstrictor to reduce the blood supply to the area, thereby limiting systemic absorption and reducing systemic toxicity.

2. Distribution. After absorption, local anesthetics are distributed throughout the body. Highly vascular organs have higher concentrations of anesthetics. Local anesthetics cross the placenta and blood-brain barrier. Lipid solubility of a particular anesthetic affects the potency of the agent. For example, bupivacaine, used as a 0.5% solution, is about 10 times more lipid soluble than lidocaine, used as a 2% solution.

3. Metabolism. Local anesthetic agents are metabolized differently, depending on whether they are amides or esters. The esters are hydrolyzed by plasma pseudocholinesterase and liver esterases. Procaine is hydrolyzed to *para*-aminobenzoic acid (PABA), a metabolite that may be responsible for its allergic reactions. Some patients have an atypical form of pseudocholinesterase that does not allow them to hydrolyze these esters.

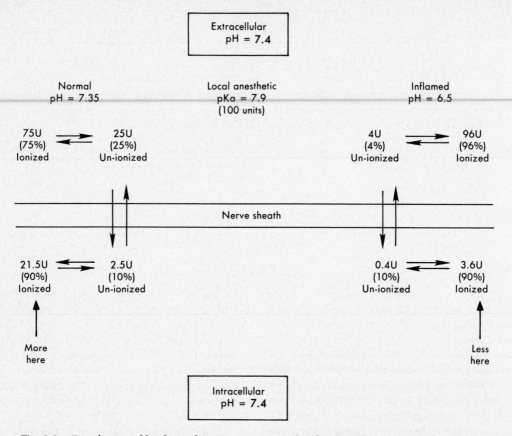

Fig. 9-2. Distribution of local anesthetic agent in normal and inflamed tissue. More local anesthetic reaches its site of action (intracellular ionized) in the normal tissue than in the inflamed tissue. (From Holroyd, S.V., Wynn, R.L., and Requa-Clark, B.: Clinical pharmacology in dental practice, ed. 4, St. Louis, 1988, The C.V. Mosby Co.)

This results in an increase in systemic toxicity if an ester is administered.

Amide local anesthetics are metabolized primarily by the liver. In severe liver disease amides may accumulate and produce systemic toxicity. A small amount of prilocaine is metabolized to orthotoluidine, which can produce methemoglobinemia if given in very large doses. By reducing hepatic blood flow, cimetidine can interfere with the metabolism of the amides.

4. Excretion. The metabolites and some of the unchanged drug of both the esters and amides are excreted by the kidneys. With end-stage renal disease, both parent drug and metabolites can accumulate.

PHARMACOLOGIC EFFECTS

1. Peripheral nerve conduction. The main clinical effect of the local anesthetics is the reversible blockage of peripheral nerve conduction. These agents inhibit the movement of the nerve impulse along the fibers, at sensory endings, at myoneural junctions, and at synapses. Therefore they may have wide-reaching effects on many kinds of

nerves. Since they do not penetrate the myelin sheath, they affect the myelinated fibers only at the nodes of Ranvier. The local anesthetics affect the small, unmyelinated fibers first and the large, heavily myelinated fibers last. This is probably related to the ability of these agents to penetrate to their site of action. The losses of nerve function are in the following order:

a. Autonomic   f. Pressure
b. Cold   g. Vibration
c. Warmth   h. Proprioception
d. Pain   i. Motor
e. Touch

Although this is generally the order in which the senses are lost, there is some individual variation in different patients. In some patients the pain sensation is lost before cold sensation. The individual nerve functions return in reverse order.

2. Cardiovascular system. Local anesthetics have a direct effect on the cardiac muscle by blocking cardiac sodium channels and by depressing abnormal cardiac pacemaker activity, excitability, and conduction. They also depress the strength of cardiac contraction and produce arteriolar dilation, leading to hypotension. They are used intravenously (IV) as antiarrhythmic agents.

ADVERSE REACTIONS

Considering the widespread use of these agents, their potential for danger must be minimal. Deaths from local anesthetics are difficult to document, but dentally related mortality is even rarer. Table 9-2 lists the maximum safe dose for common local anesthetics. Factors that influence toxicity include the following:

- Drug. Both the inherent toxicity of the particular local anesthetic and the amount of vasodilation it produces can contribute to toxicity.
- Concentration. The higher the concentration injected, the more drug that enters the systemic circulation.
- Route of administration. Inadvertent IV injection can produce extremely high blood levels. Even topical administration can produce high blood levels and lead to toxicity.

- Rate of injection. The faster the injection is made, the less chance that the local area can accept the volume injected. The operator, who has control over this variable, may find that counting the seconds is helpful.
- Vascularity. The presence of inflammation, infection, or vasodilation produced by the agent will increase the vascularity and therefore the systemic toxicity.
- Patient's weight. The same dose administered to a child and an adult, because of their differences in weight, will produce different blood levels.
- Rate of metabolism and excretion. Amides may accumulate with liver disease; both amides and esters and their metabolites may accumulate in renal disease.

Children, the elderly, and debilitated persons are more susceptible to the adverse reactions of local anesthetic agents. Symptoms of an overdose of the local anesthetic agents are directly proportional to the blood level attained. The two main systems affected by local anesthetic toxicity are the CNS and the cardiovascular system.

1. CNS effects. CNS stimulation resulting in restlessness, tremors, and convulsions can be seen. CNS depression, respiratory and cardiovascular depression, and coma follow.

2. Cardiovascular effects. The cardiovascular system can produce myocardial depression and cardiac arrest with peripheral vasodilation. The usual concentrations achieved with dental anesthesia would not be expected to result in any of these adverse reactions although deaths have been reported with the use of lower doses of anesthetic. It is postulated that the effect of these agents on heart conduction may have produced a fatal arrhythmia.

3. Local effects. Local effects can occur with the administration of local anesthetic agents. This is most commonly due to physical injury caused by the injection technique or the administration of an excessive volume too quickly to be accepted by the tissues. Occasionally a hematoma may be produced.

4. Malignant hyperthermia. Malignant hyper-

Table 9-2. Maximum safe dosage for some local anesthetic agents

Drug	mg/kg	mg	Usual concentration (%)	ml	No. of cartridges
Procaine (Novocaine)	15–20	400	2	20	11.1
Lidocaine (Xylocaine, Octocaine)	4.4–7.0*	300	2	15	8.3
Mepivacaine (Carbocaine, Isocaine)	6.6	400	2	20	11.1
Prilocaine (Citanest)	7.9	600	4	15	8.3
Propoxycaine (in Ravocaine)	6.6	30 (400†)	0.4 2.4†	7.5 17†	4.2 9.4†
Bupivacaine (Marcaine)	2	90‡ 175–225	0.5	18	10.0
Etidocaine (Duranest)	4	300–400*	0.5§	60?	33?

*Higher number with vasoconstrictor.
†Total of two agents.
‡Dental use.
§Medical use.

thermia is an inherited disease that is transmitted as an autosomal dominant gene with reduced penetrance and variable expressivity. Its symptoms include an acute rise in calcium producing uscular rigidity, metabolic acidosis, and extremely high fever. Its mortality is about 50%. Its treatment includes supportive measures and the administration of dantrolene (Dantrium). Halothane, the inhalation anesthetic, and succinylcholine, the neuromuscular blocking agent, are most commonly precipitating agents. Amides are suspected to be able to precipitate an attack also.

5. Pregnancy and nursing. Elective dental treatment should be rendered before a patient becomes pregnant. If dental treatment is needed, however, most sources suggest that both lidocaine and mepivacaine may be administered to a pregnant woman. Fetal bradycardia has been reported when larger doses are administered near-term to the mother. Both lidocaine and prilocaine are Food and Drug Administration (FDA) pregnancy category B, whereas mepivacaine and bupivacaine are category C. If a local anesthetic is needed, lidocaine, in the smallest dose that is effective, should be used. Usual doses of local an-

esthetic given to nursing mothers will not affect the health of the normal nursing infant.

6. Allergy. Allergic reactions from local anesthetics have been reported, ranging from rash to anaphylactic shock. An allergic history should be elicited from each patient before selecting a local anesthetic agent. Esters have a much greater allergic potential; in fact, there is some question whether amides can produce allergic reactions at all. Cross-allergenicity exists between the esters, but does not seem to occur between the amides in the xylidine and toluidine groups (see Table 9-1). When a patient gives a history of allergies to all local anesthetic agents they may be "tested" by giving them an amide by injection. Trained emergency personnel, equipment, and drugs must be available at all times. Use of skin testing to determine local anesthetic allergies is unreliable. Another approach is to use the antihistamine, diphenhydramine (Benadryl) as an alternative for providing some local anesthetic action.

Some past histories of allergic reactions to local anesthetics may have been due to the inclusion of a preservative, methylparaben. It is no longer present in any local anesthetic dental cartridge.

Local anesthetics with vasoconstrictors also contain a sulfite as an antioxidant. This sulfite may produce an acute asthmatic attack in sensitive patients.

COMPOSITION OF LOCAL ANESTHETIC SOLUTIONS

In addition to the local anesthetic agent, local anesthetic solutions usually contain several other ingredients such as the following:

1. A vasoconstrictor (epinephrine) to retard absorption
2. An antioxidant (sodium metabisulfite, sodium bisulfite, or acetone sodium bisulfite) to retard oxidation
3. An alkalinizing agent (sodium hydroxide) to adjust the pH to between 6 and 7
4. Sodium chloride to make the solution isotonic *No sting*
5. An antiseptic (methylparaben) is only used in multiple-dose vials. No dental cartridges contain methylparaben. *Not used any more*

INDIVIDUAL LOCAL ANESTHETICS

There are many local anesthetic agents available with similar pharmacologic and clinical effects and systemic toxicity. Commonly used local anesthetics are discussed below. Table 9-3 lists the concentrations, duration, and chemical class of some of the local anesthetic agents.

Amides

Lidocaine

Lidocaine (Xylocaine, Octocaine) is an amide derivative of xylidine. Introduced in 1948, it quickly became an anesthetic standard with which other local anesthetics are compared. It has a rapid onset, which is related to its tendency to spread well through the tissues. Lidocaine 2% with vasoconstrictor provides profound anesthesia of medium duration.

No cross-allergenicity between lidocaine and the esters or other available amides has been documented. Some patients appear to experience some sedation with lidocaine, and in toxic reactions one is likely to observe CNS depression initially rather than the CNS stimulation characteristic of other local anesthetics.

Lidocaine is used for topical, infiltration, block, spinal, epidural, and caudal anesthesia. It is also used intravenously to treat cardiac arrhythmias during surgery.

In dentistry 2% lidocaine is used for infiltration and block anesthesia with 1:50,000 or 1:100,000 epinephrine. *everyday use* It is used for topical anesthesia as a 5% ointment, a 10% spray, and a 2% viscous solution. Its onset is rapid (2 to 3 minutes). Lidocaine with epinephrine provides a 1- to 1½-hour duration of pulpal anesthesia. Soft tissue anesthesia is maintained for 3 to 4 hours. Lidocaine containing epinephrine 1:50,000 is used for hemostasis during surgical procedures. Rebound vasodilation (beta effect) can be expected after the alpha effect (vasoconstriction) has occurred.

Mepivacaine

Mepivacaine (Carbocaine, Isocaine) is an amide derivative of xylidine. Introduced in 1960, its rate of onset, duration, potency, and toxicity are similar to lidocaine. No cross-allergenicity between mepivacaine and the esters or other currently available amides has been documented.

Mepivacaine is not effective topically but is used for infiltration, block, spinal, epidural, and caudal anesthesia. The usual dosage form in dentistry is a 2% solution with 1:20,000 levonordefrin (Neo-Cobefrin) as the vasoconstrictor. Because mepivacaine produces less vasodilation than does lidocaine, it is used as a 3% solution without vasoconstrictor for short procedures. *use w/ HBP* Caution should be exercised when increased concentrations of a local anesthetic are used to eliminate the vasoconstrictor. Except in unusual cases, the benefit of a shorter duration does not warrant eliminating the vasoconstrictor, especially when the concentration of the drug is increased.

Prilocaine

← means stronger
Prilocaine (Citanest, Citanest Forte) is related chemically and pharmacologically to lidocaine and mepivacaine. Chemically lidocaine and mepiva-

Table 9-3. Commonly used dental local anesthetics

Local anesthetic	Concentration (%)	Vasoconstrictor	Concentration	Duration (hr)	Chemical class
Lidocaine (Xylocaine,	2	Epinephrine	1:50,000	3	Amide
Octocaine)	2	Epinephrine	1:100,000	3	
Mepivacaine (Carbocaine,	3			1	Amide
Isocaine)	2	Levonordefrin	1:20,000	3	
Prilocaine (Citanest,	4			1	Amide
Citanest Forte)	4	Epinephrine	1:200,000	3	
Bupivacaine (Marcaine)	0.5	Epinephrine	1:200,000	3–10	Amide
Etidocaine (Duranest)	0.5	Epinephrine	1:200,000	3–10	Amide
Propoxycaine (available only	0.4	Levonordefrin	1:20,000	2	Ester
mixed with 2% procaine)	0.4	Levoarterenol	1:30,000	2	
(Ravocaine)					

From Holroyd, S.V., Wynn, R.L., and Requa-Clark, B.: Clinical pharmacology in dental practice, ed. 4, St. Louis, 1988, The C.V. Mosby Co.

caine are xylidine derivatives, whereas prilocaine is a toluidine derivative. Prilocaine appears to be less potent and less toxic than lidocaine and has a slightly longer duration of action. It has been shown to produce satisfactory local anesthesia with low concentrations of epinephrine and without epinephrine.

Although prilocaine toxicity is 60% of that of lidocaine, several cases of methemoglobinemia have been reported after its use. Large doses of prilocaine, metabolized to orthotoluidine, induce methemoglobinemia. A very large dose (greater than the maximum safe dose) would be required to produce symptoms—cyanosis of the lips and mucous membranes and occasionally respiratory or circulatory distress. Although the small doses required in dental practice are not likely to present a problem in healthy, nonpregnant adults, prilocaine should not be administered to patients with any condition in which problems of oxygenation may be especially critical. Methemoglobinemia can be reversed by IV methylene blue.

Prilocaine is used for infiltration, block, epidural, and caudal anesthesia. It is available in dental cartridges as a 4% concentration both with and without 1:200,000 epinephrine. Its use in dentistry are for cases when a slightly longer duration of action is required or when the lowest concentration of epinephrine is desired (1:200,000).

Bupivacaine

Bupivacaine (Marcaine) is an amide-type local anesthetic related to lidocaine and mepivacaine. It is more potent but is less toxic than the other amides. The major advantage of bupivacaine is its prolonged duration of action. It is indicated in prolonged dental procedures when pulpal anesthesia of greater than 1½ hours is needed or when postoperative pain is expected (e.g., endodontics, periodontics, and oral surgery). After "feeling" begins to return, a period of reduced sensation (analgesia) may last several hours. When compared with lidocaine with epinephrine, the onset of bupivacaine with epinephrine is slightly longer, but its duration is at least twice that of lidocaine. It is available in dental cartridges as a 0.5% solution with 1:200,000 epinephrine. It should not be used in patients prone to self-mutilation (mental patients or children under 12 years old). During its use in anesthesiology and obstetrics cardiac arrests have occurred that were not resuscitable, even with adequate management. Because much lower maximal doses are recommended for dental procedures, these adverse reactions are unlikely to occur in dental

practice. Bupivacaine has been used for infiltration, block, and peridural anesthesia.

Etidocaine

Etidocaine (Duranest) is another amide-type local
anesthetic related to lidocaine and mepivacaine.
It has a rapid onset of action and a duration of
anesthesia comparable to that of bupivacaine. It is
available as a 1.5% solution with 1:200,000 epinephrine.

Esters

Procaine

Procaine (Novocain) is a PABA ester available
only in combination with propoxycaine. It has a
slow onset and a toxicity and potency of about half
that of lidocaine. It causes marked vasodilation
and thus has a relatively short duration of action
unless used with a vasoconstrictor. Rapid hydrolysis in plasma to PABA and diethylaminoetha-
nol makes it one of the safest local anesthetics
known.

Procaine is not effective topically but is used
for infiltration, block, spinal, epidural, and caudal
anesthesia. It is also used intravenously in the
treatment of cardiac arrhythmias and seizures of
status epilepticus. It is also used as an antifibril-
latory agent (procainamide) and is combined with
penicillin to form procaine penicillin G. It is the
drug of choice in the management of an arterial
spasm produced by intraarterial injection. The
principal use of procaine hydrochloride in dentistry today is as a 2% solution combined with the
more potent local anesthetic, propoxycaine.

Propoxycaine

Propoxycaine (Ravocaine), another ester of PABA,
is combined with procaine. It is slightly less potent and less toxic than tetracaine and also has a
long duration of action. Propoxycaine's rapid onset of action when injected and its lack of topical
activity are its principal clinical differences from
tetracaine. It is used for infiltration and block
anesthesia. Dental cartridges contain 0.4% propoxycaine and 2% procaine with 1:20,000 levonordefrin or 1:30,000 levarterenol.

Tetracaine

Tetracaine (Pontocaine), an ester of PABA, has a
slow onset and long duration and is generally estimated to have at least 10 times the potency and
toxicity of procaine. In view of this drug's high
toxicity and the rapidity with which it is absorbed
from mucosal surfaces, great care must be exercised if it is used for topical anesthesia. A maximal
dose of 20 mg is recommended for topical administration. Tetracaine is available in various sprays,
solutions, and ointments for topical application.
The concentration of tetracaine in most topical
preparations is 2%.

Vasoconstrictors in local anesthetics

Vasoconstrictors are included in local anesthetic
solutions to (1) prolong and increase the depth of
anesthesia by retaining the anesthetic in the area
injected, (2) reduce the toxic effect of the drug by
delaying its absorption into the general circulation, and (3) render the area of injection less hemorrhagic.

Eliminating the vasoconstrictor

Whenever a local anesthetic solution does not
contain a vasoconstrictor, the anesthetic drug will
be removed from the injection site and into systemic circulation faster than if the solution did
contain a vasoconstrictor. This will provide a
shorter duration of action and allow a more rapid
buildup of a systemic blood level of the anesthetic. Any advantage gained by eliminating the
vasoconstrictor (shorter duration and negated possible systemic effect of the vasoconstrictor) must
be weighed against the potential for adverse effects.

Concentration of the vasoconstrictor

How much vasoconstrictor is needed in a local anesthetic solution? A sufficient concentration
should be present to allow anesthesia of adequate
depth, duration, and safety. There is no justification for the use of epinephrine in a concentration
greater than 1:100,000 or even 1:200,000, except
in those cases in which 1:50,000 is necessary to
provide local hemostasis.

Vasoconstrictors in patients with cardiovascular disease

In the 1940s the literature stated that dental local anesthetics containing vasoconstrictors should not be used in patients with cardiovascular disease. This recommendation stemmed from the fear that the vasoconstrictor would elevate the blood pressure too much. It is now known that a patient can produce endogenous epinephrine far in excess of that administered in dentistry in the presence of inadequate anesthesia that sometimes occurs when vasoconstrictors are avoided. Medical consults often recommend that the use of epinephrine be avoided because physicians are used to thinking of the medical (0.5 to 1.0 mg) rather than the dental dose (0.018 mg/cartridge of 1:100,000 concentration) of epinephrine.

Patients with uncontrolled high blood pressure, hyperthyroidism, angina pectoris, or cardiac arrhythmias, as well as those who have had a myocardial infarction or cerebrovascular accident in the past 6 months, should make a later appointment for elective dental treatment. Those undergoing general anesthesia with a halogenated hydrocarbon inhalation anesthetic should be monitored for arrhythmias if epinephrine must be used for its hemostatic effect.

In conclusion, cardiovascular patients who are able to withstand elective dental treatment, excluding patients with uncontrolled arrhythmias, should receive epinephrine-containing local anesthetic agents. They should be administered in the lowest possible dose using the best technique to minimize systemic absorption including aspiration and very slow injection. Maximum cardiac doses should not be exceeded. Table 9-4 lists the maximum safe dose of epinephrine for the healthy patient (0.2 mg) and the amount for the cardiac patient (0.04 mg); the number of cartridges that each of these doses represent is included. For example, the cardiac patient may be given two cartridges of epinephrine 1:100,000 without exceeding the cardiac dose.

Drug interactions

Selected drug interactions of epinephrine are listed in Table 9-5. The most commonly mentioned interactions occur with the tricyclic antidepressants and the nonselective β-blockers. With the tricyclic antidepressants, an exaggerated increase in pressor response (increased blood pressure) may be seen and with the nonselective β-blockers, hypertension and reflex bradycardia may be exhibited. These are not absolute contraindications to the use of epinephrine, but patients taking these agents should be monitored for symptoms of these drug interactions. For example, blood pressure monitoring is especially important for these patients. Because epinephrine is not eliminated primarily by the enzyme monoamine oxidase (MAO), the MAO inhibitors (MAOI) can be given with epinephrine.

Other additives

Methylparaben. This preservative was added to dental cartridges in the past. Allergic reactions attributable to a local anesthetic agent could have been due to this agent. No dental cartridge currently contains methylparaben.

Sulfiting agents. Local anesthetic agents that contain vasoconstrictors also contain an antioxidant such as sodium bisulfite to prolong shelf life. Certain restaurant foods, such as foods in salad bars, contain sulfites to prevent browning. Deaths from hypersensitive asthmatics who ate in restaurants has been reported. Asthmatic dental patients who are given local anesthetic agents with vasoconstrictor, and also containing sulfiting agents, should be watched for symptoms of wheezing or tightness in the chest.

Electrolytes. Sodium chloride provides isotonicity to the injectable solution. Sodium hydroxide is used to alkalinize or adjust the pH of the solution.

CHOICE OF LOCAL ANESTHETIC

Each practitioner should choose a few local anesthetic solutions to use, depending on the duration of anesthesia desired. Below is a list of suggestions for anesthesia of various durations of action:

A. About 30 minutes
   1. Mepivacaine plain
   2. Prilocaine plain

learn # of cartridges used for ea drug

Table 9-4. Vasoconstrictors

Drug	Concentration	Relative pressor potency	Maximum safe dose				Approximate % of (α/β) activity
			Normal adult		Cardiac patient		
			mg	No. of cartridges	mg	No. of cartridges	
Epinephrine (Adrenalin)	1:50,000	1	0.2	5	0.04	1	50/50
	1:100,000		0.2	11	0.04	2	
	1:200,000		0.2	22	0.04	4	
Levonordefrin (Neo-Cobefrin)	1:20,000	1/5	1.0	11	0.2	2	75/25
					1.0*	11*	

*Data taken from Malamed, S.F.: Handbook of local anesthesia, ed. 2, St. Louis, 1986, The C.V. Mosby Co.

Table 9-5. Drug interactions with epinephrine

Interacting drug group	Example(s)	Outcome
Tricyclic antidepressants	Elavil, Tofranil	The use of IV epinephrine has resulted in a two- to fourfold increase in pressor response to epinephrine; some dysrhythmias reported.
β-blockers	Inderal	Administering epinephrine to patients pretreated with a β-blocker results in α-receptor predominance. This has resulted in hypertension and a reflex increase in vagal tone producing bradycardia; selective β_1-blockers may have less problems.
Antidiabetic agents	Insulin, Orinase, Diabinase	Epinephrine increases blood glucose by inhibiting glucose uptake by peripheral tissues and promoting glycogenolysis. The increase in blood sugar may require an increased dose of antidiabetic agent.
Antihypertensives	Guanethidine (Apresoline)	Reduces effects of guanethidine; increased effect of epinephrine (α-receptor); development of severe HTN (? mechanism)
Anticonvulsants	Hydantoins (Dilantin)	Effect of IV epinephrine may be decreased
Antimanics	Lithium (Lithobid)	Decreases effect of epinephrine (α-receptor); decreased pressor response
General anesthetics (halogenated hydrocarbons)	Halothane, (Fluothane)	Some general anesthetics sensitize the myocardium to the arrhythmogenic action of epinephrine.
Phenothiazines	Thorazine, Mellaril	Because phenothiazines are α-blockers, IV epinephrine given to raise blood pressure could cause even more hypotension (predominance of β-response)
Monoamine oxidase inhibitors (MAOI)	Parnate	Termination of epinephrine activity is not primarily dependent on MAOI; small enhancement of epinephrine activity may be due to "denervation supersensitivity."

B. 30 to 60 minutes
1. Lidocaine or mepivacaine with vaso-constrictor
2. Propoxycaine/procaine with vasocon-strictor
C. 60 to 90 minutes
1. Prilocaine with vasoconstrictor
2. Agents listed in *B*, above may be ef-fective
D. Longer than 90 minutes
1. Bupivacaine with vasoconstrictor
2. Etidocaine with vasoconstrictor

TOPICAL ANESTHETICS

Benzocaine, an ester, is the most commonly used topical anesthetic; lidocaine, an amide, is second.

Benzocaine

Benzocaine (Hurricaine), an ester of PABA, can-not be converted to a water-soluble form for in-jection. Because it is poorly soluble, it is poorly absorbed and lacks significant systemic toxicity. It can produce local contact dermatitis if the opera-tor does not wear gloves. It is available in dental products as well as in many over-the-counter products for teething, sunburn, hemorrhoids, or insect bites (up to 20%).

Lidocaine

Lidocaine (Xylocaine) is available as the base or hydrochloride salt. The base is poorly water sol-uble but the salt is more water soluble, can pen-etrate better, and has greater potential for sys-temic toxicity. Concentrations range from 2% to 5%. Viscous lidocaine (2%) is available for oral rinse to manage aphthous lesions or reduce gag-ging.

Cocaine

Cocaine, a naturally occurring ester of benzoic acid, is potent and extremely toxic. It is a vaso-constrictor and its CNS effects are discussed in Chapter 26. It has no dental application.

Precautions in topical anesthesia

Some local anesthetics are absorbed rapidly when applied topically to mucous membranes. To avoid toxic reactions from surface anesthesia, the dental hygienist should consider the following:
1. Know the relative **toxicity** of the drug being used.
2. Know the **concentration** of the drug being used.
3. Use the **smallest volume** and the **lowest concentration** of the **least toxic** drug that will satisfy the clinical requirements.
4. Limit the **area of application** as much as possible.

ANTIHISTAMINES AS LOCAL ANESTHETICS

Antihistamines, because of their similarity in structure to local anesthetics, have some local an-esthetic action. Diphenhydramine (Benadryl) given by injection to produce a block, may be used in a patient who is allergic to all usual local anesthetic agents. The concentration of 1% is rec-ommended plus 1:100,000 epinephrine.

DOSAGE

The amounts of local anesthetic and vasoconstric-tor contained in a certain volume of solution can be calculated from the concentration of that solu-tion. The local anesthetic percent, for example 2%, may be expressed as 2 gm/100 ml. The va-soconstrictor ratio, for example 1:100,000, may be expressed as 1 gm/100,000 ml. The dental hy-gienist should be able to determine the number of milligrams of both local anesthetic and vasocon-strictor given in a clinical situation. The maximum safe dose for both components should not be ex-ceeded.

Each dose should be recorded in the patient's chart as soon as possible after injection. The in-formation placed in the chart should include the strength of both ingredients as well as the volume of solution used. The number of milligrams of each may be recorded as an alternative. For ex-ample, if a patient were given one cartridge of lidocaine 2% with 1:100,000 epinephrine the chart would read:

lidocaine 2% with epinephrine 1:100,000–1.8 mls, or

lidocaine 36 mg with epinephrine 0.018 mg

One reason for including this information in the chart is to minimize questions that might arise later if the chart were incomplete.

REVIEW QUESTIONS

1. Name the properties of the ideal local anesthetic.
2. Differentiate between the two major chemical groups of local anesthetic agents.
3. Contrast the allergenicity and metabolism of the ester and amide local anesthetics.
4. List the systemic adverse reactions to the local anesthetics.
5. List five injectable local anesthetic agents and give their composition.
6. Explain the presence of agents other than the local anesthetic in a dental cartridge.
7. State the rationale for the inclusion of vasoconstricting agents in local anesthetic solution.
8. Give the maximum recommended dose of three common local anesthetics.
9. State the maximum safe dose of the two vasoconstrictors used in dentistry for both the normal and the cardiac patient.
10. Explain how to determine the amounts of vasoconstrictor and local anesthetic agent present in a given solution. State the reason for recording this information in the chart.
11. Name an agent that could be used as a local anesthetic if a patient is allergic to both esters and amides.

Chapter **10**

Antianxiety agents

Both the dental hygienist and the dentist recognize the value of having a relaxed patient. Often patient anxiety is sufficiently reduced by a calm, confident, and understanding attitude on the part of the dental health team. However, individual responses to dentistry vary widely, ranging from complete calmness to severe apprehension. Each patient should be provided with the most pleasant experience possible within the limits of safety. When the patient is relaxed, appointments can be more productive and both the hygienist and patient benefit.

Many patients who require dental care never go to the dental office because of fear and apprehension. A more liberal use of antianxiety agents might increase the percentage of patients requiring dental treatment to seek it.

The dental hygienist is often in a position to assess the patient's anxiety on the first visit. By questioning and observing the patient, the hygienist can make a determination concerning the need for an antianxiety agent. Thus the patient can feel comfortable and relaxed during subsequent dental appointments. The hygienist should remember that subgingival scaling and periodontal probing can produce a stress reaction in some patients.

The dental team will most commonly use orally administered drugs to provide relaxation for the anxious patient. Intravenous (IV) administration is usually avoided because it requires more training and experience than the general dentist possesses. Even though orally administered sedatives do not usually provide consistent or highly predictable results, practitioners should stay with one or two drugs, know these well, and use them repeatedly. In the long-run this practice will produce greater benefits than "jumping" from one drug to another.

The dose of a particular antianxiety agent employed for a patient will depend on the degree of that patient's anxiety and the procedure to be performed. A sedative dose of these agents is not expected to produce calmness in a patient undergoing dental treatment, but the hypnotic dose can often produce the desired degree of sedation.

This chapter deals with some of the agents that can be used to allay anxiety—the benzodiazepines primarily. Nitrous oxide, one agent that is useful in decreasing apprehension, is discussed in Chapter 11. Some drugs with antihistamine properties like hydroxyzine and promethazine are discussed in Chapter 18.

DEFINITIONS

The sedative-hypnotic agents can produce varying degrees of central nervous system (CNS) depression depending on the dose administered. A small dose will produce mild CNS depression described as sedation (reduction of activity and simple anxiety). A somewhat larger dose of the same drug will produce greater CNS depression resulting in hypnosis (sleep). Thus the same drug may be either a sedative or a hypnotic depending on the dose administered.

The name "tranquilizer" refers to two quite different groups of agents—the minor tranquilizers, whose action is very similar to that of the sedative-hypnotics, and the major tranquilizers, which possess antipsychotic activity. Table 10-1 lists some differences between the minor and major tranquilizers. Note that the major tranquilizers or antipsychotic agents are useful in the treatment of psychoses, whereas the minor tranquiliz-

120

ers are useful in the treatment of anxiety or neuroses. In larger doses the minor tranquilizers produce more sedation and finally anesthesia, whereas the major tranquilizers can cause convulsions. The adverse effects of the major tranquilizers include extrapyramidal (parkinson-like) and anticholinergic effects. The major tranquilizers are discussed in detail in Chapter 17.

This chapter discusses both the minor tranquilizers (the benzodiazepines and meprobamate) and the classic sedative-hypnotic agents (the barbiturates and chloral hydrate). The benzodiazepines are discussed first since they have become used most frequently.

BENZODIAZEPINES

There are 8 different benzodiazepines currently listed in the top 200 most commonly prescribed drugs (see Appendix). For years diazepam has been in the top 10 and now new benzodiazepines are following suit. They are used for either daytime sedation or anxiety control, as well as treatment of insomnia. They differ mainly in the onset, duration, dose, and dosage form. Some classify them as minor tranquilizers.

Chemistry

The benzodiazepines are so called because of their structure—a 1,4-benzodiazepine nucleus. Chlordiazepoxide (Librium), the first derivative, was synthesized in 1955. After its success thousands of other benzodiazepine derivatives were screened for psychopharmacologic activity. As a result of this search, diazepam (Valium) was synthesized in 1959 and marketed in 1963. It is currently one of the most frequently prescribed drugs in the United States. Many other derivatives are now available (Table 10-2).

When an additional ring was added to the original nucleus, another high-potency benzodiazepine, triazolam was synthesized. Next two imidazobenzodiazepines, midazolam and RO 15-1788, were synthesized. Interestingly, midazolam is a potent water-soluble benzodiazepine, whereas RO 15-1788 is a benzodiazepine antagonist without any pharmacologic action of its own.

Table 10-1. Some pharmacologic effects that differentiate the tranquilizers

Sedative-hypnotics ("minor" tranquilizers)	Antipsychotics ("major" tranquilizers)
Used in neuroses and anxiety	Used in psychoses (e.g., schizophrenia)
Cause sedation, ataxia, anesthesia	Patient is easily awakened
Anticonvulsant	Cause convulsions
Physical dependence and habituation	No dependence
Voluntary muscle relaxant	Cause extrapyramidal (parkinson-like) effects
Respiratory depressant	Anticholinergic

Adapted from Meyers, F.H., Jawetz, E., and Goldfien, A.: Review of medical pharmacology, ed. 6, Los Altos, Calif., 1978, Lange Medical Publications.

Pharmacokinetics

The benzodiazepines are well absorbed when administered by the oral route. They are available in tablets, capsules, and injectable forms (Table 10-2). The intramuscular route, for benzodiazepines other than midazolam, gives slow, erratic, and unpredictable results, whereas the intravenous route, for those available parenterally, produces a rapid, predictable response. Once a benzodiazepine is absorbed, the rate at which it crosses to the cerebrospinal fluid (CSF) through the blood-brain barrier is dependent on protein binding, lipid solubility, and the ionization constant of the compound. Most benzodiazepines are highly protein bound and are present in the unionized, lipid-soluble form. Therefore they cross the blood-brain barrier readily. After absorption the benzodiazepines are metabolized by dealkylation, hydroxylation, and lastly the hydroxylated metabolite is conjugated with glucuronic acid. The glucuronide is eliminated mainly in the urine. The metabolites in some cases are active and in other cases inactive. The metabolites are excreted with half-lives that range from 2 to 200 hours. The biologic half-lives do not correlate well with duration of action of the benzo-

Table 10-2. Benzodiazepines

Drug name	Usual hypnotic dose (mg)	Onset	$t_{1/2}$ (hr)
Triazolam (Halcion)	0.25–0.5	Fast	2–3
Oxazepam (Serax)	15–30	Int–Slow	5–13
Lorazepam (Ativan)	2–4	Int	10–18
Temazepam (Restoril)	15–30	Slow	8–38
Alprazolam (Xanax)	0.25–0.5	Int	12–15
Chlordiaz-epoxide (Librium)	5–20	Int	5–30 (up to 200)
Diazepam (Valium)	2–10	Very fast	20–50 (up to 200)*
Chlorazepate (Tranxene)	7.5	Fast	Up to 200*
Flurazepam (Dalmane)	5–30	Int	Up to 100
Midazolam (Versed)	(IV)	Fast	1–12

Int, Intermediate.
*$t_{1/2}$ of active metabolite.

diazepines. Repeated administration can result in drug cumulation.

In the presence of hepatic disease, the half-lives of some benzodiazepines, such as diazepam and chlordiazepoxide, are prolonged. Benzodiazepines that are already hydroxylated, such as lorazepam and oxazepam, are much less affected by hepatic disease. The process of glucuronidation, requiring glucuronyl transferase that is present in many tissues, is not as sensitive to the presence of liver disease. Kidney disease causes cumulation of the glucuronide metabolites, but these have no pharmacologic effect. However, patients with renal disease, because of proteinuria, require reduced doses of these agents.

Mechanism of action

The benzodiazepines exert their effects in the CNS. α-γminobutyric acid (GABA), a major in-

hibitory transmitter in the CNS, and the benzodiazepines produce similar clinical effects. In the mid-1970s it was found that the benzodiazepines facilitated GABAergic transmission. Therefore, the benzodiazepines probably increase the affinity of GABA for its receptor. Researchers then postulated the presence of a neurotransmitter that may increase (agonist) or decrease (inverse agonist) the GABAergic system. Recently, a peptide that has inverse agonist effects has been found in human and animal brains.

Pharmacologic effects

The pharmacologic effects of the benzodiazepines have qualitatively similar actions but vary in potency.

1. Behavioral effects. The effects of the benzodiazepines on behavior have been determined mainly through animal studies and may differ greatly from the actual effects in humans. In animals these agents are able to suppress behavior motivated by punishment, restore behavior suppressed by lack of regard, and alter behavior accompanying stress and frustration. They also have the ability to reduce aggression and hostility in animals. The clinical effects of these agents in humans are anxiety reduction at low doses and production of drowsiness at higher doses.

2. Anticonvulsant effects. The benzodiazepines, particularly diazepam, have anticonvulsant activity (i.e., they increase the seizure threshold). Diazepam has been shown to be an effective anticonvulsant for the prevention of seizures associated with local anesthesic toxicity and for the treatment of status epilepticus. The benzodiazepines prevent the spread of seizures in tissues surrounding the anatomic seizure focus (when such a focus exists) but have little effect on the discharges at the focus itself.

3. Muscle relaxation. Like all CNS depressants, the benzodiazepines can produce relaxation of skeletal muscles. Some studies show the benzodiazepines to be superior to other skeletal muscle relaxants (e.g., methocarbamol) for relief of musculoskeletal pain; other studies show it to be no better than aspirin or placebo. The benzodiaze-

pines are effective for muscle spasticity secondary to a pathologic state, such as cerebral palsy or paraplegia.

Adverse reactions

In general the benzodiazepines have a wide margin of safety. They all have similar adverse effects, but differ in their frequency. Agents with long elimination half-lives tend to cumulate and produce more side effects.

1. CNS effects. The most common side effect attributed to the benzodiazepines is CNS depression manifested as fatigue, drowsiness, muscle weakness, and ataxia. These side effects are more likely to occur in elderly persons and less likely to occur in heavy cigarette smokers. The patient may also have lightheadedness and dizziness.

Paradoxical CNS stimulation producing talkativeness, anxiety, nightmares, tremulousness, hyperactivity and increased muscle spasticity can occur. This reaction is more common in psychiatric patients and the benzodiazepines should be discontinued if this reaction occurs.

a. Amnesia. It has been documented that parenteral benzodiazepines such as diazepam and midazolam can produce amnesia. In fact, this is used to therapeutic advantage in a patient who is to have an unpleasant dental procedure rendered. Recent anecdotal reports have linked the use of triazolam orally, both with and without concurrent alcohol, to episodes of amnesia that sometimes last several hours.

2. Respiratory effects. Usual doses of benzodiazepines have no adverse effect on respiration. However, doses of diazepam administered for outpatient dental procedures have been occasionally reported to produce respiratory depression. An isolated case of apnea after IV diazepam has also been seen. These respiratory effects are more common in the elderly patient.

3. Cardiovascular effects. Therapeutic doses of the benzodiazepines have no adverse effect on circulation. The relief of anxiety may result in a fall in blood pressure and pulse rate. The pulse rate has also been reported to rise and then return to normal after a few minutes.

With parenteral use apnea, hypotension, bradycardia, and cardiac arrest has been reported. These are more frequent with rapid administration. Equipment for respiratory and cardiovascular assistance must be available if these agents are to be used parenterally (e.g., conscious sedation in the dental office).

4. Visual. The benzodiazepines are contraindicated in angle-closure glaucoma and can produce other visual changes such as diplopia, nystagmus, and blurred vision.

5. Dental. The benzodiazepines have been reported to produce xerostomia, increased salivation, swollen tongue, and bitter or metallic taste.

6. Other effects. The benzodiazepines can affect the gastrointestinal tract and genitourinary tract and produce allergic reactions.

7. Phlebitis. Given parenterally, diazepam can produce phlebitis. This is caused by the vehicle, propylene glycol, used to solubilize diazepam. The incidence is lower when the IV infusion is given in the antecubital space rather than the dorsum of the hand. Midazolam has less propensity to produce this effect.

8. Pregnancy and lactation. An increased risk of congenital malformation in infants of mothers taking benzodiazepines in the first trimester has been reported. Cleft lip and palate, microencephaly, and gastrointestinal and cardiovascular abnormalities were greater in the benzodiazepine-taking group. These agents are classified as Food and Drug Administration (FDA) pregnancy category D and some even category X (triazolam and temazepam).

Near-term administration of the benzodiazepines to the mother has resulted in floppy infant syndrome. This syndrome includes hypoactivity, hypotonia, hypothermia, apnea, and feeding problems. Since these agents are seldom absolutely needed (except for epilepsy), they should be avoided in women who are or who may be pregnant and in nursing mothers.

Abuse and tolerance

The benzodiazepines can be abused and the development of physical dependence and tolerance has been documented. Physiologic addiction can occur if large doses are taken over an extended period of time. However, their abuse and addiction potential is less than that of the other sedative-hypnotic agents.

Prolonged intake of large doses of the benzodiazepines can result in a degree of CNS tolerance. Cross-tolerance also exists between the benzodiazepines and other CNS depressants. This may explain the fact that the benzodiazepines, traditionally chlordiazepoxide, can be substituted for ethyl alcohol to relieve the symptoms of delirium tremens precipitated by acute alcohol withdrawal. One of the great advantages of the benzodiazepines over the barbiturates is their wider range of "safe" dosage. Overdose poisoning with these drugs has been rare and appears to be difficult to achieve, although apnea has been reported. In most instances excessively large doses must be ingested to produce respiratory or central vasomotor depression. The addition of alcohol can result in coma, respiratory depression, hypotension, or hypothermia.

Drug interactions

Like all other anxiety agents, benzodiazepines interact in an additive fashion with other CNS depressants, notably alcohol, barbiturates, and phenothiazines. Benzodiazepines may reduce the effectiveness of levodopa and parkinsonism has been exacerbated. Cimetidine and disulfiram may produce an increase in benzodiazepine effect, while the benzodiazepines may increase the effect of digoxin and primidone.

Uses

Medical

The benzodiazepines are useful in treating anxiety, insomnia, seizures, alcohol withdrawal, and some neuromuscular disease. They also have selected uses in anesthesia and surgery.

1. Anxiety control. Neurotic anxiety is the most common indication for the use of benzodiazepines in general medicine. Anxiety produces a physiologic response resembling fear with manifestations including restlessness, tension, tachycardia,

and dyspnea. Most well-controlled clinical trials have shown that the antianxiety effect of the benzodiazepines is better than those of placebo, barbiturates, and meprobamate. They also produce less sedation than the classic sedative-hypnotic agents.

2. Treatment of insomnia. If insomnia is a manifestation of anxiety, sleep will usually improve when a benzodiazepine is administered at bedtime as an antianxiety drug. Flurazepam, specifically indicated as a hypnotic, reduces insomnia as effectively as the barbiturate hypnotics. The benzodiazepines are preferable to the barbiturates as hypnotics because the risk of physical addiction or serious poisoning is much less. The efficacy of the benzodiazepines in the treatment of chronic insomnia has not been shown past 1 month.

3. Treatment of epilepsy (seizures). Diazepam is the drug of choice for the treatment of repetitive, intractable seizures (status epilepticus) that require intravenous therapy. It is also used for the treatment of seizures caused by local anesthetic toxicity. Orally administered diazepam is of little value, even as a maintenance anticonvulsant. Clonazepam, orally, is used as an adjunct to other anticonvulsants for some difficult to control seizure types.

4. Treatment of alcoholism. The benzodiazepines are used in the treatment of the alcohol withdrawal syndrome. Administration of an adequate amount of a benzodiazepine can prevent the emergence of the signs and symptoms of acute alcohol withdrawal, such as agitation and tremor. It has not been shown that they prevent hallucinations or delirium tremens (DTs).

5. Control of muscle spasms. Benzodiazepines are used to control the muscle spasticity that accompanies various diseases such as multiple sclerosis and cerebral palsy. They are used for the relief of pain and spasm of back strain. Studies have suggested that diazepam is more effective than other muscle relaxants such as methocarbamol, carisoprodol, and chlorzoxazone.

6. Premedication. The benzodiazepines, especially diazepam, have been used as premedicant

sedatives to be administered before general anesthesia, cardioversion, gastroscopy, sigmoidoscopy, and cystoscopy. They produce sedation and some amnesia concerning these procedures.

Dental

In dentistry the benzodiazepines, particularly diazepam, have been employed for their ability to reduce preoperative tension and anxiety,

Diazepam, lorazepam, or midazolam given intravenously provide muscle relaxation and a degree of amnesia during dental procedures. The amnesia produced is anterograde; that is, amnesia occurs to events after the injection. Although amnesia quickly follows the IV injection of diazepam and midazolam, it depends on several variables. Amnesia may be expected to persist for up to 45 minutes.

A double-blind trial of orally administered diazepam has shown the drug to be more effective than placebo in allaying apprehension in patients undergoing restorative procedures. One study also concluded that an initial treatment with the assistance of diazepam will increase the likelihood of subsequent successful treatment without it.

For preoperative dental anxiety, a benzodiazepine should be chosen that has a fast onset of action and a relatively short half-life. This requires less waiting by the patient and allows resumption of normal functions as soon as possible. The dose used should be in the range of the usual hypnotic dose. Examples for dental anxiety might include triazolam (fast onset and short half-life) and diazepam (very fast onset, but long half-life). Lorazepam or alprazolam (intermediate onset, but relatively short half-lives) could also be used.

Recent warnings have made review of the use of the parenteral benzodiazepines required in every outpatient dental office. In the first part of 1988, the manufacturers of midazolam sent out a warning letter stating that IV midazolam had been associated with respiratory depression and arrest when used for conscious sedation. They warned that use of IV midazolam required continuous monitoring of respiratory and cardiac function. Emergency drugs, equipment, and personnel were to be available. The maximum dose was also lowered from their previous recommendation. This warning, in conjunction with controls that various states and insurance companies are placing on the practicing dentist, is making the general dentist, and even the oral surgeon, reevaluate his or her use of IV benzodiazepines in outpatient dentistry.

Treatment of overdose

Rarely does the ingestion of a benzodiazepine alone result in severe symptoms. Supportive therapy should be undertaken if symptoms result. With recent ingestion, emesis may be induced. Activated charcoal and a saline cathartic may be administered. The patient's respiration and blood pressure should be monitored. Neither caffeine and sodium benzoate nor physostigmine, both previously recommended treatments, are now recommended.

AZASPIRODECANEDIONES

Buspirone (BuSpar) is currently the only member of this group of anxiolytics. It is discussed separately because of its unique structure and pharmacology. Its mechanism of action is unknown, but it is probably related to interactions with neurotransmitters in the CNS. It binds to serotonin and dopamine receptors, acting as an agonist.

The pharmacologic effects of buspirone are called "anxioselective" because of its selective anxiolytic action without hypnotic, anticonvulsant, or muscle relaxant properties. It produces less CNS depression and, in some patients, has been associated with nervousness or insomnia. It has no additive CNS depressant effects and so far does not appear to be addicting. Patients taking this agent should be provided with dental treatment taking into account that they may be more anxious than the normal patient.

BARBITURATES

The barbiturates, the original sedative-hypnotic agents, are chemically related agents with similar pharmacologic effects. They differ mainly in their onset and duration of action (Table 10-3). Since

Table 10-3. Classification, route of administration, and dosages of commonly used barbiturates

| Barbiturate | Route of administration | Oral adult dosage (mg) | | Onset* | Duration of action (hr) |
		Anticonvulsant (tid)	Hypnotic (single dose)		
Ultrashort acting					
Methohexital sodium (Brevital)	IV			Immediate	
Thiamylal sodium (Surital)	IV			Immediate	Few min
Thiopental sodium (Pentothal)	IV			Immediate	
Short acting					
Pentobarbital (Nembutal)	PO, IM, IV, rectal		100–200	30 min	3–4
Secobarbital (Seconal)	PO, IM, IV, rectal		100–200	30 min	3–4
Intermediate acting					
Amobarbital (Amytal)	PO, IM, IV, rectal		200	40–60 min	6–8
Butabarbital (Butisol)	PO		50–100	40–60 min	6–8
Long acting					
Phenobarbital (Luminal)	PO, IM, IV	15–30		2–3 hr	24
Mephobarbital (Mebaral)	PO	32–100		2–3 hr	24

IV, intravenous; PO, orally; IM, intramuscular.

these agents have been used for years, the problems with their use have been well documented. Although nonbarbiturate sedative-hypnotics have been developed in an attempt to overcome the problem of barbiturate abuse, these agents seem to possess little if any clinical advantage over the barbiturates. The benzodiazepines have almost completely replaced the barbiturates in clinical use except for the barbiturates' action as anticonvulsants and use to induce general anesthesia.

Chemistry

Most of the clinically useful barbiturates are formed by the substitution of R_1 and R_2 groups on the barbiturate nucleus. Another modification made by replacing the carbon-2 (X = oxygen) with sulfur creates agents that are used intravenously.

Barbiturate nucleus

Pharmacokinetics

The barbiturates are well absorbed orally and rectally. Because the injectable solutions are highly irritating, the intramuscular route is avoided and the drugs are used intravenously.

After entering the body, the short-acting and intermediate-acting barbiturates are rapidly and almost completely metabolized by the liver. The long-acting barbiturates are largely excreted through the kidneys as the free drug. Patients with liver damage may have an exaggerated response to the short-acting and intermediate-acting agents, and patients with renal impairment may have an accumulation of the long-acting agents. The intravenous agents are inactivated mainly by redistribution from their site of action in the CNS to the muscles and finally to adipose tissue.

Pharmacologic effects

1. CNS depression. The principal effects of the barbiturates are on the CNS. When small doses of these agents are administered, sedation results. With larger doses, the inhibitory fibers of the CNS are depressed, resulting in disinhibition and euphoria. If excitation occurs at this point, it is due to depression of the inhibitory pathways. Anxiety relief cannot be separated from the sedative effects. When a sufficient dose is administered, hypnosis can be produced. The administration of even higher doses can result in anesthesia, with respiratory and cardiovascular depression and finally arrest. This progressive CNS depression parallels that caused by the general anesthetics (see Chapter 11).

The CNS depression produced by the barbiturates is additive with other agents that produce this effect. For example, a patient who takes an alcoholic beverage or is given an opioid analgesic will show additive respiratory depression.

2. Analgesia. The barbiturates have no significant analgesic effects. Even doses that produce general anesthesia do not block the reflex response to pain. Patients in pain may become agitated and even delirious if barbiturates are administered without an analgesic agent.

3. Anticonvulsant effect. The barbiturates possess anticonvulsant action. The long-acting agents such as phenobarbital are routinely used in the treatment of epilepsy (see Chapter 16).

Adverse reactions

1. Sedative or hypnotic doses. In the usual therapeutic doses the barbiturates are relatively safe. However, one should be aware that CNS depression may be exaggerated in elderly and debilitated patients or those with liver or kidney impairment. In some patients, especially the elderly, the barbiturates can have an idiosyncratic effect causing stimulation instead of sedation. Barbiturates can cause fetal harm if administered to a pregnant woman.

2. Anesthetic doses. With higher doses of barbiturates, concentrations attained in the blood can be lethal. High concentrations are used for intubation or very short procedures. Coughing and laryngospasm have been reported with intravenous use of the barbiturates. High doses may reversibly depress liver and kidney function, reduce gastrointestinal motility, and lower body temperature.

3. Acute poisoning. When prescribing barbiturates, the practitioner must consider the possibility that acute poisoning can occur. Although a lethal dose can only be approximated, severe poisoning will follow the ingestion of 10 times the hypnotic dose, and life is seriously threatened when over 15 times the hypnotic dose is consumed. The cause of death when an overdose occurs is respiratory failure. The treatment includes conservative management and treatment of specific symptoms.

Chronic long-term use. Chronic use of the barbiturates can lead to physical and psychologic dependence. Long-term use produces a state similar to alcohol intoxication. The barbiturate addict becomes progressively depressed and is unable to function. Tolerance develops to most effects of the barbiturates but not to the lethal dose. There is cross-tolerance among the different barbiturates and between the barbiturates and the nonbarbiturate sedative-hypnotic agents. Chapter 2 discusses the abuse of barbiturates.

Contraindications

The use of barbiturates is absolutely contraindicated in patients with intermittent porphyria or a positive family history of porphyria. This is because the barbiturate can stimulate and increase the synthesis of porphyrins, which are already at an excessive level in this metabolic disease.

Drug interactions

Because the barbiturates are potent stimulators of liver microsomal enzyme production, they are involved in many drug interactions. These enzymes are responsible for the metabolism of many drugs, so that an increase in these enzymes could increase the rate of drug destruction and decrease the duration of action. For example, an epileptic patient who is currently receiving phenytoin (Dilantin) is subsequently given phenobarbital. The phenobarbital stimulates the liver microsomal enzymes to destroy the phenytoin more rapidly, which could cause convulsions. This drug interaction requires repeated doses and is not significant with a single dose. Some barbiturate drug interactions are listed in Table 10-4.

Uses

The uses of the barbiturates are determined by their duration of action (see Table 10-3).

1. The ultrashort-acting agents are used intravenously for the induction of general anesthesia. For very brief procedures they may be used alone. For more extensive procedures they are used to induce stage III surgical anesthesia (see Chapter 11).

2. The short-acting and the intermediate-acting agents have little medical use. The benzodiazepines have replaced them for insomnia and anxiety relief.

3. The long-acting barbiturates are used for the treatment of epilepsy.

Table 10-4. Barbiturate drug interactions

Barbiturate reduces these drugs' effects	Barbiturate's effect enhanced by these drugs
Acetaminophen	Disulfiram
Warfarin	Monoamine oxidase
Tricyclic antidepressants	inhibitors (MAOI)
(TCAs)	Propoxyphene
β-blocker	
Birth control pills (BCP)	**Enhanced or additive**
Steroids	**CNS depressant**
Digitoxin	Alcohol
Estrogens	CNS depressants
Griseofulvin	Opioid analgesics
Chlorpromazine	
Phenytoin	
Quinidine	
Doxycycline	

NONBARBITURATE SEDATIVE-HYPNOTICS

During the last half of the nineteenth century the bromides and chloral hydrate began to replace opium, alcohol, and belladonna as drugs for the production of sedation. The barbiturates were introduced in 1904 and, until the benzodiazepines, remained the principal sedative-hypnotic drugs used in dental and medical practice.

The nonbarbiturate sedative hypnotic drugs offer no advantage over the barbiturates. Preoperative sedation in dental practice can usually be adequately obtained with a properly selected dose of a benzodiazepine. Only because of tradition does the use of chloral hydrate for children persist in dentistry.

Chloral hydrate

Chloral hydrate ($CCl_3CH[OH]_2$) is an inexpensive, orally effective sedative-hypnotic drug with a rapid onset (20 to 30 minutes) and fairly short duration of action (about 4 hours). Therapeutic doses do not produce pronounced respiratory or cardiovascular depression. An exaggerated effect occurs in patients with advanced liver or kidney disease. Large doses or long-term use may produce peripheral vasodilation and hypotension with some degree of myocardial depression. Gastric irritation can be minimized by taking chloral hydrate in diluted solutions with milk or food. The highly irritating effect of this drug on mucosa is illustrated by a report of laryngospasm in a child that was believed to be caused by the aspiration of chloral hydrate.[1] The disagreeable odor and taste of chloral hydrate can be partially masked in a flavored syrup. As with all the sedative-hypnotic agents, psychologic or physical dependence may follow the prolonged use of this drug.

Chloral hydrate has been used successfully in dentistry for the preoperative sedation of children. The child's hypnotic dose of chloral hydrate, when used alone, is 50 mg/kg, up to a maximum of 1 gm.

Meprobamate

Meprobamate (Equanil, Miltown) was developed to enhance the central muscle-relaxing action of mephenesin. Its assumed potential to relieve anxiety furthered its rapid acceptance, but abuse of this agent quickly followed.

Although meprobamate's action is difficult to differentiate from that of the barbiturates, it is classed by some as a minor tranquilizer. It has sedative properties and anticonvulsant action. With increasing dosage, the relief of anxiety is accompanied by a longer reaction time and a definite slowing of learning. Meprobamate has some muscle-relaxing properties.

In the usual therapeutic doses meprobamate has few side effects. With an acute overdose, meprobamate produces excessive CNS depression manifested as unconsciousness, cardiovascular collapse, respiratory depression, and death. As with the barbiturates, the treatment of an overdose is supportive and symptomatic.

Chronic long-term administration of meprobamate can lead to CNS tolerance, compulsive use, and physical dependence. When the drug is abruptly stopped, the withdrawal syndrome can occur.

The use of meprobamate with other CNS depressants will produce an additive effect. With chronic use, cross-tolerance develops between meprobamate and other sedative-hypnotics, including alcohol.

Minor tranquilizers such as meprobamate have been associated with an increased risk of congenital malformations during the first trimester of pregnancy. Their use in pregnant women should be avoided. Meprobamate crosses the placenta and is present in the fetal circulation as well as in breast milk.

Meprobamate is occasionally used for the treatment of anxiety and as a daytime sedative or nighttime hypnotic. It is used in combination products (Equagesic [meprobamate plus aspirin]) and has been employed in dentistry as an antianxiety agent and muscle relaxant. No current clinical trials are available.

Ethchlorvynol, glutethimide, and methyprylon

Ethchlorvynol (Placidyl), glutethimide (Doriden), and methyprylon (Noludar) are nonbarbiturate sedative-hypnotics that have no advantage over the barbiturates. Since development of the benzodiazepines, these agents have no clinical use.

CENTRALLY ACTING MUSCLE RELAXANTS

Drugs classified as centrally acting muscle relaxants exert their effects on the CNS to cause skeletal muscle relaxation.

Pharmacologic effects

Some degree of sedative effect is exhibited by all the CNS muscle relaxants. In some clinical tests the sedative effects have been shown to predominate over the selective muscle relaxant activity. When administered intravenously in humans, these agents have been shown to be useful in treating muscle spasm and producing muscle relaxation for certain orthopedic procedures. When these agents are given orally, they do not produce the flaccidity obtainable with intravenous administration. Thus, until better studies are produced, the beneficial effects of these drugs can be logically ascribed to their sedative action.

Individual CNS muscle relaxants

Carisoprodol (Soma), chlorzoxazone (Para-flex), methocarbamol (Robaxin), orphenadrine (Norflex), and cyclobenzaprine (Flexeril). These five agents probably exert their muscle relaxing properties indirectly by producing CNS depression. They act in the CNS and have no direct effect on striated muscle, the motor endplate, or nerve fibers. They do not directly relax tense skeletal muscles. They are all indicated as an adjunct to rest and physical therapy for relief of muscle spasm associated with acute painful musculoskeletal conditions. Questions about their efficacy still linger in the literature. Carisoprodol, is a relative of meprobamate, while cyclobenzaprine is structurally related to the tricyclic antidepressants. They all produce sedation as a side effect (cyclobenzaprine, 40%). Carisoprodol produces allergic or idiosyncratic reactions occasionally. Postural hypotension and gastric upset are also side effects. Chlorzoxazone produces gastric disturbances and may discolor the urine purple-red. Both cyclobenzaprine and orphenadrine pro-

Educate Pt

duce dry mouth and dizziness. Diazepam, a benzodiazepine, also possesses muscle relaxant properties as discussed previously. The four agents mentioned first have been classified as "possibly effective," and cyclobenzaprine has yet to be evaluated by the National Academy of Sciences–National Research Council.[2] These drugs are used in the treatment of TMJ with varying and poorly documented success.

Baclofen (Lioresal). Baclofen inhibits both monosynaptic and polysynaptic reflexes at the spinal level. It also inhibits GABA, but whether this is related to its action is unknown. It is indicated for spasticity from multiple sclerosis or spinal cord injuries or diseases. Although not an FDA-approved indication for it, baclofen has been used to treat trigeminal neuralgia. Drowsiness, weakness, headache, and insomnia have been reported. Nausea, dry mouth, taste disorder, and urinary frequency have been seen. Lowering of the seizure threshold and an increase in ovarian cysts in rats have also occurred.

Dantrolene (Dantrium). Dantrolene affects the contractile response of the skeletal muscle directly on the muscle itself. It dissociates the excitation-contraction coupling, probably by interfering with the release of calcium from the sarcoplasmic reticulum. It is indicated in the treatment of spasticity from upper motor neuron disorders such as spinal cord injury, cerebral palsy, or multiple sclerosis. It is also used orally to prevent, and intravenously to treat malignant hyperthermia brought on by inhalation general anesthetics. The hepatotoxicity it produces is more common with higher doses, and in older female patients taking concomitant medications. This agent may cause drowsiness or photosensitivity.

SEDATIVE-ANALGESIC COMBINATIONS

The use of a combination product to provide concomitant sedation and analgesia is rational for the following reasons:

1. Relief of both anxiety and pain is frequently required in one patient.
2. Sedatives potentiate analgesic agents.
3. Sedatives may induce excitation when given

without an analgesic to patients with uncontrolled pain.

Both sedation and analgesia can be obtained from the opioid analgesics alone. However, it is not desirable to prescribe an opioid to add sedation to analgesia unless the analgesic potency is required. When analgesia can be adequately obtained with a nonopioid analgesic, these drugs and a sedative can be prescribed separately. Some fixed-dosage combinations of analgesics with sedative-hypnotic agents such as Fiorinal (contains butalbital) are used in dentistry. When more complete pain relief is required with sedation, a narcotic analgesic agent can be used with a sedative.

SPECIAL CONSIDERATIONS

Certain generalizations should be kept in mind when discussing the use of the antianxiety agents. The dental hygienist plays an important role in making the patient understand the possible effects of the drugs used to allay anxiety. The patient often feels more comfortable talking with the hygienist and commonly raises questions about these agents.

Drugs are no substitute for patient management. The practitioner should not rely exclusively on drugs to provide a calm and cooperative patient. The dental team's confident but relaxed manner and a pleasant, soothing office atmosphere are of great importance in relaxing an anxious patient. Drugs should not be substituted for patient education or for the proper psychologic approach to patient care.

When an agent for anxiety relief is required, the selection of the specific drug should be based on a knowledge of the advantages and disadvantages of the agents available and an understanding of the needs and contraindications related to the case at hand.

CAUTIONS

Regardless of the antianxiety agent selected, the following precautions pertain:

1. Patients with impaired elimination may experience exaggerated effects of medication. These

persons include the young, the elderly, the debilitated, and those with liver or kidney disease.

2. Depression caused by all sedative-hypnotics will add to depression caused by other depressants that the patient may be taking. The patient should be made aware of this, particularly in regard to alcohol; over-the-counter (OTC) sleep aids may also be a potential source of hazard.

3. The patient should understand that the drug prescribed may make it unsafe to perform acts requiring full alertness and muscle coordination, such as driving a car. The patient should be accompanied by a responsible adult who can drive them home. The patient should be warned against signing any important papers or documents. These cautions are particularly important if the patient has not taken the drug previously and his or her response to it is consequently less predictable.

4. Psychic and physical dependence has been observed with almost all drugs used to allay anxiety. The dentist should realize that these drugs have abuse potential and should limit their use accordingly. This is particularly important in regard to the treatment of chronic conditions or persons with a history of addiction.

5. Suicide is commonly attempted by taking sedative-hypnotic drugs. Consequently, the amount of drug prescribed should be limited to the minimum required to accomplish the therapeutic objective.

6. These drugs should never be administered to pregnant women or those who may be pregnant unless the potential benefit to the mother outweighs the risk to the fetus. Rarely, if ever, is this the case. Epilepsy is often an exception.

7. Sedatives do **not** provide analgesia. In fact, the use of a sedative without adequate pain control may cause the patient to become highly excited and act irrationally. However, sedatives may potentiate the effect of an analgesic taken concomitantly.

REVIEW QUESTIONS

1. Define the following terms:
   a. Sedative
   b. Hypnotic
   c. Minor tranquilizer
   d. Major tranquilizer
2. State four differences between the major and minor tranquilizers.
3. Name two major pharmacologic effects of the barbiturates.
4. List the four groups of barbiturates and state what differentiates these groups from one another.
5. Describe the major adverse reactions of the barbiturates.
6. Name the one absolute contraindication to the use of the barbiturates.
7. Describe the mechanism of the most important drug interaction of the barbiturates. Explain its clinical implication with an example.
8. Explain the important differences between the barbiturates and the nonbarbiturate sedative-hypnotic agents.
9. Name four benzodiazepines, two that are shorter acting and two that are longer acting.
10. State the major differences between the benzodiazepines and the barbiturates.
11. Explain why the sedative-hypnotic agents are controlled substances and how their abuse determines on what Schedule (II, III, or IV) they are listed.
12. Describe the adverse effect that can occur with intravenous administration of diazepam but not with oral administration.
13. Describe the parenteral use of diazepam and midazolam in dentistry. State a benefit over oral use.
14. State three uses of the benzodiazepines.
15. Review the following terms:
    a. Tolerance
    b. Withdrawal

REFERENCES

1. Granoff, D.M., McDaniel, D.B. and Borkowf, S.P.: Cardiorespiratory arrest following aspiration of chloral hydrate, Am. J. Dis. Child. **122**:170, 1971.
2. National Academy of Sciences–National Research Council: Drug efficacy study, Washington, D.C., 1969.

Chapter 11

General anesthetics

General anesthesia is produced by a heterogeneous group of potent central nervous system (CNS) depressants. They produce a reversible loss of consciousness and insensibility to painful stimuli. Contemporary general anesthetic techniques employ a balanced combination of drugs to minimize adverse reactions, taking into account the patient's physical status as well as preanesthetic and postanesthetic needs. Respiratory depression and loss of protective reflexes are associated with general anesthesia; thus the patient must be constantly monitored and evaluated. Because of the variety of anesthetic agents and techniques employed, special training and a complete working knowledge of the pharmacology of each anesthetic is essential.

The hospital operating room provides the optimum setting for general anesthetic procedures because of the ready availability of monitors for vital signs, resuscitative equipment, and trained anesthesia personnel. However, oral and maxillofacial surgeons have used general anesthetic drugs in their offices for many years with an excellent safety record. Nitrous oxide, although not useful alone as a general anesthetic, is commonly employed in the dental office setting to allay patient anxiety. Other general anesthetic drugs, in less than anesthetic doses, are now used in dental office conscious-sedation techniques. In today's practice the dental health team should have a knowledge of general anesthesia because it is an indispensable tool for the total needs of special patients, as well as for extensive oral and maxillofacial surgery.

HISTORY

Dentists have played a significant role in the development of general anesthesia. Horace Wells recognized nitrous oxide's potential use in dentistry. In 1884, he attended a demonstration of nitrous oxide's effects. During the program Wells noted that one of the participants who had inhaled nitrous oxide did not notice the pain when he gashed his leg. The next day Wells had one of his own teeth extracted without pain after administration of nitrous oxide. He then began using nitrous oxide in his own dental practice. He finally persuaded William T. G. Morton, a former dental partner studying medicine at Harvard University, to arrange a demonstration of nitrous oxide before the medical faculty. During the demonstration the patient awoke too soon and began screaming. Nitrous oxide's low potency accounted for its failure. After much unjust criticism, Wells became insane and committed suicide.

In the following months Morton demonstrated the use of ether as an effective general anesthetic before the same Harvard University group. Morton attempted to patent ether and spend the remainder of his life futilely trying to collect claims for compensation from the U.S. government. Even though the accomplishments of neither of these dentists were recognized during their lifetimes, the medical and dental professions today applaud their contribution to the alleviation of pain.

METHODS OF ADMINISTRATION

The method employed for administering a general anesthetic agent is determined by the choice of agent.

1. Open drop. Volatile liquids such as ether and chloroform can be administered by simply dripping the agent onto a gauze-covered wire mask placed over the patient's face. This is a seldom-used method that may be observed primarily

in animal anesthesia or under dire circumstances.

2. Inhalation. In this method anesthetic vapors of gases are blown into the respiratory tract. An anesthetic machine is required to meter the gas flow and vaporize the volatile agents. This technique is useful when a mask cannot be used, as in dental procedures.

3. Nonrebreathing. This method involves the administration of fresh anesthetic agent and oxygen to the patient with each breath. The exhalation is channeled into the atmosphere.

4. Partial and total rebreathing. The demand for patient safety, explosive-free operating rooms, and a more suitable means of controlling volume flow of gases to the patient resulted in the development of sophisticated machines that allow some rebreathing or full rebreathing of anesthetic gases. The excess carbon dioxide is removed by the absorber system. Explosive gases require this closed type of system.

5. Intravenous route. The intravenous route is commonly employed for the rapid induction of unconsciousness by the sedative-anxiolytic drugs such as the ultrashort-acting barbiturates. This is also the most common route of administration for general anesthetic drugs in the dental office. Muscle relaxants and other adjunctive drugs necessary during anesthesia are also given by this route.

MECHANISM OF ACTION

Many theories have been proposed to explain the mechanism of action of the various general anesthetic agents, but, unfortunately, none of them does so completely. It may seem relatively simple to say that these drugs are CNS depressants. However, the way in which they depress the normal functions of the CNS is a matter complicated by lack of knowledge of the physiologic and biochemical events of arousal and unconsciousness.

Stages and planes of anesthesia

The degree of CNS depression produced by general anesthetics must be carefully adjusted to avoid excessive cardiorespiratory depression. In 1920, Guedel described a system of stages and planes to quantitate the effects of anesthetics (Fig. 11-1). While Guedel's classification applied to the effects produced by ether using the open drop method of administration, modern anesthetic techniques seldom show these exact stages. However, the four stages are briefly described because Guedel's terminology is still used to describe the depth of anesthesia.

1. Stage I—analgesia. This stage is characterized by the development of analgesia or reduced sensation to pain. The patient is conscious and can still respond to command. Reflexes are present, and respiration remains regular. Some amnesia may also be evident. The end of this stage is marked by the loss of consciousness.

2. Stage II—delirium or excitement. This stage begins with unconsciousness and is associated with involuntary movement and excitement. Respiration becomes irregular, and there is increased muscle tone. As the depth of anesthesia increases, the patient begins to relax and progresses to the next stage. This can be an uncomfortable time for the patient because emesis and incontinence can occur. Sympathetic stimulation produces tachycardia, mydriasis, and hypertension.

Induction is progressing through stages I and II. For the patient's comfort and safety it is important to have a smooth and rapid induction. The ultrashort-acting barbiturates accomplish this readily. When balanced anesthesia is used, the patient rapidly passes through stages I and II into stage III or surgical anesthesia without signs of stage II.

3. Stage III—surgical anesthesia. This is the stage in which most major surgery is performed. Its onset is typically characterized by the return of regular respiratory movements, muscle relaxation, and normal heart and pulse rates. Conjunctival and eyelid reflexes disappear. This stage is further divided into four planes that are differentiated on the basis of eye movements, depth of respiration, and muscle relaxation. Plane 3 is associated with decreased skeletal muscle tone, dilated pupils, tachycardia, and hypotension. The progression to plane 4 is characterized by inter-

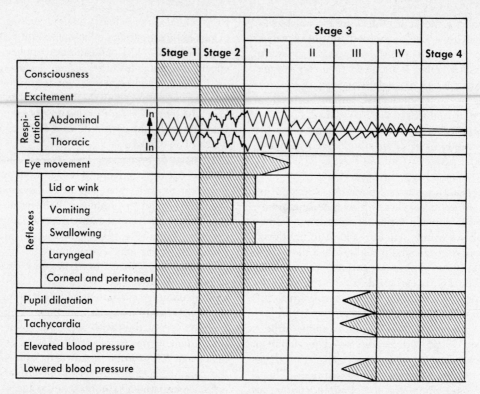

Fig. 11-1. Stages and planes of anesthesia. *In,* inspiration. (Reproduced, with permission, from Meyers, F.H., Jawetz, E., and Goldfien, A.: Review of medical pharmacology, ed. 7. Copyright 1980 by Lange Medical Publications, Los Altos, California.)

costal muscle paralysis (diaphragmatic breathing remains), absence of all reflexes, and extreme muscle flaccidity. If the depth of anesthesia is allowed to increase, the patient will rapidly progress to the last stage with cessation of all respiration.

4. Stage IV—respiratory or medullary paralysis. Stage IV is characterized by complete cessation of all respiration and subsequent circulatory failure. At this point pupils are maximally dilated, and blood pressure falls rapidly. If this stage is not reversed immediately, death of the patient will occur.

Modern anesthetic techniques now employ more rapidly acting agents than those associated with the four stages of Guedel. A more recent ap-

proach used to describe the level of anesthesia is suggested by Flagg:

1. Induction. This phase encompasses all the preparation and medication necessary for a patient up to the time the operation begins, including preoperative medications, adjunctive drugs to anesthesia, and anesthetics required for induction.

2. Maintenance. This phase begins with the patient at a depth of anesthesia sufficient to allow surgical manipulation and continues until completion of the procedure.

3. Recovery. This phase begins with the termination of the surgical procedure and continues through the postoperative period until the patient is fully responsive to the environment.

ADVERSE REACTIONS

The goals of surgical anesthesia are good patient control, adequate muscle relaxation, and pain relief. It should be remembered that to produce anesthesia, potent CNS depressants are given in relatively high doses, and many combinations of drugs are employed in balanced anesthesia.

The hazards encountered with the administration of general anesthetics include the following:

1. Cardiovascular system
   a. Cardiovascular collapse and cardiac arrest can occur if the concentration of the anesthetic is too high.
   b. Arrhythmias, including ventricular fibrillation, are a risk with any anesthesia. The halogenated hydrocarbons are prone to cause these effects, especially in the presence of catecholamines such as epinephrine.
   c. Hypertension or hypotension can result from different stages of anesthesia (Fig. 11-1).
2. Respiratory system
   a. If the stage of anesthesia is deep enough, respiration will be depressed (stage III) or will cease (stage IV).
   b. The ultrashort-acting barbiturates can cause laryngospasm, which can occlude the airway. Intubation and neuromuscular blocking agents may be required to manage this problem.
   c. A "boardlike" chest can occur under the influence of the neuroleptanalgesia produced by fentanyl and droperidol (Innovar).
3. The potential for explosions and flammability with cyclopropane and ether has been reduced by the introduction of halogenated hydrocarbons.
4. Teratogenicity. The potential for teratogenicity has been a more recent concern associated with anesthetic agents. Because of their constant exposure, dental personnel are more likely than patients to be affected. Current data suggest that waste anesthetic gases found to contaminate surgical suites are a potential health hazard. In a survey of operating room personnel an increase in spontaneous abortions was noted in the wives of exposed male dentists.
5. Liver disease. A significant increase in liver disease has been discovered in operating room personnel exposed to anesthetic gases. Also, several of the general anesthetic agents are known to be hepatoxic, especially with repeated or prolonged exposure.
6. Other complaints in this survey included headache, fatigue, and irritability. Current knowledge dictates that dental offices using inhalation anesthetics should adopt methods to minimize exposure to the operator including scavenging systems, adequate ventilation, good technique, and safe equipment.

CLASSIFICATION OF ANESTHETIC AGENTS

The general anesthetic agents are usually categorized in the following classes according to their route of administration (Table 11-1):

1. Inhalation agents. These agents can be divided into gases and volatile liquids. The liquids are vaporized and carried to the patient in the form of gas. The inhalation agents are often used in combination with one another using oxygen as a carrier gas.
2. Intravenous agents. Although most injectable general anesthetics are administered intravenously, one agent, ketamine, can be given intramuscularly too. The IV agents are used for anesthesia induction, in balanced anesthesia techniques, for conscious sedation, or occasionally as the only anesthetic agent.

Inhalation anesthetics
Physical factors

The depth of anesthesia produced is a function of the tension (partial pressure) of the anesthetic agent in the brain. The most important physical factors that influence brain anesthetic tension are the tension of the anesthetics in the inspired gases, the rate and volume of delivery of anesthetics to the lungs, and anesthetic solubility in body tissues. Induction can be hastened with high initial anesthetic concentrations and hyperventilation. As anesthesia depth develops, both the concentration and rate of delivery are reduced to maintenance levels. The less soluble the anes-

Table 11-1. Classification of general anesthetics by route of administration

Inhalation agents		Intravenous agents
Gases	**Volatile liquids**	
Nitrous oxide	Halogenated hydrocarbons	Barbiturates
	Chloroform*	Methohexital sodium (Brevital)
Cyclopropane*	Trichloroethylene*	Thiamylal sodium (Surital)
	Halothane (Fluothane)	Thiopental sodium (Pentothal)
		Dissociative
	Halogenated ethers	Ketamine (Ketalar, Ketaject)
	Methoxyflurane (Penthrane)	Opioids
	Enflurane (Ethrane)	Morphine
	Isoflurane (Forane)	Fentanyl (Sublimaze)
		Sufentanil (Sufenta)
		Alfentanil (Alfenta)
	Ethers	Neuroleptic
	Diethyl ether (ether)*	Fentanyl with droperidol (Innovar)
		Benzodiazepines
		Diazepam (Valium)
		Midazolam (Versed)
		Others
		Etomidate (Amidate)

From Holroyd, S.V., Wynn, R.L., and Requa-Clark, B.: Clinical pharmacology in dental practice, ed. 4, St. Louis, 1988, The C.V. Mosby Co.
*Historical interest only.

[Handwritten margin notes: N₂O Delivery — O₂ 100% 2-3 min then N₂O 5-10% Range 10-50% N₂O onset 3-5 min, terminate w/ 100% 3-5 min.]

thetic is in body tissues, the more rapid the onset and recovery. The low solubility of nitrous oxide correlates well with its rapid onset and recovery. These physical factors allow the anesthesiologist to quickly adjust the desired level of anesthesia.

The term minimum alveolar concentration (MAC) is used to compare the potency of general anesthetic inhalation agents. MAC is defined as the minimal alveolar concentration of an anesthetic, at 1 atmosphere, required to prevent 50% of the patients from responding to a supramaximal surgical stimulus. The MAC of nitrous oxide is greater than 100, whereas halothane has an MAC of 0.77, isoflurane 1.15, and enflurane 1.68. The lower MAC values indicate the more potent anesthetics. The volatile anesthetics are given in combination with nitrous oxide to reduce the concentration of each while improving MAC values.

Gases (nitrous oxide)

Nitrous oxide, N_2O, is a colorless gas with little to no odor and is the least soluble in blood of all the inhalation anesthetics. Because of its low potency (MAC greater than 100), nitrous oxide is unsatisfactory as a general anesthetic agent when used alone. However, if anesthesia is first induced with a rapidly acting intravenous agent and nitrous oxide–oxygen (N_2O-O_2) administered in combination with a volatile anesthetic, excellent balanced anesthesia is produced. This synergistic combination permits the use of reduced doses of the more potent inhalation anesthetics.

Nitrous oxide has become a primary part of dental office conscious-sedation procedures. This use should not be confused with general anesthesia, because the intent is to provide for a lightly sedated and relaxed patient. When nitrous oxide is properly administered, the patient remains conscious with the protective reflexes intact. Nitrous oxide provides anxiety relief coupled with analgesia. Thus, the N_2O-O_2 sedation technique may be adopted to offer increased patient cooperation and comfort in a wide range of dental office procedures. The dental hygienist should be thoroughly familiar with this use of nitrous oxide. In fact, in some states the hygienist may legally administer nitrous oxide.

The N_2O-O_2 sedation technique involves varying the concentration of nitrous oxide to titrate the patient to a desired level of sedation. The gas mixture is delivered to the patient by flowmeters that control both the volume flow and the ratio of nitrous oxide and oxygen. Starting with 100% oxygen for 2 to 3 minutes, nitrous oxide is gradually added in 5% to 10% increments until the patient response indicates a desired level of sedation. Once the nitrous oxide is added, onset occurs rapidly within 3 to 5 minutes. Table 11-2 shows the typical responses observed with increasing concentrations of nitrous oxide. The percent of nitrous oxide required for patient comfort is variable and may range from 10% to 50%. At the termination of an N_2O-O_2 sedation procedure, the patient should be placed on 100% oxygen for at least 5 minutes. Recovery occurs rapidly as nitrous oxide is quickly removed from the tissues. If the mask is removed without the oxygen recovery period and the patient allowed to breathe room air, a phenomenon known as diffusion hypoxia might result. This occurs because of the rapid outward flow of nitrous oxide accompanied by oxygen and carbon dioxide. The loss of carbon dioxide, a stimulant to respiratory drive, could decrease ventilation with resultant hypoxia. Patients may complain of headache or other side effects if this occurs. Recovery with 100% oxygen avoids this problem.

Advantages. As has been implied, the N_2O-O_2 technique has sufficient advantages to recommend its consideration in many dental procedures. Among its advantages are the following:

1. Rapid onset. Owing to the poor solubility of nitrous oxide in blood, it has a rapid onset of action (less than 5 minutes).

know

Table 11-2. Signs and symptoms in response to nitrous oxide and oxygen conscious-sedation

Concentration N$_2$O	Response
10% to 20%	Body warmth
	Tingling of hands and feet
20% to 30%	Circumoral numbness
	Numbness of thighs
20% to 40%	Numbness of tongue
	Numbness of hands and feet
	Droning sounds present
	Hearing distinct but distant
	Dissociation begins and reaches peak
	Mild sleepiness
	Analgesia (maximum at 30%)
	Euphoria
	Feeling of heaviness or lightness of body
30% to 50%	Sweating
	Nausea
	Amnesia
	Increase sleepiness
40% to 60%	Dreaming, laughing, giddiness
	Further increased sleepiness, tending toward unconsciousness
	Increased nausea and vomiting
50% and over	Unconsciousness and light general anesthesia

From Bennett, C.R.: Conscious-sedation in dental practice, St. Louis, 1974, The C.V. Mosby Co.

2. Easy administration. No injection is required to obtain an effect. The patient merely breathes through his or her nose.

3. Close control. The proper depth of sedation can be maintained by adjusting the percentage of nitrous oxide administered.

4. Rapid recovery. Recovery is rapidly effected with full return to presedative psychomotor capacity. Thus the need for the patient to be accompanied to the dental appointment can often be eliminated. a couple of minutes

5. Acceptability for children. Nitrous oxide is a valuable adjunct in managing some apprehensive children. However, it cannot be used when a child's behavior is openly defiant or hysterical,

and it is not a substitute for good behavioral management technique.

6. Relaxed dental team. The N_2O-O_2 technique will not only offer comfort to the patient and increase the acceptance of dental procedures but will also afford more relaxed treatment; that is, the dental team should be less tense and fatigued at the end of the office day.

Safety. Invariably, the complications that have occurred with the use of N_2O-O_2 techniques have been the result of misuse or faulty installation of equipment. Obviously, an installation that crossed oxygen and nitrous oxide lines could be disastrous if nitrous oxide were given under the assumption that it was oxygen!

All cylinders are now colored in a standard manner. Nitrous oxide cylinders are blue, and oxygen cylinders are green. The cylinders are also "pin coded" to prevent inadvertent mixing of cylinders and lines.

Equipment with built-in safety features is now available. Features that every dental office's inhalation administration equipment should have include a limit to the percentage of nitrous oxide that can be administered and a "fail-safe" system that shuts down the nitrous oxide if the oxygen runs out.

The combination of nitrous oxide with other sedative regimens can increase the potential danger of causing a general anesthetic state. The limits of this sedation technique must be understood by every member of the dental health team. If inhalation sedation is combined with other modes of sedation, the entire dental staff must be trained and prepared for the eventuality that general anesthesia might be produced.

Contraindications

1. Respiratory obstruction. Since the nasal passages are used for gaseous exchange, upper respiratory obstruction or a stuffy nose is an absolute contraindication to this technique. Other respiratory diseases must also be carefully evaluated.

2. Chronic obstructive pulmonary disease (COPD). The use of an N_2O-O_2 combination in the patient with emphysema (COPD) is contraindicated. Respiration in these patients is driven by

the lack of oxygen rather than an elevated carbon dioxide level. Thus these patients could cease to breathe if more than the room-air percentage of oxygen is administered.

3. Emotional instability. Since patients experience euphoria or an altered sensorium with nitrous oxide analgesia, a patient's emotional instability is a relative contraindication to its use. Patients taking psychotherapeutic medication must be carefully evaluated before nitrous oxide is used. These medications include phenothiazines, tricyclic antidepressants, and lithium. Since fanciful dreams occurring during a procedure may be interpreted on recovery as having actually occurred, a female staff member must be in attendance when a female patient is being treated by a male dentist or dental hygienist and nitrous oxide is used. Aberrant sensations may lead to unfounded accusations unless this requirement is strictly enforced.

4. Pregnancy. The safety of the use of nitrous oxide in pregnant patients or administration by pregnant operators is in question. Although no direct correlation has yet been found, several epidemiologic studies cast doubt on the safety of exposure to nitrous oxide during pregnancy. The incidence of spontaneous abortion or miscarriages is higher in female operating personnel chronically exposed to anesthetic agents or in wives of male operators. This is especially important to female dentists and dental hygienists, since dental operatories have been found to have higher concentrations of gases than even hospital operating rooms.

Pharmacologic effects

1. CNS effects. The main pharmacologic effect of nitrous oxide is on the CNS, resulting in analgesia and amnesia. Although there is sensory depression, auditory perception is not affected to the same degree. Therefore a tranquil, quiet environment is required for N_2O-O_2 analgesic procedures.

2. Circulatory effects. The circulatory system is not significantly affected except that peripheral vasodilation may occur. This property may facilitate venipuncture should an intravenous route be desired.

3. Respiratory effects. The respiratory system is not significantly affected.

4. Gastrointestinal effects. The incidence of nausea and vomiting with N_2O-O_2 analgesia is low. The patient should be requested to eat a light meal before the appointment but should be warned to avoid a large meal within 3 hours of the appointment time.

When nitrous oxide is administered slowly, its effects may be evaluated according to Table 11-2. Note the following responses to nitrous oxide's administration:

1. The best indicator of the degree of sedation is the patient's response to questions. The patient may exhibit slurred speech or a slow response.

2. The patient is relaxed and cooperative and reports a feeling of euphoria. Local anesthetic injections elicit little response at this time. Analgesia produced by nitrous oxide is variable but can be significant in some patients.

3. The patient is easily able to maintain an open-mouth position in the desired plane.

4. The patient's eyes may be closed but can be easily opened.

5. The respiration, pulse rate, and blood pressure are within normal limits.

In addition to the features already mentioned, the patient often indicates that the time frame the procedure occupied in his or her consciousness has been dramatically decreased. The operating time may appear to the patient to be one third or one half as long as it is in reality. This can be especially beneficial in long procedures.

Abuse. The dental hygienist should be knowledgeable about the hazards associated with the abuse of nitrous oxide. The literature cites several examples of nitrous oxide–induced neuropathy as a common finding with the chronic self-administration of nitrous oxide. Symptoms include numbness and paresthesia of the hands or legs that progresses to more severe neurologic symptoms with continued abuse. Nitrous oxide has also been shown to reduce the activity of methionine synthetase, the enzyme involved with the function of vitamin B_{12}. Thus it appears that the chronic abuse of nitrous oxide and attendant neurologic symptoms may be related to its effect on the utilization of vitamin B_{12}. Liver and kidney problems have also been mentioned in association with nitrous oxide abuse.

Volatile anesthetics

The volatile general anesthetics are liquids that evaporate easily at room temperature because of their low boiling points. They are classified chemically as halogenated hydrocarbons because they contain fluorine, chlorine, or bromine in their structure. These are potent agents with limited solubility in body tissues and they have successfully replaced the use of ether in anesthesia. Both methoxyflurane and halothane are used infrequently; enflurane and isoflurane are the most popular agents in current use.

Halogenated hydrocarbons

Halothane (Fluothane). Halothane has a fruity, pleasant odor, and is nonflammable and nonexplosive. Both induction and recovery are relatively rapid. The MAC for halothane is 0.77 but is improved to 0.29 when combined with 70% nitrous oxide. Because halothane is nonirritating to bronchial mucous membranes, it is considered safe to use for asthmatics. As with the other volatile agents, the halothane dose must be carefully regulated to prevent overt respiratory depression. Muscle relaxation is incomplete and peripheral neuromuscular blocking drugs such as d-tubocurarine are required. Halothane also depresses renal function and can cause uterine muscle relaxation.

Halothane's effects on the cardiovascular system are manifested by increased vagal activity, with bradycardia and peripheral vasodilation that lowers the blood pressure. It sensitizes the myocardium to the cardiac stimulatory effects of injected epinephrine and norepinephrine, leading to serious cardiac arrhythmias such as ventricular fibrillation.

Evidence indicates a causal relationship between halothane use and postanesthetic hepatitis. Some 12% to 20% of halothane is metabolized in the liver and these metabolites have been suggested as a cause of liver damage. Even though halothane has proved to be a reliable and effective general anesthetic for many years, the occurrence of this adverse effect has diminished its popularity. For this reason, halothane is contraindicated in patients when a previous exposure to halothane or other halogenated hydrocarbons has been followed by postanesthetic liver toxicity.

Enflurane (Ethrane). Enflurane is a halogenated ether anesthetic with a pleasant smell. Induction and recovery are rapid owing to its low tissue solubility. The MAC is 0.57 when combined with nitrous oxide. Enflurane depresses respiration but this effect is controlled with assisted ventilation. It provides good analgesia and muscle relaxation but supplemental muscle relaxants are still required. The heart is depressed and blood pressure is reduced. Myocardial sensitization to injected epinephrine is generally believed to be less than that associated with halothane.[1]

Adverse effects associated with enflurane use include alteration in electroencephalographic activity; thus, excessive motor activity may occur during anesthesia. Careful regulation of anesthetic depth prevents such muscular activity. Enflurane is metabolized less than other volatile agents, which may account for the absence of hepatotoxicity. Enflurane also produces a transient depression of renal function.

Isoflurane (Forane). Isoflurane is chemically related to enflurane. Its low tissue solubility allows for rapid induction and recovery. Isoflurane has a slightly pungent smell limiting the induction concentration that otherwise could provoke coughing. The MAC, when combined with 70% nitrous oxide, is 0.5. The pharmacologic effects of isoflurane are similar to the other halogenated ethers including respiratory depression, reduced blood pressure, and muscle relaxation. Only a small amount of isoflurane undergoes metabolism and liver toxicity does not seem to be a problem. Limited myocardial sensitization to injected epinephrine occurs. Nausea, vomiting, and shivering on recovery are comparable to other anesthetic agents. The most undesirable side effect is respiratory acidosis associated with deeper levels of anesthesia. Isoflurane has proved to be a useful and popular drug for general anesthesia.

Intravenous anesthetics

The intravenously administered general anesthetics are a diverse group of CNS depressants that include the opioids, the ultrashort-acting barbiturates, etomidate and, according to many sources, the benzodiazepines. These drugs find their greatest utility in induction of general anesthesia, but may occasionally be used as single agents for short procedures. While they offer the advantage of convenience, the depth and duration of anesthesia is less easily controlled in comparison to the inhalation agents. Certain drugs of this group are used in less than anesthetic doses to produce conscious sedation.

Ultrashort-acting barbiturates

The ultrashort-acting barbiturates used include methohexital sodium (Brevital), thiopental sodium (Pentothal) and thiamylal sodium (Surital). Although the basic pharmacology of the barbiturates is discussed in Chapter 10, certain facts about these drugs are discussed here.

These ultrashort-acting agents have a rapid onset of action (about 30 to 40 seconds) when given intravenously. If repeated doses are given, as is often the case during anesthesia, the drug accumulates in body tissues, resulting in prolonged recovery.

If these drugs are employed as the sole anesthetic for short procedures, the patient will respond to painful stimuli. Because no analgesia is observed with doses that allow the patient to breathe spontaneously, the intravenously administered barbiturates function more effectively when used with a local anesthetic agent as part of a balanced anesthetic technique.

A serious complication with the use of the intravenous barbiturates occurs when the solution is accidentally injected extravascularly or intraarterially. Symptoms with extravascular infiltration can range from tissue tenderness to necrosis and sloughing. Intraarterial injection is extremely dangerous and can lead to arteriospasm associated with ischemia of the arm and fingers and severe pain.

Other complications with the ultrashort-acting

barbiturates include laryngospasm and broncho-spasm. In some patients hiccoughs, increased muscle activity, and delirium occur on recovery. Premedication with atropine or the opioids has proved reasonably effective in reducing these recovery problems.

The absolute contraindications to the use of the ultrashort-acting barbiturates include an absence of suitable veins for administration, status asthmaticus, porphyria, and known hypersensitivity. The dosage should be adjusted and caution should be taken in patients with asthma or hepatic, renal, or cardiovascular impairment. Because these drugs are potent anesthetics, they should be administered only by qualified individuals, with resuscitative equipment readily available.

Dissociative anesthesia

Ketamine. Ketamine (Ketalar) is related chemically to phencyclidine (PCP), a hallucinogen. The anesthetic state ketamine produces has been given the name "dissociative anesthesia" because ketamine appears to disrupt association pathways in the brain.

Ketamine may be given intravenously or intramuscularly, with a rapid (1 to 2 minutes) onset of action occurring with either route. Pharyngeal and laryngeal reflexes remain unaffected, and there is little respiratory change. Because excessive salivation is a common finding with ketamine, atropine is a necessary premedication. Muscle tone may increase during its use.

The principal drawback to the use of ketamine is the occurrence of emergence reactions including delirium and hallucinations during recovery. This happens most often in adults, older children, and drug abusers. Reactions of this type can be minimized if visual and auditory stimuli are reduced during recovery. Small doses of an ultrashort-acting intravenously administered barbiturate has been employed to control the recovery problem.

Specific contraindications include a history of cerebrovascular disease, hypertension, and hypersensitivity to the drug. Psychologic problems present a relative contraindication. Since protective reflexes of the pharynx and larynx are active, care should be taken not to stimulate the pharynx.

Opioids

The opioids have long been used as adjunctive drugs to general anesthesia in preanesthetic medication and to provide analgesia during and after a surgical procedure. Now opioids are used as anesthetic agents as well. The opioids used include morphine, fentanyl (Sublimaze), sufentanil (Sufenta), and alfentanil (Alfenta). These drugs do not significantly alter cardiovascular function or peripheral resistance. Prolonged respiratory depression is the major disadvantage and requires careful attention to ventilatory function throughout the anesthetic period. Reversal of this depression can be produced by the antagonist naloxone.

Neuroleptanalgesia

The term neuroleptanalgesia refers to a so-called wakeful anesthetic state produced by the combination of a neuroleptic drug, droperidol (Inapsine) and a potent opioid analgesic, fentanyl (Sublimaze). Droperidol produces marked sedation and a catatonic state. The combination of drugs is marketed as Innovar and is usually given intravenously for a rapid onset. Adding nitrous oxide results in neuroleptanesthesia. Return to consciousness appears to be rapid, but the effects of droperidol are long-lasting and recovery is slow.

The adverse effects can be quite serious and are those that would normally be associated with the opioids and major tranquilizers. Respiratory depression and extrapyramidal tremors have occurred. This combination of drugs should be used with great care, especially in patients with pulmonary insufficiency and parkinsonism. A board-like chest, associated with intercostal muscle paralysis and requiring ventilatory support, has occurred in some patients. Fentanyl is sometimes employed as a sole agent for sedation.

Benzodiazepines

The anxiolytic benzodiazepines have been an integral part of conscious sedation and preanesthetic medication for years. With the advent of midazolam (Versed), this group of drugs has become more important in induction of anesthesia. Midazolam is water soluble and has a short duration of action giving it some advantages over the often used diazepam (Valium). Both of these drugs produce excellent sedation and amnesia. The benzodiazepines find their greatest application as adjunctive drugs in the balanced anesthesia technique.

REVIEW QUESTIONS

1. Name and describe the four stages of anesthesia.
2. Differentiate between the three routes of administration of the general anesthetics.
3. State the pharmacologic effects of the general anesthetics.
4. Describe the effects observed with varying concentrations of nitrous oxide.
5. Explain the rationale for the use of several agents during general anesthesia.
6. List the contraindications to the use of nitrous oxide.
7. State the potential hazards associated with the general anesthetic agents.

REFERENCES

1. Johnston, R.R., Eger, E.I., II, and Wilson, C.: A comparative interaction of epinephrine with enflurane, isoflurane, and halothane in man, Anesth. Analg. **55:**709, 1976.

Chapter 12

Fluorides

The effectiveness of fluorides in the prevention of dental caries has long been recognized and accepted by the dental profession. However, renewed interest has focused on fluoride's potential antiplaque and antigingivitis properties. Its relationship with dentinal hypersensitivity, cemental caries, and alteration in the loss of alveolar bone density associated with osteoporosis are also of interest. Fluorides may also be used as effective therapeutic agents in selected nonsurgical periodontal therapies, as well as in the active treatment of ongoing carious lesions.

Maximum anticaries effectiveness is achieved by frequent exposure of the teeth to low fluoride concentrations. Therefore, the primary site of fluoride therapy is in the patient's home. Oral self-care programs include the simultaneous use of a variety of fluoride products based on the concept of low concentration and high frequency. Recommendations for fluoride products are dependent on the patient's age, caries history, caries susceptibility, and fluoride history. The informed and concerned dental hygienist is in a position to assist the patient and the public in undertaking a preventive and therapeutic program to achieve the maximum desirable benefits of fluoride.

Both the dental professional and the consumer easily can become confused by the wide variety of available fluoride products and by the advertising claims of manufacturers. Products that have received the American Dental Association (ADA) Seal of Acceptance have been officially reviewed and evaluated for safety and efficacy in the prevention of dental caries. The concerned professional should periodically check the most current list of accepted products developed by the ADA Council on Dental Therapeutics. These reports are published in the *Journal of the American Dental Association* on a frequent basis, or may be obtained by calling the ADA number at 1-800-621-8099.

TERMINOLOGY

ppm F: Refers to the *parts per million* of *fluoride*, for example, 1 ppm F means one part of fluoride to one million parts of water (equivalent to 1 mg/L).

fluoride concentration: Concentration of the fluoride salt expressed as a percent, or concentration of the fluoride ion alone expressed as a percent or in ppm. For example, 0.02% NaF = 0.01% F^- = 100 ppm F^-.

optimum level: Concentration of fluoride in the drinking water which provides the maximum protection against dental caries with the minimum risk of enamel fluorosis.

fluoridation: Community water supply is adjusted to an optimum fluoride concentration appropriate for the climate.

defluoridation: Process to reduce excessive fluoride content in community water supplies to the recommended level.

fluoridization: The application of fluoride solutions to the exposed surfaces of the erupted teeth.

CLASSIFICATION

Fluorides are generally classified according to the method of administration: (1) systemically administered fluorides, and (2) topically administered fluorides, which are directly applied to the teeth. Systemic and topical fluoride products may be used alone or in combination.

SOURCES AND INGESTION OF FLUORIDE

Fluoride (F), the thirteenth most common element in the earth's crust, is present in almost all foods and water supplies. The amount of fluoride ingested varies with the climate. The optimum fluoride level in the water supply in moderate climates is 1 ppm F (in cold climates it is 1.2 ppm F, and in warm climates it is 0.6–0.8 ppm F).

Certain foods (especially seafoods) are rich sources of fluoride. Tea leaves and processed fish products that include bones also contain high levels of fluoride.

The concentration of fluoride in fruits and leafy, green vegetables depends on soil, watering conditions, and the fluoride content of the water utilized in their preparation. This source of fluoride is not a major factor elevating fluoride intake in the normal diet, but it does contribute to the total daily level of fluoride.

PHARMACOKINETICS

1. Absorption. Transport of the fluoride ion depends only on its concentration. Ingested fluorides are therefore absorbed through the wall of the gastrointestinal tract by the process of simple diffusion across a semipermeable membrane. This occurs primarily in the stomach and small intestine.

The amount of fluoride absorbed is proportional to its water solubility. Relatively soluble compounds, such as sodium fluoride or the fluoride ions present in drinking water, are more completely absorbed than less soluble fluoride compounds. Fluoride found in fluids is more rapidly absorbed than fluoride in solids. Calcium, magnesium, or aluminum ions interfere with fluoride absorption because they form insoluble compounds with fluoride.

2. Distribution. Fluoride is absorbed into the circulating blood and tissue fluids and then is rapidly deposited in the bones and teeth. The amount of fluoride deposited in hard tissues depends on the person's age and past ingestion of fluoride. Greater fluoride deposition will occur in persons with growing bones and mineralizing teeth than in mature adults. Fluoride steadily accumulates in the human skeleton during most of the lifetime and reaches a plateau at approximately 50 to 60 years of age. The amount of fluo-

ride deposited in bone is directly related to the amount of fluoride ingested.[1] Studies indicate that the urinary output of fluoride increases with age.

The concentration of fluoride in teeth is greatest at the enamel surface. The dentinoenamel junction contains the next highest concentration. The outer surface of enamel continues to take up fluoride during the preeruptive period after calcification is completed and after eruption. Fluoride concentrations in saliva and crevicular fluid are low, but they do function topically on erupted teeth by promoting enamel remineralization. This is an important aspect when considering the benefits of fluoridated water supplies for adults as well as children.

3. Excretion. The major route of fluoride excretion is the urine. It is also excreted in the feces, by the sweat glands and, in a limited amount, in the milk of nursing mothers. An overview of fluoride metabolism related to primary dental consideration is presented in Fig. 12-1.[2]

TOXICITY

Toxicity is the dose or concentration of an agent that elicits harmful responses or produces death. Toxic reactions may be either acute, resulting from a single large dose, or chronic, resulting from long-term ingestion.

Acute fluoride toxicity

A single ingested dose of 2.5 gm (5 gm of sodium fluoride) may be lethal to an adult. An LD50 dose in adults is estimated to range between 50 and 225 mg/kg (depending on age, sex, and weight); a dose of 25 to 50 mg/kg may produce acute gastroenteritis.[3] Fatalities in infants have occurred with the ingestion of only 0.25 gm. Death has resulted from the incorrect preparation and excessive administration of professional fluoride treatments to a child.[4] In terms of fluoridated water, a 9 lb baby would have to consume 26 gal of water containing 1 ppm F at one sitting to equal a toxic dose. The equivalent amount for an average-sized adult is more than 450 gal of water consumed at one time.[5]

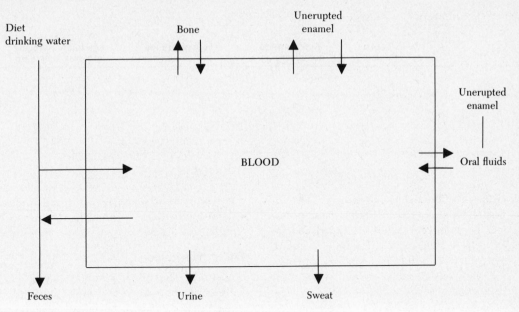

Fig. 12-1. Fluoride metabolism overview. (From Horowitz, H.S.: Fluorides to prevent dental decay: an update, Proc. Min. Conf. Dent. Caries Prev. Pub. Health Programs, June 18-19, 1982.)

When administering or recommending fluorides, the dental hygienist must inform parents or supervising adults about the prevention of fluoride toxicity in children. Initial symptoms of acute fluoride toxicity are salivation, nausea, abdominal pain, vomiting, and diarrhea. Other symptoms may include muscle hyperirritability or convulsions, hypotension, diaphoresis, and mucoid discharge from the nose and mouth.

When acute fluoride poisoning is suspected, an emergency situation exists and medical assistance must be summoned immediately. Death has been reported to occur within 1 hour after ingestion of a large toxic dose. Immediately administer milk, which acts as a demulcent to protect the upper gastrointestinal tract from chemical burns and also serves as a fluoride binder. Perform gastric lavage repeatedly with limewater (0.15% calcium hydroxide).

Chronic fluoride toxicity

The most frequently observed effect of chronic fluoride toxicity is endemic fluorosis or mottled enamel. This occurs when fluoride in the drinking water ranges between 2 and 8 ppm and is ingested continually during crown formation of the permanent teeth. Fluorosis is a hypoplastic defect resulting from a disturbance of ameloblastic activity during tooth development. The condition ranges from white opaque spots or flecking of the enamel to moderate or severe pitting, or brownish staining of enamel as the fluoride concentration in the drinking water increases.

The teeth most frequently observed with fluorosis have the longest exposure time to body fluids between the onset of enamel formation and their eruption into the oral cavity. The permanent canines, premolars, and second molars are the teeth most commonly affected (Table 12-1).[6] Teeth lowest in fluorosis potential are the incisors and the first molars. Once crown formation is completed, no amount of fluoride, either topically applied or systemically administered, will cause fluorosis.

The safety of community water fluoridation at 1 ppm F has been studied extensively. Water fluor-

Table 12-1. Fluorosis incidence factors

Teeth	Fluorosis incidence	Age crown is completed (yr)	Total years for crown completion	Age tooth emerges into oral cavity (yr)
Canines	High	6–7	4.6–5.7	9–12
Premolars	High	5–7	3.0–5.0	10–12
Second molars	High	7–8	4.0–5.5	12–13
Incisors	Low	4–5	3.0–4.7	6–9
First molars	Low	2.5–3.0	2.5–3.0	6–7

idation, despite "claims" to the contrary, has not been found to be related to cancer, kidney dysfunction, heart disease, allergies, blood anomalies, arthritis, osteoporosis, Down's syndrome, poor eyesight, or harmful effects on fish. The unequivocal safety of water fluoridation has been frequently documented in the literature.

MECHANISM OF ACTION

Fluoride's mechanism of action for caries reduction is not completely understood. Previously, the primary effect of fluoride was thought to be the conversion of hydroxyapatite crystals to fluorapatite, resulting in improved crystalline structure and decreased enamel solubility. However, recent studies indicate that the presence of fluoride enhances remineralization and accelerates the growth of enamel crystals. The larger crystals have more surface area and are less soluble. Fluoride deposits may also be redistributed during the caries process and it has been suggested that the lesion itself may act as a fluoride reservoir.[7]

High fluoride levels can occur in plaque; fluoride then has the capability of being antienzymatic or antibacterial. This antibacterial effect has the potential for reducing not only dental caries, but periodontal disease as well.

SYSTEMIC FLUORIDES

Systemic fluorides provide benefits to both developing and erupted teeth. Extensive research has documented the anticaries properties of systemic fluoride. The fluoride concentration of water supplies at which dental decay is minimal and no tooth staining occurs is approximately 1 ppm F.

Water fluoridation

Adjustment of community water supplies to the optimum level of fluoride is an economically feasible, reliable, and effective means of reducing dental caries among large population groups. Currently, approximately 50% of the people in the United States receive the benefits of fluoridated drinking water. Table 12-2 shows that lifelong exposure to water fluoridation produces a caries reduction in permanent teeth that increases with age. A significant reduction in root surface caries has been demonstrated among adults who have been lifelong residents in communities with fluoridated water supplies.

Community water fluoridation

Since the 1940s, numerous studies have been conducted among large population groups showing a 50% to 65% caries reduction in the permanent teeth of children who have ingested fluoridated water from birth.

Various fluoride compounds, such as hydrofluoric acid, fluosilicic acid, sodium fluoride, and sodium silicofluoride, may be added to community water supplies to achieve the optimum level. When these compounds are dissolved, fluoride ion is produced in the water. It is impossible to differentiate, either chemically or in anticaries activity, between naturally present and artificially added fluorides.[8] The amount of fluoride con-

Table 12-2. Effect of lifetime exposure to water fluoridation on caries in permanent teeth

Child's age (yr)	Reduction in caries per child*
6	0.6–1.2
7	0.3–2.0
8	0.9–2.5
10	1.3–2.4
11	0.8–3.4
12	4.6
16	6.3

Adapted from British Dental Association: Fluoridation of water supplies: questions and answers, London, 1976, The Association; and Davies, G.N.: Br. Dent. J., **135**:79, 1973.
*Decayed, missing, or filled teeth.

Table 12-3. Supplemental fluoride dosage schedule*

Age (yr)	Concentration of fluoride in water (ppm)		
	0–0.3	0.3–0.7	>0.7
0–2	0.25	0	0
2–3	0.50	0.25	0
3–13	1.00	0.50	0

*Recommended daily dosage of fluoride in mg/day. 1 mg of fluoride is equivalent to 2.2 mg sodium fluoride.
Adapted from American Dental Association Council on Dental Therapeutics: Accepted dental therapeutics, ed. 40, Chicago, 1984.

sumed is dependent on both the level in the drinking water and the air temperature.

School water fluoridation

In areas where the fluoridation of public water supplies is not feasible, 4.5 times the optimal fluoride level for the area's climate has been tested in school water systems. This regimen is based on the fact that children are in school only part of the time and higher levels of fluoride can be given to children at least 5 years old when the permanent teeth are well into the process of enamel maturation. This exposure to fluoride has resulted in a 30% to 50% reduction in caries.[2]

Oral fluoride supplements

Oral fluoride supplements are available by prescription as liquid drops, tablets, or in combination with vitamin preparations. It is suggested that children swish with the fluoride drops or chew the tablets before swallowing so that both topical and systemic benefits will occur. Since pediatricians as well as dental professionals may prescribe dietary supplements, caution must be exercised to ensure that the recommended level of fluoride is not exceeded. A patient's age, stage of tooth development, and concentration of fluoride

in the water supply are essential factors in recommending fluoride supplements (Table 12-3).

Research on the effect of prenatal fluoride exposure on developing dentition has been inconclusive. Some clinical reports indicate that prenatal fluoride supplementation results in cariostatic benefits,[9] but additional, more well-designed studies are necessary. In the past there was a question whether fluoride crossed the placenta, but recent evidence has demonstrated its presence in the fetal skeleton. Based on these findings, fluoride administration at controlled levels may be beneficial not only to the fetal skeleton but also to teeth. There is no evidence that adverse reactions may occur if recommended levels are observed.

Only trace amounts of fluorides have been found in human breast milk. Infants who are solely breast-fed, or whose formulas are prepared with fluoride-deficient water, should receive oral fluoride supplements according to the recommended schedule (Table 12-3).

TOPICAL FLUORIDES

The wide array of topical fluoride products currently available are classified according to the method of delivery to the patient; that is, professionally applied or self-applied. These topical fluoride products are further categorized by the vehicle utilized, such as solutions, gels, pastes, dentifrices, or rinses.

There are only four fluoride compounds that have been incorporated into the products available to the public or the dental profession (Table 12-4). Fluoride-containing dentifrices, mouthrinses, or professionally applied products differ greatly in their fluoride concentrations (Table 12-5).

Professionally applied topical fluorides
Solutions and gels

The fluoride compounds available for professional in-office use include 1.23% acidulated phosphate fluoride (APF), 2% sodium fluoride (NaF), and 8% stannous fluoride (SnF_2). Many preparations have been accepted by the Council on Dental Therapeutics.

Modes of application and treatment therapy are different for each of the active agents. The products administered in the dental office have been formulated in either solution or gel vehicles and contain between 10,000 and 20,000 ppm F. These products have been shown to produce a 30% to 40% reduction in dental caries. Additional benefits recently cited may include decreased dentinal hypersensitivity, decreased gingivitis, and an antiplaque effect. Professionally applied topical fluorides are beneficial for children and adults, especially those residing in nonfluoridated communities, and those who may be at high risk of caries because of factors such as rampant decay, xerostomia, orthodontic appliances, overdentures, and exposed root surfaces.

APF solutions and gels are commonly preferred because of patient acceptability and stability. Recent reports that APF gels or solutions may dull the surface of porcelain or composite restorations or have a detrimental effect on exposed cementum warrant consideration when selecting an appropriate fluoride agent.

A two-part sequential rinse (APF/stannous fluoride) is available but has not as yet been accepted by the American Dental Association as effective in the prevention of dental caries.

Prophylaxis pastes

Fluorides in prophylaxis pastes have a very limited effect on the prevention of dental caries and are not recommended as the sole topical fluoride. However, the fluoride may replenish that removed from the fluoride-rich outer layer of enamel by the abrasiveness of the cleaning agent. Prophylaxis pastes containing fluoride are contraindicated for use before dental bonding procedures, such as pit and fissure sealants, asthetic bonded restorations, and bonded orthodontic appliances.

Self-applied topical fluorides
Dentifrices

The fluoride compounds most commonly used in dentifrices and their concentrations are sodium monofluorophosphate (MFP) 0.76%, sodium fluoride (NaF) 0.22%, and stannous fluoride (SnF_2) 0.4%.

Several research studies have shown that the

Table 12-4. Fluoride compounds administered topically

Compound	Advantages	Disadvantages
Stannous fluoride (SnF_2)	Both cation and anion are effective	Unstable; staining potential; inherent taste
Sodium fluoride (NaF)	Used at neutral pH; stable in solution	Not compatible with many abrasives
Acidulated phosphate fluoride (APF)	Agent of choice for professional applications; stable in solution; nonirritating to gingiva	Acid pH may affect cementum; not available in dentifrices
Sodium monofluorophosphate (MFP)	Stable at various pHs and with many abrasives; most widely tested in products	Not available in mouthrinses or professionally applied products

Table 12-5.   Oral fluoride levels after product use

Product	Fluoride concentration (ppm F)	Amount used	Fluoride concentration in oral cavity per use (mg)	Suggested use
Dentrifrice	1000	1 gm	1.0	2–3 per day
Mouthrinse	100	10 ml	1.0	2 per day
	250	10 ml	2.5	1 per day
	1000	10 ml	10.0	1 per week
Professional gel	12,300–12,500	1 gm	12.3–12.5	1 per 6 months

fluoride ion may become insoluble and unable to interact with the teeth when combined with the abrasive agent (calcium or phosphate) in a dentifrice. The acceptance by the ADA of the individual formula of each dentifrice provides assurance that the bioavailability of the fluoride has been evaluated as effective.

Most major dentifrices contain MFP as the effective caries-preventive ingredient. Products with MFP, such as Aim, Aquafresh, Colgate, Dentagard, Macleans, and others, have been accepted by the Council on Dental Therapeutics as being effective in preventing dental decay.

Crest dentifrice contains sodium fluoride with silica as the abrasive system. This formula has been accepted as an effective anticaries agent by the Council on Dental Therapeutics.

Stannous fluoride was one of the early agents in dentifrices shown to be effective in the reduction of decay. At the present time, however, there are no commercially available stannous fluoride dentifrices which carry the ADA Seal of Acceptance.

Dentifrices contain approximately 1100 ppm F. A single layer of toothpaste placed on a brush head will equal approximately 1 gm, which provides 1 mg of fluoride. Studies have shown that this concentration, used at least once a day, will provide 20% to 30% caries reduction.

A home care program for all patients, including adults whether residing in a fluoridated or nonfluoridated community, should include the daily use of a fluoride dentifrice since the continuous presence of a low concentration of fluoride will enhance remineralization. In addition to the anticaries effect, fluoride dentifrices appear to have antiplaque and desensitizing properties as well.

It is desirable for adults to supervise all children under 6 years of age while brushing and to carefully monitor the amount of dentifrice used. Recent studies among young children have demonstrated that a mild mottling of the enamel may be caused by the ingestion of large quantities of fluoride over an extended period of time. Commonly, youngsters will swallow toothpaste while brushing and can often ingest up to 0.3 mg of fluoride during a single sequence of brushing. A small dab placed on the end of the brush is sufficient for the preschooler. All dentifrices should be stored beyond children's reach.

Mouthrinses

Self-applied fluorides in the form of diluted mouthrinses are an effective and cost-efficient method for preventing dental caries. While a variety of fluoride compounds have been developed, the most commonly used are sodium fluoride (NaF) mouthrinses prepared at concentrations of either 0.05% (250 ppm F) for daily use or 0.2% (1000 ppm F) for weekly use. Stannous fluoride rinses have also been effective in reducing the incidence of dental decay. Recent research has emphasized the antiplaque properties of the tin ion (Sn) and has focused attention on the impact of stannous fluoride rinses in the prevention of gingivitis.

Several low-potency mouthrinses (100 to 250 ppm F) are available as nonprescription over-the-counter (OTC) products. Those that are currently accepted by the ADA include ACT, Fluorigard, Kolynos, and Reach. The manufacturer's directions indicate that after brushing a 10 ml dose (2 tsp) be swished around the mouth for 60 seconds and then expectorated. Maximum benefit may be derived if no eating or drinking is permitted for 30 minutes after rinsing. A product with the lower concentration of 100 ppm F is to be used twice a day.

Several fluoride mouthrinse products with concentrations of 1000 ppm F are dispensed by prescription only and have been approved by the ADA. These mouthrinses are used weekly or biweekly, and have been found to be as effective as the OTC products used daily. Approximately 35% reduction in dental caries can be achieved with regular use of fluoride mouthrinses. The anticaries effectiveness is increased when fluoride mouthrinses are used in combination with a fluoride dentifrice.

Individuals in both fluoridated and nonfluoridated communities will benefit from the use of fluoride mouthrinses. Mouthrinses are recommended especially for patients who are undergoing orthodontic therapy, have overdentures, or suffer from a high rate of caries or dentinal hypersensitivity.

Although studies indicate that fluoride mouthrinses provide the greatest benefit to newly erupted teeth, rinses are to be considered only for children with mixed dentitions (over 6 years of age) with appropriate supervision. Swallowing of the product is to be avoided. Therefore, fluoride rinses are not recommended for children under 6 years of age.

In addition to age, the alcohol (ethanol) content must be carefully considered when selecting dental products. The Committee on Drugs of the American Academy of Pediatrics recommends that no ethanol be used in medicinal products intended for use by children. Patients experiencing xerostomia also should avoid products containing ethanol.

Gels

Several fluoride gels have been developed for patients to use at home. The fluoride compounds used and their concentrations are 0.5% acidulated phosphate fluoride (APF), 1.1% sodium fluoride (NaF), and 0.4% stannous fluoride (SnF).

The gels containing APF and NaF are available by prescription only. There are two recommended methods for applying these gels:

1. The custom tray method
2. The brushing method

The dental hygienist may consider recommending self-applied fluoride gels to achieve caries control for patients who exhibit one of the following conditions: xerostomia, radiation therapy, overdentures, rampant or recurrent decay, exposed root surfaces, dentinal hypersensitivity, or orthodontic appliances. Self-applied fluoride gels are not recommended for children under the age of 6. For older children, adult supervision is advisable until the teenage years are reached.

REVIEW QUESTIONS

1. State the recommendations and rationale for adjusting the levels of fluoride in the water supplies according to the average maximum daily temperatures.
2. List the various sources of ingested fluorides and explain how these are related to daily fluoride intake.
3. Define acute and chronic toxic reactions.
4. List recommended actions to take in the treatment of an acute toxic reaction to fluoride.
5. Describe the major symptom of chronic fluoride toxicity.
6. Discuss the mechanisms of action of fluorides related to the prevention and control of dental caries.
7. Identify methods of similarity between naturally and artificially fluoridated community water supplies.
8. State the rationale and recommendations for fluoridating water supplies within school systems.
9. Compare levels of fluoride available in the oral cavity following the use of dentifrices and mouthrinses.
10. Identify by name the four fluoride compounds that are incorporated into the current available topical fluoride products.
11. Describe the reason that some dentifrices containing fluoride may not be effective in the reduction of dental caries.
12. List the main factors to consider in the recommendation of fluoride oral supplements.

13. State the prevailing concept of fluoride therapy in relation to dosage and administration.
14. Discuss the rationale for recommending fluoride oral supplements to breast-fed infants.

REFERENCES

1. Ekstrand, J., et al.: Relationship between fluoride in the drinking water and the plasma fluoride concentrations in man, Caries Res. **12:**123, 1978.
2. Horowitz, H.S.: Fluorides to prevent dental decay: an update. In Frazier, J., editor: Proceedings of the Minnesota Conference on Dental Caries Prevention in Public Health Programs, June 18-19, 1982, State of Minnesota, Department of Health, 1983.
3. Fry, B.W.: Toxicology of fluorides. In Picozzi, A., and Smudski, J., editors: Pharmacology of fluorides, First Symposium of the Pharmacology, Therapeutics and Toxicology Group, International Association of Dental Research, Atlanta, 1974.
4. Church, L.E.: Fluorides—use with caution, J. Maryland State Dent. **19:**106, August, 1976.
5. British Dental Association: Fluoridation of water supplies: question and answers, London, 1976, The Association.
6. Myers, H.M.: Fluorides and dental fluorosis, Monogr. Oral Sci. **7:**1, 1978.
7. Silverston, L.M.: Fluorides and remineralization. In Wei, S.H., editor: Clinical uses of fluorides, Philadelphia, 1985, Lea & Febiger.
8. Burt, B.B., Eklund, S.A., and Loesche, W.J.: Dental benefits of limited exposure to fluoridated water in childhood, J. Dent. Res. **61:**1332, 1986.
9. Kula, K., and Wei, S.H.Y.: Supplements and dietary sources of fluoride. In Wei, S.H., editor: Clinical uses of fluorides, Philadelphia, 1985, Lea & Febiger.

Vitamins and minerals

The vitamins are a group of low molecular weight organic compounds that are essential in small quantities for the maintenance of cell structure and metabolism. These agents may be employed to treat problems not associated with vitamin deficiency. When used as such they are regarded as drugs. However, there are few situations in which proof that vitamins are useful for the treatment of any condition except vitamin deficiency exists.

The vitamins are classified into two large groups: water soluble and fat soluble. The water-soluble vitamins include mainly the B vitamins and vitamin C. The fat-soluble vitamins are vitamins A, D, E, and K. Although the functions of the water-soluble vitamins are somewhat understood, the functions of the fat-soluble vitamins are unclear. Vitamin C, a water-soluble vitamin, plays a role in biologic oxidation and reduction for cellular restoration. Table 13-1 lists the common names of the vitamins and their deficiencies.

RECOMMENDED DIETARY ALLOWANCE (RDA)

The recommended daily dietary allowance (RDA) is a standard based on scientific facts. These values for intake of essential nutrients are high enough to meet the needs of almost everyone. They are used to plan and obtain nutritionally adequate food supplies for populations. They are determined by scientists in nutrition interpreting current scientific information. They are then used to determine policy. In 1985-1986, the National Academy of Sciences/National Research Council (NAS/NRC) rejected the recommendations of the 10th Committee on RDAs because of some vague need for "new directions." Their recommendations included a reduction in the RDA of nu-

trients and a debate raged over the levels for others. For these reasons, the most recent RDA information reflects the latest released information, unfortunately published in 1980. When the RDA is listed in this text, the recommendations of the Academy (Table 13-2) are being quoted.

WATER-SOLUBLE VITAMINS
Ascorbic acid

Ascorbic acid (vitamin C) chemically is a sugar acid that readily undergoes oxidation to form dehydroascorbic acid. Because of this ability, ascorbic acid is an effective reducing agent.

Source. Good natural sources of ascorbic acid include citrus fruits, green peppers, tomatoes, strawberries, broccoli, raw cabbage, baked potatoes, and papaya. A number of food products are fortified with vitamin C. Because of its ability to be easily oxidized, ascorbic acid is readily destroyed through cooking, and as much as 50% of the ascorbic acid content of foods can be lost in this manner.

Recommended dietary allowance. The RDA of ascorbic acid for the normal adult is 60 mg. The unaccepted new RDA is 40 mg. Smoking and stress are said to increase the need for this vitamin.

Role. The metabolic role of ascorbic acid is probably related to the fact that ascorbic acid and dehydroascorbic acid form a readily reversible oxidation-reduction system. It is thought that this vitamin plays a role in biologic oxidations and reductions in cellular respirations. Ascorbic acid also plays a definite role in connective tissue metabolism, since it is required for the formation of collagen. The function of ascorbic acid can be dramatically demonstrated in the wound healing

Table 13-1. Vitamins and their deficiencies

Vitamin	Name	Disease caused by deficiency
Water soluble		
B_1	Thiamine	Beriberi
B_2	Riboflavin	
B_3	Niacin (nicotinic acid)	Pellagra
B_6	Pyridoxine	
B_{12}	Cyanocobalamin	Pernicious anemia
	Folacin (folic acid)	Megaloblastic anemia
	Pantothenic acid	
	Biotin	
C	Ascorbic acid	Scurvy
Fat soluble		
A	Retinoic acid, retinal, retinol	Night blindness
D	Cholecalciferol	Rickets
E	Tocopherol	
K	Phytonadione, menadione	Bleeding

process. Scorbutic wounds have a decrease in mature collagen fibrils associated with an accumulation of mucopolysaccharides or ground substance around a matrix of precollagenous fibers. The absence of mature collagen results in abnormal healing that reduces the tensile strength of the wound.

Deficiency. A deficiency of ascorbic acid produces a condition termed **scurvy.** The manifestations of scurvy occur because of the inability of the connective tissue to produce and maintain intercellular substances such as collagen, bone matrix, dentin, cartilage, and vascular endothelium. As a result of defective connective tissue formation, persons with a vitamin C deficiency demonstrate alterations in bone formation, tissue, and wound healing. The following are manifestations of defective connective tissue formation in vitamin C deficiency:

Poor wound healing
  Lack of collagen
  Inadequate response to infections

Alterations in the integrity of capillary walls, manifested as hemorrhages in
  Skin
  Mucous membranes
  Muscles
  Lungs
  Joints
  Gingivae (spongy, edematous, inflamed)
Lack of formation of bone matrix, resulting in
  Disorganization of epiphyseal line
  Weakening of bones
  Pathologic fractures
  Resorption of alveolar bone with loosening and loss of teeth

Since humans and other primates cannot synthesize vitamin C, they must obtain it daily from their diet. Diets completely deficient in vitamin C are unusual, and there are few cases of serious vitamin C deficiency (scurvy). After a prolonged period of time (4 to 5 months) without vitamin C, humans have symptoms of weakness, anorexia, suppressed growth, anemia, lower resistance to infection and fever, swollen and inflamed gums, loosened teeth, swollen wrists and ankle joints, petechial hemorrhages, fracture of ribs at costochondral junctions, and hemorrhaging owing to capillary fragility in joints, muscle, and intestines.

Clinical considerations. As long ago as 1942, it was suggested that vitamin C could be therapeutically beneficial in preventing the common cold. Linus Pauling, reviewing available data, indicated that vitamin C has a substantial beneficial effect in preventing and treating the common cold. Other investigators, reviewing the data, concluded that little evidence existed to suggest the effectiveness of vitamin C in either preventing or treating the common cold. Based on current evidence, unrestricted use of ascorbic acid for these purposes could not be advocated.

Another Pauling hypothesis suggested that large quantities of vitamin C may suppress neoplastic cellular proliferation. He indicated that vitamin C should be used in the management of all types of cancer. Other investigators have been unable to verify this claim. In conclusion, well-controlled, prospective clinical trials are needed

Table 13-2. Recommended daily dietary allowances[a]

		Weight		Height			Fat-soluble vitamins			Water-soluble vitamins	
	Age (years)	kg	lbs	cm	in	Protein (g)	Vitamin A (μg R.E.)[b]	Vitamin D (μg)[c]	Vitamin E (mg α T.E.)[d]	Vitamin C (mg)	Thiamine (mg)
Infants	0.0-0.5	6	13	60	24	kg $\times$ 2.2	420	10	3	35	0.3
	0.5-1.0	9	20	71	28	kg $\times$ 2.0	400	10	4	35	0.5
Children	1-3	13	29	90	35	23	400	10	5	45	0.7
	4-6	20	44	112	44	30	500	10	6	45	0.9
	7-10	28	62	132	52	34	700	10	7	45	1.2
Males	11-14	45	99	157	62	45	1000	10	8	50	1.4
	15-18	66	145	176	69	56	1000	10	10	60	1.4
	19-22	70	154	177	70	56	1000	7.5	10	60	1.5
	23-50	70	154	178	70	56	1000	5	10	60	1.4
	51+	70	154	178	70	56	1000	5	10	60	1.2
Females	11-14	46	101	157	62	46	800	10	8	50	1.1
	15-18	55	120	163	64	46	800	10	8	60	1.1
	19-22	55	120	163	64	44	800	7.5	8	60	1.1
	23-50	55	120	163	64	44	800	5	8	60	1.0
	51+	55	120	163	64	44	800	5	8	60	1.0
Pregnant						+30	+200	+5	+2	+20	+0.4
Lactating						+20	+400	+5	+3	+40	+0.5

From Food and Nutrition Board: Recommended dietary allowances, ed. 9, Washington, D.C., 1980, National Academy of Sciences-National
[a]The allowances are intended to provide for individual variations among most normal persons as they live in the United States under usual ments have been less well defined.
[b]Retinol equivalents. 1 Retinol equivalent = 1 μg retinol or 6 μg carotene.
[c]As cholecalciferol. 10 μg cholecalciferol = 400 I.U. vitamin D.
[d]α tocopherol equivalents. 1 mg d-α-tocopherol = 1 αT.E.
[e]1 NE (niacin equivalent) is equal to 1 mg of niacin or 60 mg of dietary tryptophan.
[f]The folacin allowances refer to dietary sources as determined by *Lactobacillus casei* assay after treatment with enzymes ("conjugases") to
[g]The RDA for vitamin B_{12} in infants is based on average concentration of the vitamin in human milk. The allowances after weaning are based
[h]The increased requirement during pregnancy cannot be met by the iron content of habitual American diets nor by the existing iron stores different from those of nonpregnant women, but continued supplementation of the mother for 2-3 months after parturition is advisable in

to assess the value of ascorbic acid in the management of both the common cold and the cancer patient.

Untoward effects have been reported with the use of megadoses of vitamin C. A daily intake of 1 gm of the vitamin may cause precipitation of oxalate stones in the urinary tract. For this reason, unwarranted use of large quantities of vitamin C is discouraged.

A rebound scurvy has been reported in adults and infants who received megadoses that were then stopped abruptly. Megadoses of ascorbic acid can destroy vitamin B_{12}, reduce copper absorption, and increase plasma cholesterol. The

implications of these effects have not yet been elucidated. Vitamin C enhances the absorption of iron, a fact that may be used to advantage in iron deficiency anemia.

B-complex vitamins

The water-soluble vitamins, except for vitamin C, are known as the B-complex vitamins. On a functional basis these vitamins may be subdivided into three classes:

1. Those that primarily release energy from carbohydrates and fats (thiamine, pyridoxine, niacin, riboflavin, pantothenic acid, biotin)

Water-soluble vitamins					Minerals					
Riboflavin (mg)	Niacin (mg N.E.)[e]	Vitamin B_6 (mg)	Folacin[f] (μg)	Vitamin B_{12} (μg)	Calcium (mg)	Phosphorus (mg)	Magnesium (mg)	Iron (mg)	Zinc (mg)	Iodine (μg)
0.4	6	0.3	30	0.5[g]	360	240	50	10	3	40
0.6	8	0.6	45	1.5	540	360	70	15	5	50
0.8	9	0.9	100	2.0	800	800	150	15	10	70
1.0	11	1.3	200	2.5	800	800	200	10	10	90
1.4	16	1.6	300	3.0	800	800	250	10	10	120
1.6	18	1.8	400	3.0	1200	1200	350	18	15	150
1.7	18	2.0	400	3.0	1200	1200	400	18	15	150
1.7	19	2.2	400	3.0	800	800	350	10	15	150
1.6	18	2.2	400	3.0	800	800	350	10	15	150
1.4	16	2.2	400	3.0	800	800	350	10	15	150
1.3	15	1.8	400	3.0	1200	1200	300	18	15	150
1.3	14	2.0	400	3.0	1200	1200	300	18	15	150
1.3	14	2.0	400	3.0	800	800	300	18	15	150
1.2	13	2.0	400	3.0	800	800	300	18	15	150
1.2	13	2.0	400	3.0	800	800	300	10	15	150
+0.3	+2	+0.6	+400	+1.0	+400	+400	+150	h	+5	+25
+0.5	+5	+0.5	+100	+1.0	+400	+400	+150	h	+10	+50

Research Council.
environmental stresses. Diets should be based on a variety of common foods in order to provide other nutrients for which human require-

make polyglutamyl forms of the vitamin available to the test organism.
on energy intake (as recommended by the American Academy of Pediatrics) and consideration of other factors such as intestinal absorption.
of many women; therefore the use of 30-60 mg of supplemental iron is recommended. Iron needs during lactation are not substantially
order to replenish stores depleted by pregnancy.

2. Those that, among other functions, catalyze the formation of red cells (folic acid, vitamin B_{12})
3. Those that have not been shown to be required in human nutrition (choline and inositol)

A close interrelationship among the B-complex vitamins exists. If a deficiency of one of them occurs, it will impair the utilization of others. Also, the signs and symptoms of a deficiency of individual B vitamins are similar. This is probably because a deficiency of a single member of the B complex seldom occurs. A diet deficient in one B vitamin is usually lacking in other B vitamins.

Thiamine

Thiamine (vitamin B_1) is an essential water-soluble vitamin in humans. It is converted in the liver to its active coenzyme form, thiamine pyrophosphate (TPP).

Source. Thiamine is present in foods of both animal and vegetable origin. The best sources are pork, whole-grain and enriched breads, cereals and pastas, seeds of legumes such as peas, dried brewer's yeast, and wheat germ. Since the vitamin tends to be destroyed if heated to about 100° C; significant amounts of this vitamin may be lost if foods are cooked too long above this temperature.

Recommended dietary allowance. The requirement for thiamine is related to caloric intake. The RDA is 0.5 mg/1000 kcal with an additional 0.4 mg daily during the last two trimesters of pregnancy and 0.5 mg daily during lactation.

Role. TPP plays a principal role in intermediary metabolism. It is a coenzyme required for the oxidative decarboxylation of α-keto acids. In this role TPP is sometimes referred to as cocarboxylase.

Deficiency. A severe deficiency of thiamine leads to a condition known as beriberi. Characteristics of beriberi are peripheral neuritis, muscle weakness, paralysis of the limbs, enlargement of the heart, tachycardia, and edema (typical of wet beriberi). Gastrointestinal tract effects including loss of appetite, intestinal atony, and constipation may also be present. The symptoms of mild thiamine deficiency are less characteristic. They include tiredness and apathy, loss of appetite, moodiness and irritability, pain and paresthesias in the extremities, slight edema, decreased blood pressure, and lowered body temperature. Possible oral manifestations of thiamine deficiency are burning tongue, loss of taste, and hyperesthesia of the oral mucosa.

The most common cause of thiamine deficiency in the United States is alcoholism. Both poor appetite and the effect of alcohol on the nerves may exacerbate this problem. Both Wernicke's syndrome and Korsakoff's syndrome can result if a severe deficiency exists.

Riboflavin

Riboflavin (vitamin B$_2$) is a water-soluble vitamin composed of flavin and D-ribitol.

Source. Riboflavin occurs abundantly in both plants and animals. However, dairy products and meat are the best sources of this vitamin. Riboflavin is relatively stable to heat, and cooking will not cause an appreciable loss of it. It is destroyed by ultraviolet radiation.

Recommended dietary allowance. The requirements for riboflavin are related to caloric intake, with the minimum requirement established

at 0.6 mg/1000 kcal. The RDA for riboflavin is between 1.2 and 1.7 mg.

Role. Riboflavin carries out its functions in the body as a component of two flavoprotein coenzymes, riboflavin phosphate (flavin mononucleotide, FMN) and flavin adenine dinucleotide (FAD). Flavoprotein coenzymes in turn are proteins that act as electron acceptors and are involved in a variety of oxidation-reduction reactions.

Deficiency. Symptoms of riboflavin deficiency usually involve the lips, tongue, and skin. Sore throat and angular stomatitis (cheilosis) appearing as an ulceration with painful fissuring at the corners of the mouth are early and frequent findings. The lips may be either unusually red or whitish because of desquamation. Later, glossitis can occur with the dorsum of the tongue becoming pebbly or granular. Contact with food or drink may produce pain or a burning sensation on the tongue. In some instances the tongue may become magenta-colored or purplish red. Excessive salivation and enlargement of the salivary glands may occur. Skin manifestations include a greasy, scaling inflammation around the nose, cheeks, and chin. Involvement of the scrotum and the vulva is frequent. Other manifestations of riboflavin deficiency are anemia and neuropathy.

Clinical considerations. Riboflavin deficiency is most likely to be seen in alcoholics, economically deprived individuals, or patients with severe gastrointestinal disease that causes loss of appetite, vomiting, and malabsorption syndromes. The manifestations of riboflavin deficiency are difficult to distinguish from those of other B vitamin deficiencies because of the similarities in syndromes.

Niacin and niacinamide

Niacin (nicotinic acid) and niacinamide (nicotinamide) are water-soluble organic compounds that have the ability to alleviate a deficiency syndrome known as pellagra (It., *pelle* skin; *agra* rough). Niacin, in the form of niacinamide, is a component of two coenzymes that participate in biologic oxidation-reduction reactions. These coenzymes are nicotinamide adenine dinucleotide (NAD) and nicotinamide adenine dinucleotide phosphate (NADP).

Source. Good sources of niacin are lean meats, liver, poultry, and legumes. Pellagra was at one time a common disease of the southeastern United States among persons subsisting on a diet exclusively of corn products because corn is extremely low in tryptophan, a precursor of this vitamin.

Recommended dietary allowance. The niacin requirement in the diet is somewhat dependent on both caloric and protein intake. Since tryptophan, an amino acid found in dietary protein, is metabolized to niacin in the body, the intake of protein would reduce the amount of vitamin needed in the diet. Sixty milligrams of tryptophan is approximately equivalent to 1 mg of niacin.

The minimum requirement of niacin, including that formed from tryptophan, to prevent pellagra is approximately 4.4 mg/1000 kcal. A 50% margin of safety has been added to this minimum to arrive at the recommended niacin allowance of 6.6 mg/1000 kcal. A minimum intake of between 9 and 13 mg is suggested to prevent pellagra. The RDA of niacin in the adult male is as great as 19 mg of niacin equivalent.

Role. The role of niacin is similar to that of riboflavin. It plays a key role in metabolism by participating in a variety of oxidation-reduction reactions (transfer of electrons)

Deficiency. The clinical syndrome produced by niacin deficiency is called pellagra. Early symptoms are an erythematous cutaneous eruption on the back of the hands, glossitis, and stomatitis. In advanced stages pellagra can be diagnosed by the classic "three D's": dermatitis, diarrhea, and dementia. The dermatitis consists of redness, thickening, and roughening of the skin followed by scaling desquamation and depigmentation. Diarrhea is caused by atrophy of the gastrointestinal tract mucosal epithelium, followed by inflammation of the mucosal lining of the esophagus, stomach, and colon. The dementia results from regressive changes in the ganglion cells

of the brain and tracts of the spinal cord. Death may also result.

During the course of pellagra, symptoms are evident in the oral cavity. A burning sensation occurs throughout the oral mucosa. The lip and lateral margins of the tongue are initially reddened and swollen. In the later stages the entire dorsal surface of the tongue becomes red and swollen. In acute stages vascular hyperemia, proliferation, hypertrophy, atrophy, and extinction occur successively in the papillae. Papillary loss may ultimately become complete, with the tongue surface becoming beefy red. Deep penetrating ulcers may appear on the tongue surface. In the gingiva desquamative epithelial degeneration may occur, exposing the tissue to infection, inflammation, and fibrinous exudation. Gingivitis caused by pellagra is characterized by ulcers in the interdental papillae and marginal gingiva. There is also excessive salivary secretion with enlargement of the salivary glands.

Niacin deficiency occurs most frequently in the poverty-stricken areas of the world because of inadequate intake. Deficiency may also arise from chronic alcoholism, gastrointestinal disturbances, pregnancy, hyperthyroidism, and infections.

Clinical considerations. Niacin, or nicotinic acid, is used not only as a vitamin but also in the treatment of certain cardiovascular conditions. It reduces plasma cholesterol, triglycerides, very low density lipoproteins (VLDL), low density lipoproteins (LDL), and chylomicrons. These effects are dose dependent. Side effects, from these larger doses, include cutaneous flushing, pruritus, and gastrointestinal distress. It can also be used in combination with other lipid-lowering agents so that a lower dose of each may be used.

Pyridoxine

Pyridoxine is one of three different pyridoxine derivatives known as vitamin B_6. The other two derivatives, pyridoxal and pyridoxamine, are chemically similar.

Source. Vitamin B_6 is present in most foods of both plant and animal origin. Good sources of this vitamin include whole-grain cereals, meat, egg yolk, and some vegetables.

Recommended dietary allowance. The RDA for vitamin B_6 is 2 mg daily for adults, with an additional 0.6 and 0.5 mg during pregnancy and lactation, respectively. The newest rejected recommendation for vitamin B_6 is 2 mg for men and 1.7 mg for women.

Role. To exert physiologic activity, all three forms of vitamin B_6 are converted to pyridoxal phosphate in the body. Pyridoxal phosphate is the active coenzyme form of vitamin B_6 and participates in all metabolic reactions that require the vitamin. Pyridoxal phosphate acts as a coenzyme in a variety of metabolic transformations of amino acids, including transamination and decarboxylation.

Deficiency. Vitamin B_6 deficiency is rare because of the widespread distribution of this vitamin in food. The characteristics of vitamin B_6 deficiency resemble those of riboflavin, niacin, and thiamine deficiencies. These include angular cheilosis, stomatitis, dermatitis, and erythema of the nasolabial folds. The dorsal mucosa of the tongue seems to be unusually sensitive to a single deficiency or mixed deficiencies of the B vitamins. Specifically, glossitis resulting from pyridoxine deficiency has been described in which the tongue's surface is smooth, slightly edematous, painful, and purplish.

Clinical considerations. Vitamin B_6 can interact with other therapeutically useful drugs. For example, isoniazid (INH), a drug used to treat tuberculosis, inhibits the action of vitamin B_6 by blocking both the formation and the reaction involving pyridoxal phosphate, the active coenzyme. Isoniazid-induced vitamin B_6 deficiency can be prevented or treated by the administration of pyridoxine.

Vitamin B_6 administration can cancel the therapeutic and side effects of levodopa, a drug used to treat Parkinson disease. A pyridoxine-free vitamin preparation (Larobec) has been produced for use as a vitamin supplement in patients receiving levodopa. If a peripheral decarboxylase inhibitor such as carbidopa is administered simultaneously with levodopa (the combination is called Sinemet), pyridoxine may be administered concomitantly. In practice, Sinemet is currently used almost exclusively rather than levodopa alone.

Estrogenic steroids can produce vitamin B_6 deficiency in women. About 20% of women taking oral contraceptive agents can be shown to have a biochemical pyridoxine deficiency. Usual RDAs seem to be enough to prevent this situation and women on birth control pills should routinely be encouraged to take supplemental pyridoxine.

Folic acid

Folic acid (pteroylglutamic acid) is made up of a pteridine heterocycle, p-aminobenzoic acid (PABA), and glutamic acid. It is metabolized by dihydrofolate reductase to various folates. It is sparingly soluble in water and is destroyed by heating in neutral or alkaline solution. Although commonly the terms "folacin," "folic acid," and "folate" are used interchangeably, technically folate is a general group of substances that give rise to folacin in the body.

Source. Significant sources of folic acid include glandular meats such as liver, some fruits and vegetables, wheat germ, and yeasts. Since its availability from foods is highly variable, there is a wide margin of safety for differences in availability from foods. Synthetic folic acid is much better absorbed than that supplied from foods.

Recommended dietary allowance. The World Health Organization recommends a dietary folate intake of 400 μg for adults, while the RDA is 400 μg daily for adults.

Role. The biologically active form of folic acid is the reduced derivative tetrahydrofolic acid (THFA), which is formed enzymatically in the body. THFA functions primarily in the transfer and utilization of one-carbon groups.

Certain microorganisms synthesize their own folic acid from PABA. The sulfonamides exert their bacteriostatic effect by antagonizing PABA and thereby interfere with the biosynthesis of folic acid in these organisms. This has no effect on humans because they require preformed folic acid and do not synthesize their own.

Deficiency. Folic acid deficiency, the most common deficiency in the United States, results in megaloblastic anemia, which is indistinguishable from that caused by vitamin B_{12} deficiency. Other symptoms include weakness, weight loss, loss of skin pigmentation, and mental irritability. As with riboflavin deficiency, oral manifestations of folic acid deficiency include glossitis, angular cheilosis, and gingivitis. The glossitis begins with swelling and pallor of the tongue followed by desquamation of the papillae and accompanied by minute ulcers with fiery red borders.

Some causes of folic acid deficiency are inadequate diet, pregnancy, malabsorption syndrome, and chronic alcoholism. Pregnant women need supplemental synthetic folacin and should not rely solely on dietary sources. The absorption of folate decreases during pregnancy and in patients taking oral contraceptives.

Several drugs have been reported to produce folic acid deficiencies including the anticonvulsants, oral contraceptives, and some cancer chemotherapy agents (folic acid antagonists). The anticonvulsants produce a deficiency by interfering with the conversion of folate to a form of the vitamin that can penetrate the brain.

Clinical considerations. Although the administration of folic acid will cause remission of the hematologic effects of pernicious anemia, it will not prevent the neurologic effects caused by a deficiency of vitamin B_{12}. Therefore folic acid can mask a vitamin B_{12} deficiency. For this reason the FDA has limited the dose of folic acid per tablet that can be purchased as a nonprescription supplement to 0.4 mg, or 0.8 mg for pregnant or lactating women.

Vitamin B_{12}

Vitamin B_{12} or cyanocobalamin is a chemically complex substance that contains an extensively substituted pyrole ring system surrounding an atom of cobalt. A cyanide molecule is attached to the cobalt; hence the name "cyanocobalamin." Vitamin B_{12} is heat stable at a neutral pH but is readily destroyed by heat at an alkaline pH.

Source. The only source of vitamin B_{12} in nature are certain microorganisms that synthesize the vitamin. When vegetable produce is contaminated with these microorganisms they possess the vitamin. Animals depend on synthesis within their own gastrointestinal tracts. Human vitamin B_{12}, synthesized within the gastrointestinal tract, is unavailable for absorption.

Foods of animal origin are good sources of vitamin B_{12}, with liver and kidney serving as the best sources and milk, cheese, and eggs serving as adequate sources. Strict vegetarians can become deficient because they do not eat these foods. In recent years some vegetable products such as soy milk have been fortified with vitamin B_{12}.

Vegetarians rarely exhibit a vitamin B_{12} deficiency because legumes often are contaminated with the vitamin B_{12}-producing bacteria.

Vitamin B_{12} is inadequately absorbed from the gastrointestinal tract without the presence of intrinsic factor, a protein-binding factor that aids in the absorption of vitamin B_{12}.

Pernicious anemia is a conditional vitamin B_{12} deficiency disease caused by a lack of intrinsic factor in the gastric mucosa. It can be treated by the intramuscular injection of vitamin B_{12}, since intrinsic factor is not required for absorption from an intramuscular site.

Recommended dietary allowance. A daily intake of 0.6 to 1.2 μg will sustain modest body stores of vitamin B_{12} in normal adults. The World Health Organization recommends a daily dietary intake for adults of 2 μg; this amount allows for 60% to 80% absorption from food. The RDA is 3 μg of vitamin B_{12} with an additional 1 μg during pregnancy and lactation.

Role. Vitamin B_{12} serves as a coenzyme for the hydrogen transfer and isomerization process required in the conversion of methylmalonyl-CoA to succinyl-CoA. Thus vitamin B_{12} is important in the metabolism of fats and carbohydrates.

Deficiency. The symptoms of vitamin B_{12} deficiency include inadequate hematopoiesis, gastrointestinal tract disturbances, inadequate myelin synthesis, and generalized debility. The lack of this vitamin affects the cells that are most actively dividing, such as those in the bone marrow and gastrointestinal tract. The erythroblasts do not undergo proper division, resulting in anemia. Atropic changes occur in the alimentary canal. There is also myelin degeneration of the spinal cord. The patient suffers from weakness, numbness, and difficulty in walking, symptoms that fluctuate with remission and relapses. The skin may have a distinctive lemon-yellow hue.

The most common cause of vitamin B_{12} deficiency is pernicious anemia. In this disease mucosal cells do not produce intrinsic factor, and thus vitamin B_{12} is not absorbed. With a gastrectomy, usually for the treatment of peptic ulcer, intrinsic factor secretion ceases. Then it takes 3 to 6 years for a vitamin B_{12} deficiency to develop. Other causes of vitamin B_{12} deficiency include inadequate dietary intake and malabsorption syndromes.

Pernicious anemia results in a number of oral manifestations. Recurrent attacks of soreness and burning of the tongue occur followed by glossitis, at the peak of which the tongue is extremely painful and red. Atrophy of the filiform and fungiform papillae is a common occurrence. Involvement of the circumvallate papillae may cause diminution of taste. Painful, bright red lesions may occur in the buccal and pharyngeal mucosa and undersurface of the tongue.

Clinical considerations. As mentioned previously, patients who are vegetarians (rarely) or who have had a gastrectomy can exhibit the symptoms of vitamin B_{12} deficiency.

Ingestion of other agents can alter the absorption of vitamin B_{12}. For example, vitamin C may have an effect on the vitamin B_{12} levels in food. Pregnancy and use of the sweetener sorbitol increase vitamin B_{12} absorption. Absorption of vitamin B_{12} is decreased in persons with pyridoxine deficiency, iron deficiency, or hypothyroidism.

Vitamin B_{12} has also been used, without any proof of efficacy, to treat trigeminal neuralgia, psychiatric disorders, and tiredness.

Pantothenic acid

Pantothenic acid is another compound required to form acetyl-CoA. The active form of pantothenic acid is a component of the more complex compound, coenzyme A.

Source. Pantothenic acid is a part of all living material. Egg yolk and beef liver are excellent sources.

Recommended dietary allowance. It is suggested that a daily dietary intake of 4 to 7 mg is completely adequate for adults.

Role. The physiologically active form of pantothenic acid is coenzyme A, which serves as a coenzyme in various metabolic reactions, some of which involve the transfer of acetyl (two-carbon) groups. Both pantothenic acid and thiamine are required for the oxidative decarboxylation of pyruvate to produce acetyl-CoA. Pantothenic acid also functions as part of a glucose-carrier system to facilitate absorption through the intestinal mucosa.

Deficiency. Since clinical deficiencies of pantothenic acid are extremely rare in humans, deficiencies are produced experimentally in humans only by using a pantothenic acid antagonist. The symptoms of pantothenic acid deficiency include fatigue, headache, malaise, nausea, abdominal pain, "burning" of hands and feet, and cramping of leg muscles.

Clinical considerations. Pantothenic acid has been used to treat gastrointestinal tract paralysis after surgery. It apparently promotes gastrointestinal motility. Even though a deficiency of pantothenic acid produces gray hair in black rats, there is absolutely no evidence that it reduces gray hair in humans.

Biotin

Biotin was initially demonstrated to be an essential growth factor for yeast, and it was later isolated from both yeast and egg yolk.

Source. Although biotin is present in almost all foods, good sources include liver, cow's milk, egg yolk, and yeast. It is also synthesized by the microflora in the intestinal tract, so that the amount of biotin excreted in the feces can actually exceed the intake.

Recommended dietary allowance. Although no minimum daily requirement of biotin has been established, the suggested adequate daily dietary intake for adults is between 100 and 200 μg.

Role. Biotin is a coenzyme required in metabolism in carbon dioxide fixation reactions (carboxylations).

Deficiency. A biotin deficiency can be induced by eating large quantities of raw egg white. Avidin, a component of egg white, can combine with biotin in the gastrointestinal tract and prevent its absorption. If the egg white is cooked, avidin is denatured and has no activity.

Biotin deficiency is extremely rare in humans. When it is induced experimentally by concurrent administration of large amounts of raw egg white containing avidin, symptoms include loss of appetite, mental depression, hyperesthesia of the skin, nausea, and malaise.

Clinical considerations. Since the amount of biotin synthesized in the intestines is related to the number of microorganisms present, antiinfective agents such as the sulfonamides or tetracyclines can produce a biotin deficiency. Two types of infant dermatitis respond to biotin therapy.

Other B vitamins

"Vitamin B_{15}" and "vitamin B_{17}," also known as pangamic acid and laetrile respectively, have been shown to be neither vitamins nor to be important in human nutrition.

Choline and inositol. Neither choline nor inositol have been demonstrated to be required in the human diet. They serve as lipotropic agents and prevent fatty infiltration of the liver. Choline serves as a precursor to acetylcholine. In humans, no deficiency for either choline or inositol has been demonstrated. Deficiencies of choline (in rats) and inositol (in mice) have been produced.

FAT-SOLUBLE VITAMINS
Vitamin A

Vitamin A is an essential fat-soluble compound necessary for normal growth and for maintaining the health and integrity of certain epithelial tissues. The term "vitamin A" represents vitamin A_1 (retinol), vitamin A_2 (3-dehydroretinol), and the carotenes. By cleavage of the carotene molecule, two molecules of vitamin A aldehyde (retinal) are formed.

Source. Vitamin A_1 occurs naturally in saltwater fish and animal tissues. Vitamin A_2 is found in freshwater fish. Preformed vitamin A is found in milk, liver, and some cheeses. Margarine is fortified with vitamin A. However, the carotenes are the best source of vitamin A. The carotenes are found in various pigmented fruits such as apricots, peaches, tomatoes, and watermelon and in vegetables such as carrots, pumpkins, broccoli, spinach, and sweet potatoes. A dark green, yellow, or orange color indicates that a vegetable or fruit has carotene.

Recommended dietary allowance. The adult RDA for vitamin A is 800 to 1000 retinol equivalents (R.E.) One retinol equivalent is equal to 1 μg of retinol or 6 μg of carotene. During pregnancy and lactation an increased intake of 200 and 400 R.E., respectively, of vitamin A is required. The rejected RDA was to be 700 R.E. for men and 600 for women.

Role. Vitamin A is essential for the maintenance of normal vision and certain epithelial surfaces such as the mucous membranes of the eye and the mucosa of the respiratory, gastrointestinal, and genitourinary tracts.

Vitamin A may play a significant role in maintaining the integrity and possibly the normal permeability of the cell membrane and the membrane subcellular particles. Vitamin A deficiency decreases the activity of osteoblasts and odontoblasts, thereby reducing the growth of bones and teeth. In contrast, excessive doses of vitamin A accelerate bone and cartilage resorption and new bone formation.

Deficiency. Since the human liver may store

enough vitamin A to meet physiologic demands for as long as a year, a deficiency of this vitamin is rare. Deficiencies generally result from inadequate intake of the vitamin, a malabsorption syndrome, especially biliary tract disease, and severe liver disease. Deficiency of the vitamin leads to impaired vision in dim light called night blindness (nyctalopia). It also results in keratinization of mucosa and cornea. Corneal keratinization leads to impairment of vision called xerophthalmia. Irritation and inflammation may occur on the cornea, a condition called keratomalacia. Keratinization may also occur in the oral cavity and mucosa. The normal defense mechanism of ciliary movement and mucous production is impaired, producing irritation and inflammation of these surfaces. A loss of the senses of taste and smell also occurs in vitamin A deficiency. A deficiency of vitamin A during pregnancy and infancy contributes to the development of enamel hypoplasia and caries in primary teeth.

Toxicity. An excessive intake of vitamin A results in a toxic condition called **hypervitaminosis A.** The characteristics of this toxic reaction include itching skin, desquamation, coarse or absent hair, painful subcutaneous swellings, gingivitis, hyperirritability, and limitation of motion. Hyperostosis in the bone is easily demonstrated on radiography. In infants, headache from increased intracranial pressure, gastrointestinal distress, jaundice, and heptomegaly may occur. Since the margin of safety of vitamin A intake is large, a toxic reaction can occur only after the long-term daily ingestion of more than 50,000 R.E.

Acute poisoning has been reported in both infants and adults. When the Vikings landed in Iceland they ingested polar bear liver, a rich source of vitamin A, and died from acute poisoning. Following the ingestion of lesser amounts by infants increased intracranial pressure with bulging fontanel and vomiting has been reported.

Vitamin A relatives used therapeutically

Tretinoin (Retin-A) is a topical product of retinoic acid. It causes skin peeling and is used to treat acne. Its newest use is in the treatment of wrinkles. Erythema, desquamation, and unusual sun sensitivity can occur.

Isotretinoin (13-*cis*-retinoic acid, Accutane) is used orally for treatment of severe cystic acne. Side effects include pseudotumor cerebri, corneal opacities, abnormal liver function tests, and elevated plasma triglycerides. It is highly teratogenic and should not be used without adequate birth control measures. Remission can remain after the drug has been withdrawn.

Vitamin D

Source. "Vitamin D" is a collective term used to refer to both vitamin D_2 and vitamin D_3, two closely related sterols. Vitamin D_3 (cholecalciferol) is produced in the skin of mammals by the action of sunlight (ultraviolet rays) on its precursor, 7-dehydrocholesterol. Cholecalciferol is also present in some foods. Vitamin D_2 (calciferol) is produced by the commercial irradiation of ergosterol.

Recommended dietary allowance. The RDA of cholecalciferol is 10 μg (400 IU of vitamin D) for a child. Recently, an allowance for adults of between 5 and 10 μg of cholecalciferol has been recommended with an additional 5 μg for pregnant or lactating women.

Role. Vitamin D promotes the normal mineralization of the bone by stimulating intestinal absorption of calcium. Vitamin D_3 (cholecalciferol) is first hydroxylated in the liver to form 25-hydroxycholecalciferol, which is then transported to the kidney and converted to the physiologically active form, 1,25-dihydroxycholecalciferol. This active form, in conjunction with parathyroid hormone (PTH), stimulates intestinal absorption of calcium and mobilizes calcium from formed bones. These effects result in an elevation of serum calcium, which suppresses PTH secretion and secondarily 1,25-dihydroxycholecalciferol synthesis. If the calcium level rises, the thyroid gland secretes calcitonin, which reduces the formation of 1,25-dihydroxycholecalciferol and increases the production of 24,25-dihydroxycholecalciferol. Low levels of phosphorus stimulate the production of 1,25-dihydroxycholecalciferol, whereas high phosphorus levels produce more 24,25-dihydroxycholecalciferol.

Deficiency. A deficiency of vitamin D produces inadequate absorption of calcium and phosphate with a decrease in plasma calcium. PTH secretion is stimulated, which removes calcium from the bone to restore plasma levels. In children this deficiency results in rickets, a disease involving a decreased mineralization of newly formed bone and cartilage tissue. Children with rickets have bones that are unusually soft and easily bent, compressed, or fractured. Under the stress and strain of weight-bearing, the gross deformities of rickets, including spine curvature and bowing of the legs, become evident. Owing to the excess formation of osteoids a squared appearance of the head occurs. Collapse of the ribs and protrusion of the sternum (pigeon breast syndrome) are also seen. Bone pain and muscle weakness may be present.

A vitamin D deficiency during pregnancy or in young children may result in enamel hypoplasia, but the teeth may remain caries free.

In adults a vitamin D deficiency produces a disease state called osteomalacia. In general, there is decreased bone density owing to inadequate mineralization, which results in an excess of osteoid matrix. Because of the weakness of the bones, there are pathologic fractures and deformities of weight-bearing bones. This occurs most frequently during times of increased calcium usage such as pregnancy or lactation. Persons with malabsorption syndromes, alcoholics, those adhering to a low-fat diet, strict vegetarians, and those undergoing anticonvulsant therapy or using sedatives and tranquilizers are more prone to vitamin D deficiency.

Toxicity. The symptoms of hypervitaminosis D, which may result from either long-term or short-term ingestion of excessive quantities of vitamin D, are caused by abnormal calcium metabolism. The signs and symptoms of vitamin D toxicity include weakness, fatigue, headache, nausea, vomiting, and diarrhea. With prolonged hypercalcemia, calcification of the blood vessels, heart, lung, and kidney can occur. Continued ingestion of more than 50,000 units in a normal adult would be likely to produce hypervitaminosis D.

Vitamin E

Compounds possessing vitamin E activity are known chemically as tocopherols. Three such tocopherols are designated α, β, and γ. Since α-tocopherol comprises the majority of tocopherols found in animal tissue and has the greatest biologic activity, it is considered the most important. Although the metabolic role of vitamin E is not understood, it is known that this vitamin functions as an antioxidant.

Source. The best sources of vitamin E are vegetable oils such as soybean, corn, and cottonseed oils. Other sources include fresh greens and vegetables.

Recommended dietary allowance. It has been estimated that a daily intake of 10 to 30 mg of vitamin E will keep the vitamin E serum level within a normal range. The Food and Nutrition Board of the National Research Council recommends between 8 and 10 α-tocopherol equivalents for adults per day (Table 13-2). Vitamin E deficiency has not been detected in a normal healthy adult or child.

Role. As an antioxidant, vitamin E probably prevents the formation of toxic oxidation products and the oxidation of essential cellular constituents. There is also a relationship between vitamins A and E in that vitamin E increases the absorption and utilization of vitamin A and protects against hypervitaminosis A.

Deficiency. A deficiency of vitamin E can affect the reproductive, muscular, cardiovascular, and hematopoietic systems. Vitamin E deficiency in male rats has resulted in reproductive failure and sterility and in the pregnant female rat has led to fetal death and resorption. In humans vitamin E has been used for the treatment of sterility and habitual abortion, but there is no conclusive evidence that this vitamin provides any beneficial effect in these conditions. Although vitamin E has been used to treat several cardiovascular diseases, there is no scientific rationale for this use.

A deficiency of vitamin E can occur in malabsorption syndromes and in premature infants with impaired absorption ability. A deficiency of vitamin E has also been reported to cause anemia resulting from a decreased erythrocyte life span and abnormal hematopoiesis. Oxidizing agents can more easily hemolyze the erythrocytes from vitamin E–deficient animals.

Toxicity. Vitamin E is generally thought to have low toxicity. Levels of vitamin E greatly in excess of the normal dietary requirements have been administered to human subjects with no apparent adverse effect.

Clinical considerations. Vitamin E therapy has been recommended for the treatment of a wide variety of human diseases that are similar to conditions observed with vitamin E deficiency. Research is continuing into claims that vitamin E can even slow the aging process. It is also thought to relieve the symptoms of intermittent claudication and to have some protective value against certain air pollutants. Others found that vitamin E supplementation had no effect on work performance, sexuality, or general well-being. At the present time no therapeutic use of vitamin E has been proved by controlled scientific studies with the possible exception of specific, extremely rare anemias. Pharmacologic doses of vitamin E have been employed as an antioxidant in premature infants exposed to high concentrations of oxygen to reduce the incidence and severity of retrolental fibroplasia.

Vitamin K

Vitamin K was originally found to be a fat-soluble substance present in hog liver fat and alfalfa. Large quantities of the vitamin are also found in the feces of most species of animals. At least two distinct natural substances possess vitamin K activity: vitamin K_1 and vitamin K_2. Vitamin K_1 is thought to be the biologically active form; the other forms are converted in the body to vitamin K_1. Vitamin K_1 (phytonadione, phytylmenaquinone, phylloquinone) is found in plants. Vitamin K_2 (menaquinone, multiprenylmenaquinone) is synthesized by the gram-positive bacteria present in the gastrointestinal tract. The synthetic vitamin K, vitamin K_3 (menadione), possesses activity approaching that of the natural vitamin.

Source. Vitamin K_1 occurs in green vegetables such as alfalfa, cabbage, and spinach and in egg yolk, soybean oil, and liver. Vitamin K_2 is synthesized by gram-positive bacteria, and the microorganisms in the intestinal flora can provide humans with some vitamin K.

Recommended dietary allowance. There is no generally accepted figure for the human requirements for vitamin K. The amount needed must be very small and is satisfied by the average diet. The adequate daily dietary intake for adults is between 70 and 140 µg.

Role. Vitamin K is essential for the synthesis of prothrombin (factor II) and the blood clotting factors VII, IX, and X (see Fig. 15-4). Without these factors, the normal blood clotting process does not occur.

Deficiency. A vitamin K deficiency is referred to as hypoprothrombinemia. In the absence of this vitamin bleeding will result. With a severe deficiency of vitamin K, the smallest trauma may produce hemorrhage. The most common sites of hemorrhage are operative wounds, skin (petechial bleeding), mucous membranes in the intestinal tract, and serosal surfaces. Ecchymoses, epistaxis, and hematuria are also common.

Vitamin K deficiency is usually caused by inadequate intake or absorption or by decreased normal bacterial flora resulting from prolonged antibiotic use.

The naturally occurring vitamins K_1 and K_2 are essentially nontoxic in massive doses, and vitamin K_3 (menadione) must be administered in large doses before toxicity can be demonstrated. It has been implicated in producing hemolytic anemia in newborns and hemolysis in persons suffering from glucose-6-phosphate dehydrogenase (G6PD) deficiency.

Clinical considerations. Anticoagulant drugs such as warfarin act competitively to antagonize vitamin K and interfere with the production of prothrombin and factors VII, IX, and X. Vitamin K_1 in the form of phytonadione is used to treat excessive hypoprothrombinemia caused by warfarin toxicity.

SELECTED MINERALS
Iron

Although iron is widely distributed throughout the human body, it is principally found as hemoglobin. Approximately 70% of the iron in the body is functional or "essential" iron (e.g., in hemoglobin and myoglobin), whereas 30% remains as storage or "nonessential" iron.

Source. Good sources of iron include organ meats such as liver and heart, wheat germ, brewer's yeast, egg yolks, oysters, red meats, and dried beans. Breads, flours, and cereals are commonly enriched with iron. Cooking utensils made of iron can raise the iron content of foods if the foods prepared in them are acidic. The percentage of iron absorbed from foods varies considerably, with absorption from meats being better. Numerous factors affect absorption such as other foods eaten concomitantly, the bulk in the diet, the size of the dose of iron, the body's need, and the presence of achlorhydria.

Recommended dietary allowance. The body carefully conserves its iron; there is no mechanism for its excretion. The iron level is regulated by limiting its absorption from the intestinal tract. However, since iron is contained in each cell, when body cells are lost, iron is also lost. Women must replace the extra iron lost during menstruation. On the average a man requires about 1 mg of absorbed iron per day, whereas a woman needs about 2 mg of absorbed iron daily to replace losses. Replacement of a donated pint of blood would require an additional 0.7 mg of absorbed iron daily for 1 year. Since between 2% and 10% of ingested iron is absorbed, men need about 10 mg and women 18 mg of iron in their diets each day. The unapproved recommendation was 10 mg for adult men and 15 mg for menstruating women. A pregnant woman's need for iron cannot be met by the usual American diet or the 18 mg supplement recommended for women. For this reason a supplemental 30 to 60 mg of iron is recommended for pregnant women.

Role. The basic function of iron is to allow the movement of oxygen and carbon dioxide from one tissue to another. Iron accomplishes this task by being a part of both hemoglobin and myoglobin. Iron is also a component of enzymes involved in the uptake and release of oxygen and carbon dioxide, and therefore it is essential for protein metabolism.

Deficiency. Because the body is so efficient in conserving iron, a deficiency can occur only with growth, blood loss, or inadequate intake during pregnancy. The requirements of younger women cannot be easily reached without a supplement. Preschool children, adolescents, and elderly persons are also frequently found to be deficient in iron, probably because of inadequate intake.

The symptoms of iron deficiency anemia are nonspecific but include pallor, irritability, fatigue, decreased resistance to infection, and sore mouth. Anemia, a decrease in the quality or quantity of red blood cells, can be measured by laboratory tests.

Iron deficiency anemia is treated by the concurrent administration of adequate iron salt, usually in tablet form, and ascorbic acid, which increases the absorption of iron. When the hemoglobin becomes normal, which may require months, there is no reason to continue therapy if the diet has improved or the cause of the deficiency has been removed (as by control of excessive bleeding).

Although there are many salt forms of iron, no product has been shown to be superior to ferrous sulfate. Since ferrous sulfate contains about 30% iron, 200 mg tablets contain about 60 mg of iron. If side effects occur, one may substitute ferrous gluconate, 300 mg (12% iron), to administer about 36 mg of iron. Other preparations, including sustained-release products, have at best no advantage and in some cases may actually be less effective than ferrous sulfate.

Toxicity. Complaints of gastrointestinal distress are common, even with therapeutic doses of iron. However, with an acute overdose bleeding into the intestine can occur, resulting in shock or even death. Treatment of an acute overdose of iron involves removing the iron by gastric lavage and introducing phosphate into the stomach to decrease the iron's solubility. Chelating agents such as deferoxamine, which form a complex with iron, can be used if warranted.

With prolonged administration of iron, the intestinal mucosa, which normally regulates iron absorption, can be overcome. When an excess of iron accumulates, it produces hemochromatosis, a deposition of hemosiderin, in the organs. An iron overload can also occur with frequent blood transfusions. As with the treatment of acute overdose, chelating agents can be used to treat chronic toxic effects from iron.

Zinc

Only in 1961 was a zinc deficiency recognized in humans. A delay in sexual maturity, slow healing of wounds, and slowed growth are associated with this deficiency.

Source. The best sources of zinc are seafood and meat. Cereals and legumes also contain zinc but it is more poorly absorbed from these foods owing to the presence of phytic acid, which interferes with intestinal absorption.

Recommended dietary allowance. The RDA for adults is 15 mg.

Role. Zinc is required to transport carbon dioxide in the blood and eliminate it in the lungs. It is essential in the utilization of alcohol, and it rids the body of lactic acid formed during exercise. It is also a component of insulin.

At least 59 enzymes involved in digestion or metabolism contain zinc or need it to function. Zinc plays an integral part in some enzymatic reactions and is a catalyst for others.

Deficiency. In zinc-deficient rats, fetuses were either resorbed or born with congenital malformations. In humans zinc-deficient mothers gave birth to low-birth-weight infants or infants with suggested malformations of the central nervous system. Both sexes have shown retarded gonadal development, and with severe deficiency reproduction is impossible. In view of the drop in

serum zinc produced by the oral contraceptives, speculation concerning subsequent pregnancies would be natural. A deficiency of zinc also stunts growth.

Hypogeusia, anorexia, and hyposmia have been reported in conjunction with zinc deficiency. Zinc seems to be essential to the growth and differentiation of the taste buds. It may also be a part of a "growth factor" for taste buds appropriately named gustin. It may soon become routine to measure the zinc in saliva to correlate it with body zinc levels.

Toxicity. Long-term studies must be conducted concerning chronic zinc toxicity. Nausea, vomiting, fever, and diarrhea have been reported to follow acute ingestion.

Clinical considerations. Although it has long been known that zinc participates in wound healing, there is no known advantage to the administration of zinc in patients who have no zinc deficiency. The use of zinc supplements to promote wound healing is currently being studied for periodontal surgery.

Calcium

Calcium, the fifth most prevalent element in the body, is present in both bones and extracellular fluids.

Recommended daily allowance. The 1980 RDA is 800 mg for the adult. The rejected recommendations (1985) changed the women's requirement to 1000 mg and the pregnant woman's requirement to 1500 mg.

Role. Calcium is essential for the function of nerve and muscle. It is needed for muscle contraction, cardiac function, membrane integrity, and blood coagulation. The skeleton is a reservoir of calcium for the body. Parathyroid hormone (PTH), calcitonin, and vitamin D regulate calcium concentrations in the body.

Deficiency. A deficiency of calcium can occur when both calcium and vitamin D are withheld. Mobilization from the bone keeps tissue levels nearly normal. If levels in the blood fall, tetany, paresthesias, muscle cramps, and convulsions can result.

Clinical considerations. Calcium is used to treat a deficiency of calcium, as well as tetany secondary to low calcium levels. When calculating the RDA of calcium the **amount of elemental calcium,** not the total weight of the calcium salt, must be used.

REVIEW QUESTIONS

1. Name the water-soluble and fat-soluble vitamins.
2. For each of the vitamins, discuss the following, if applicable:
   a. Source
   b. Role
   c. Recommended dietary allowance
   d. Deficiency
   e. Toxicity
   f. Clinical considerations
3. For each of the vitamins, name the deficiency state and describe the major signs and symptoms.
4. Name the vitamins that have great toxicity and explain the reason for this phenomenon.
5. Describe the conditions that are likely to produce iron deficiency anemia and explain its treatment.
6. Explain the potential use of zinc in dentistry.
7. List the vitamin deficiencies that may be induced by drug therapy with oral contraceptives and anticonvulsants.
8. Describe a use for niacin involving the cardiovascular patient.

Chapter 14

10/13/93

Oral conditions and their treatment

Although the dental hygienist does not directly treat these oral conditions, patients often ask the hygienist questions about their treatment. A few comments about each condition and then the medications for their treatment are discussed.

ACTINIC LIP CHANGES

Long-term exposure of the lip to the sun can cause irreversible tissue changes. Sunscreen preparations with high (greater than 15) sun protective factors (SPF) should be applied before sun exposure and reapplied as needed. If keratotic changes have occurred the treatment is topical 5-fluorouracil (5-FU). A topical steroid (see Chapter 19) may be used to relieve the irritation produced by 5-FU.

ACUTE NECROTIZING ULCERATIVE GINGIVITIS

Acute necrotizing ulcerative gingivitis (ANUG), also called Vincent's infection and trench mouth, has both bacteriologic (spirochetes) and environmental (stress, debilitation) factors. Beginning at the interdental papillae, ANUG is a spreading ulcer associated with a distinctive odor. Good oral hygiene is the most important component of treatment, but other modalities will be mentioned. Mouthwashes, such as hydrogen peroxide, or saline rinses assist by their flushing action. If pain or elevated temperature accompanies ANUG, then aspirin or acetaminophen can be recommended. If eating is difficult then food supplements (Meritene, Nutrament, Sustagen) may be used instead of meals. Vitamin supplementation is useful only if the patient is not taking in adequate vitamins. These supplements contain the required vitamins and minerals. Routine antibiotics should be condemned. Antibiotics should be considered only if the patient is immune-suppressed or there is evidence of systemic involvement. Normal cases respond dramatically to local treatment.

HERPES INFECTIONS

Primary herpetic gingivostomatitis, or primary herpes, is caused by the herpes simplex virus and occurs principally in infants and children. Frequently associated with other infections, its painful lesions may appear throughout the oral mucosa. Ulcers with a circumscribed area of erythema appear, and systemic symptoms can develop. Systemic reactions are more severe in infants and in some cases can be life-threatening. Acyclovir, a specific antiviral antibiotic, can be helpful in shortening the course of the disease. It may be given intravenously (IV), orally, or topically. The fever may be managed by giving acetaminophen or sponging with tepid water. The painful local symptoms may be alleviated with the use of diphenhydramine (Benadryl, Benylin), viscous lidocaine, kaolin (Kaopectate), or combinations of these medications. Sodium carboxymethylcellulose paste (Orabase Emollient) may also reduce discomfort and food supplements may be used. These remedies are the same as those used for patients receiving cancer chemotherapy agents. Corticosteroids are contraindicated because they reduce immunity.

Recurrent herpes labialis involves herpes infections of the lip and are very common. Beginning

wear hat & clothes in sun.

See Erythema } pain → ? contagious
vesicle
scab

as an erythematous area, it is followed by vesicle formation and finally scabbing. Prophylactic measures include applying a sunscreen agent before exposure to the sun. Topical application of acyclovir appears ineffective, probably related to poor penetration. Oral acyclovir has been shown to be effective in the prevention of herpetic episodes, but should not be used indiscriminately. Some authors have suggested that water-soluble bioflavonoid–ascorbic acid complex (vitamins) reduce symptoms, but evidence is weak.

RECURRENT APHTHOUS STOMATITIS

Recurrent aphthous stomatitis, a common condition seen after 20 years of age, has an unknown etiology. Symptomatic control of pain with analgesics and of oral discomfort with mouthwashes, as well as dietary supplements for nutrition, is used as indicated. Topical adrenal steroids may be used for short-term application. Since steroids are contraindicated for infectious processes, a diagnosis should be assured before treatment. Tetracycline suspension is prescribed to be swished and either swallowed or expectorated. It is sometimes mixed with viscous lidocaine 1:1. With severe multiple aphthae, both topical and systemic corticosteroids beginning with a large dose and tapering is indicated.

NOT viral

must have correct diagnosis to use

CANDIDIASIS (MONILIASIS)

Fungal

Candidiasis, an infection caused by *Candida albicans*, frequently affects the oral and vaginal mucosa. Oral candidiasis occurs when some predisposing factor is present (Table 8-2). Lesions are typical or may be confirmed by culture. Angular cheilitis may occur with chronic candidiasis. Nystatin aqueous suspension, vaginal tablet, or pastille, or clotrimazole troches may be used (see Chapter 8). All are effective, but must be continued for at least 2 days after symptoms have subsided and for at least 2 weeks. Ketoconazole, administered systemically, may be used once daily.

Table 8-2

ANGULAR CHEILITIS/CHEILOSIS

Angular cheilitis may be simple redness or may include fissures, erosion, ulcers, and crusting at the angles of the mouth. They may or may not be painful. A reduced vertical dimension may exacerbate the condition. Causes may include infection, allergic reactions, trauma, and nutritional deficiency. Use of vitamins, especially those high in vitamin B, may be helpful. Alteration of vertical dimension by reestablishing an acceptable interocclusal distance is indicated. If *Candida* is present, treatment with an antifungal (see above and Chapter 8) agent is indicated. Antibiotics may be indicated if a bacterial origin is suspected. A combination of an antifungal, antibiotic, and steroid may improve the situation.

Denture worn occ. missing teeth

LICHEN PLANUS

Lichen planus, a skin condition, frequently involves the oral mucous membranes. A white network on an erythematous base is the most characteristic lesion. Slight to extreme discomfort may be present. Topical steroids, or in extreme cases, systemic steroids may be used. This treatment is similar to severe aphthous stomatitis.

BURNING TONGUE SYNDROME AND SYMPTOMATIC GEOGRAPHIC TONGUE

Sensitivity of the tongue has, at present, an unknown etiology. Systemic disturbances, such as nutritional deficiencies or allergic reactions, must be ruled out before local palliative therapy is begun. Diphenhydramine (Benadryl) may provide some symptomatic relief. Tricyclic antidepressants are used on a trial basis, adjusting the dose to minimize the side effects.

PERICORONITIS

Pericoronitis is the inflammation of tissue around the crown of the tooth. Most commonly applied to partially erupted third molars, an inflammatory response is produced when food and bacteria are trapped between the operculum and the tooth. Periodontal pockets can become painful and swell. If caught early, debridement with saline irrigation and use of warm saline rinses are indicated. With severe pericoronitis, debridement is still primary. If the affected tooth is to be extracted, extraction can prevent further episodes.

Mild analgesics can be used for the discomfort. Infection, usually managed by local treatment, may rapidly spread in debilitated patients and should be aggressively treated with antibiotics.

ALVEOLAR OSTEITIS ("DRY SOCKET")

Alveolar osteitis occurs in 2% to 3% of extractions, most commonly in the lower molar region, where the incidence is considerably higher. Alveolar osteitis is caused by loss or necrosis of the blood clot, exposing bone in the extraction socket. This exposed bone is extremely painful. Infection, swelling, elevated temperature, lymphadenopathy, and a foul odor may be present. Treatment consists of debridement, placing a pack, analgesics, antibiotics (if infection is present), and supportive therapy. Although there is some indication that local placement of antibiotics may reduce the incidence of dry socket, use of aseptic technique, proper suturing techniques, and minimal trauma should be used as prophylactic measures. Topical antibiotics should be considered in patients at high risk for infection.

XEROSTOMIA

Xerostomia may result from a disease (e.g., Sjögren's syndrome) or a drug (e.g., atropine), or aging. Radiation therapy to the head and neck affects the salivary glands so that the consistency is altered and the volume reduced. Artificial saliva may be suggested for use in these patients. Table 14-1 lists the drug groups most likely to produce dry mouth.

POSTIRRADIATION CARIES

Changes in saliva after irradiation therapy and lack of proper plaque control can rapidly accelerate the rate of dental caries. Generalized cervical decay within the first year after x-ray therapy can result. Meticulous oral hygiene, reinforced by the hygienist, and self-application of sodium fluoride gel four times daily in a bite guard is recommended.

ROOT SENSITIVITY

Sensitivity of exposed root surfaces may be precipitated by heat, cold, and sweet or sour foods.

Table 14-1. Agents that produce xerostomia (dry mouth)

Drug group	Examples
Anticholinergics*	Bentyl, Donnatal, Artane
Antihypertensives*	Aldomet, Catapres, Minipress
Antipsychotics,* phenothiazines	Haldol, Navane, Mellaril
Tricyclic antidepressants	Elavil, Norpramin
Antihistamines	Benadryl, Chlor-Trimeton, hydroxyzine
Adrenergic agents	Phenylpropanolamine, Sudafed
Diuretics	Dyazide, hydrochlorothiazide
Benzodiazepines	Xanax, Valium, Halcion

*Most likely to cause xerostomia.

Occlusal trauma may produce irritation to the exposed dentinal tubules, and occlusal adjustment is the treatment. Roots exposed by periodontal surgery, extensive root planing, or accumulation of tooth-accumulated materials are more difficult to manage. Application in the dental office of glycerin with burnishing, sodium fluoride, stannous fluoride, and adrenal steroids have been used in an attempt to reduce root sensitivity. Adequate clinical trials for these products are minimal, at best. The patient may use home brushing with concentrated sodium chloride and 0.5% stannous fluoride. Sodium fluoride gel may also be self-applied in a bite guard. Desensitizing toothpastes have been tried, but controlled clinical trials with sufficient patient populations are lacking.

REVIEW QUESTIONS

1. State the best way to prevent actinic lip changes.
2. Describe the treatment of a patient with acute necrotizing ulcerative gingivitis.
3. Compare and contrast herpes labialis and aphthous stomatitis.
4. State the treatment for oral candidiasis.
5. Name two ways to reduce alveolar osteitis.
6. Describe the management of xerostomia and state reasons for its occurrence.

Chapter **15**

9/3/10/20/93

Cardiovascular drugs

The term "cardiovascular disease" refers to a variety of diseases of the heart and blood vessels. These diseases include, among others, hypertension, angina pectoris, cerebrovascular accident, and heart failure. Although cardiovascular disease is the leading cause of death in the United States, these patients are now living longer, more productive lives because of cardiac care units, comprehensive drug therapy, and intensive screening procedures. This explains why cardiovascular disease affects such a large proportion of the dental patient population.

The dental hygienist first identifies the cardiovascular patient while taking the drug history. Often these patients use several medications for their disease(s). The importance of this group of drugs is demonstrated by the fact that 38 drugs listed in the top 200 drugs (see Appendix) are from this group. Since cardiovascular medications are frequently given for the patient's lifetime, a knowledge of their actions, problems, and effects on dental treatment is essential. Both the disease and the drugs used in its treatment can affect the management of a patient's dental care. Before each group of drugs is discussed in this chapter, the disease for which the drugs are used is briefly described. Some general considerations concerning the dental treatment of patients with cardiovascular disease is mentioned first.

cardio. pts are living longer.

DENTAL IMPLICATIONS OF CARDIOVASCULAR DISEASE
Contraindications to treatment

Although many patients with cardiovascular disease can be treated in the dental office, there are circumstances when dental treatment should not be rendered. Generally, the following are absolute contraindications to dental treatment until a consultation between the patient's physician and dentist has determined any special considerations:

1. Acute or recent myocardial infarction (MI) (within the preceding 3 to 6 months)
2. Unstable or the recent onset of angina pectoris
3. Uncontrolled congestive heart failure (CHF)
4. Uncontrolled arrhythmias
5. Significant, uncontrolled hypertension

The absolute contraindications apply only to uncontrolled or severe cardiovascular diseases. Many patients whose cardiovascular disease is under control can be treated in the dental office. The type of procedure anticipated, the stress of the procedure, and the fact that many procedures are elective must be considered. By obtaining a thorough health history, it can be determined whether the patient's physician should be consulted before dental treatment is given. **At no time should dental office personnel begin treatment on a patient with any degree of cardiovascular disease without discussing the situation with the dentist.**

✓Dentist & MD
first

Vasoconstrictor limitation

When a local anesthetic–vasoconstrictor combination is used in the treatment of patients with cardiovascular disease, the amount and type of vasoconstrictor in the solution should be considered. It must be kept in mind that endogenous release of epinephrine caused by pain thought due to inadequate anesthesia can also stimulate the heart (see Chapter 9 for a discussion of vasoconstrictor limits). The use of the aspiration technique to avoid intravascular injection can reduce the chance of vasoconstrictor adverse reactions.

Bacterial endocarditis

When a thorough history is taken and the presence of rheumatic heart disease or other valvular or degenerative diseases is discovered, the risk of inducing bacterial endocarditis must be considered. In these cases antibiotics should be given prophylactically before dental treatment. Chapter 8 discusses the prevention of bacterial endocarditis by the use of antibiotic prophylaxis.

Cardiac pacemakers

A cardiac pacemaker is an electrical device implanted in a patient's chest to regulate the heart rhythm. Electrical devices commonly used in dentistry, such as vitalometers and high-frequency electrosurgical units, may interfere with proper pacemaker activity. Before treatment of a patient with a pacemaker is begun, consultation with the patient's physician is appropriate.

CARDIAC GLYCOSIDES
Congestive heart failure

The function of the heart is to act as a pump, ensuring adequate circulation of the blood to meet the oxygen needs of all the body's tissues. When the circulation needs are increased, as in exercise, the normal heart adjusts its output to meet the increased oxygen needs. If the heart is unable to keep up with the body's needs, it becomes a "failing" heart and the pumping mechanism becomes inefficient. This occurs because the heart muscle is stretched past its maximum effectiveness by the presence of excess blood that it cannot pump out.

This inefficient pumping mechanism results in an inadequate cardiac output and unsatisfactory circulation. Various forms of injury to the heart such as myocardial infarction (heart attack), arrhythmias, and valvular disease from rheumatic heart disease can produce a failing heart.

One might think of the heart as a two-part pump with a right and left side. In congestive heart failure the blood backs up behind the part of the heart that is failing. If the right side of the heart is failing, blood backs up behind it, causing systemic congestion. This leads to edema in the extremities evidenced by pitting of the legs (pedal edema). If the left side of the heart fails, blood backs up into the pulmonary circulation (lungs), causing dyspnea and orthopnea. In many patients both sides of the heart fail, leading to pulmonary edema and dyspnea and concomitant peripheral edema.

Major drugs

The major group of drugs used in the treatment of congestive heart failure was first described by William Withering in 1785. These drugs are called cardiac or digitalis glycosides. There are several of these cardiac glycosides available for clinical use. They have the same action in the body but differ in their route of administration, onset, and duration of action. Digoxin (Lanoxin) is the most commonly used product.

Pharmacologic effects

The major effect of the cardiac glycosides on the failing heart is to increase the force and efficiency of contraction of the myocardium (termed the positive inotropic effect). It allows the heart to do more work without increasing oxygen utilization. When the contractile force of the heart is improved, the heart becomes a more efficient pump and the cardiac output increases. As a result of this improved pumping action, other changes such as a reduction in the heart size and a decrease in the heart rate occur.

Its effect on heart rate in the intact animal is bradycardia.

Digitalis also reduces the edema that occurs

with congestive heart failure. Diuresis results from an improved circulation that increases the glomerular filtration rate. The mobilization of fluid from the peripheral circulation indirectly decreases the edema. Digitalis slows atrioventricular (AV) conduction, prolongs the refractory period of the AV node, and decreases the rate of the sinoatrial (SA) node. These effects are useful in the treatment of arrhythmias.

Uses

The most common use of the cardiac glycosides is in the treatment of congestive heart failure. Digitalis is also used in the treatment of certain cardiac arrhythmias.

Adverse reactions

Because of the narrow margin of safety with the digitalis glycosides, toxic effects are not uncommon. Even slight changes in dosage, metabolism, or absorption can trigger toxic symptoms.

1. Gastrointestinal effects. Early signs of a toxic reaction to digitalis include anorexia, nausea and vomiting, and copious salivation. A reduction in dosage can decrease this toxicity.

2. Arrhythmias. If a sufficient overdose is given, severe cardiac irregularities can develop. These arrhythmias can progress to ventricular fibrillation and death. Diuretics, often used in the treatment of congestive heart failure, can produce hypokalemia, which can predispose a patient to serious arrhythmias. Note that digitalis can either cause arrhythmias or be used to treat them.

3. Neurologic effects. The neurologic signs of toxicity include headache, drowsiness, and visual disturbances (green and yellow vision, halo around lights). A pain in the lower face resembling that associated with trigeminal neuralgia has been reported as a neurologic symptom of digitalis toxicity. Weakness, faintness, and mental confusion have also been reported.

4. Drug interactions. Some important problems associated with the digitalis glycosides involve their interactions with other drugs. One example is the interaction between digitalis and the diuretics, which potentiates arrhythmias.

The sympathomimetic agents and the digitalis glycosides interact. Since agents in both groups can produce ectopic pacemaker activity, their concomitant administration can enhance the chance of arrhythmias. The epinephrine included as a vasoconstrictor in local anesthetic solutions can also increase the chance of arrhythmias in patients taking cardiac glycosides.

Dental implications

1. Gastrointestinal effects. If a patient complains of nausea or vomiting, special care must be taken to prevent emesis. These symptoms may be associated with digitalis toxicity, and the patient's physician should be consulted if the nausea and vomiting have been protracted.

2. Epinephrine administration. Because digitalis can sensitize the myocardium to arrhythmias, epinephrine should be used cautiously in patients taking digitalis. Patients taking digitalis should be questioned about toxic symptoms before epinephrine is administered.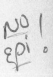

3. Pulse monitoring. Because digitalis can cause bradycardia or arrhythmias that could be exacerbated by dental treatment, the patient's pulse should be checked for a normal rate and a regular rhythm. An abnormally slow rate or an irregular rhythm should be reported to the dentist for evaluation before the patient's physician is notified.

ANTIARRHYTHMIC AGENTS
Arrhythmias

The function of the heart depends on rhythmic contractions of the cardiac muscle. The sequence of events in the contraction process requires the atrial muscle to contract before the ventricular muscle to ensure complete ventricular filling. These steps are necessary for adequate cardiac output. The contraction rhythm depends on specialized conductive fibers that constitute part of the cardiac muscle.

The SA node, located in the right atrium, normally determines the heart rate. It signals the ventricles through the AV node, which telegraphs the message to the ventricular muscle via the Purkinje fibers. These nervous impulses produce rhythmic contraction of the various parts of the heart.

The heart rate is subject to regulation by the autonomic nervous system in response to demands by the organism. Vagal nerve (parasympathetic) stimulation causes a slowing of the cardiac rate, and vigorous vagal stimulation can cause complete stoppage of the heart. Simulation of the sympathetic nervous system produces the opposite effect; it increases the heart rate.

Normal cardiac rhythm may be altered by cardiac disease or injury. The altered patterns of rhythm are referred to as cardiac arrhythmias. The causes of arrhythmias include the development of an ectopic pacemaker, blockage or alterations in the impulse-conducting systems, and abnormal pacemaker rhythms.

If a patient has a history of arrhythmias, the dental hygienist should check the patient's pulse for normal rate and regular rhythm and report the findings to the dentist.

Major drugs

The growing list of drugs now used in the management of the various arrhythmias allows the physician to select the drug best suited for a specific patient's arrhythmia (Table 15-1). Many of the antiarrhythmic drugs are used for a variety of cardiovascular diseases and other conditions as well. The antiarrhythmics are classified according to their mechanism of action. Class I drugs interfere with depolarization and are further subdivided on the basis of their effect on the myocardial action potential. Class IA drugs include quinidine and procainamide, which prolong the action potential. Class IB drugs shorten the action potential and include the local anesthetics lidocaine, tocainide, and mexiletine, as well as the

Table 15-1. Agents commonly used as antiarrhythmics

Drug	Adverse effects	Comments
Quinidine (Cin-Quin, Quinora)	Gastrointestinal symptoms, cinchonism, thrombocytopenia, rashes, hypotension, heart block, or tachyarrhythmias	Discussed in text
Procainamide (Procamide, Pronestyl)	Lupuslike syndrome common, gastrointestinal symptoms, rash, hypotension, arrhythmias, heart block	Same action as quinidine
Lidocaine (Xylocaine)	Drowsiness or agitation, disorientation, coma, seizures, paresthesias, cardiac depression, cardiac arrhythmias	Used as local anesthetic
Phenytoin (Dilantin)	Ataxia, nystagmus, drowsiness, coma, hematologic effects, cardiotoxic effects with rapid IV injection	Used as anticonvulsant
Propranolol (Inderal)	Heart block, heart failure, asthma, hypotension	Used as antihypertensive
Digoxin (Lanoxin)	Gastrointestinal symptoms, neurologic effects (yellow-green vision, halos), arrhythmias	Used to treat congestive heart failure
Bretylium (Bretylol)	Hypotension, bradycardia, PVCs, nausea, vertigo, and syncope	Used for severe ventricular arrhythmias
Verapamil (Calan)	Nausea, constipation, dizziness, hypotension, pulmonary edema, congestive heart failure	Used for angina pectoris and hypertension
Other agent Dipyridamole* (Persantine)		Used prophylactically

*Possibly effective.
PVCs, premature ventricular contractions.

anticonvulsant phenytoin. The class IC drug, fle-
cainide, slows conduction without affecting the
action potential. Class II drugs, the β-adrenergic
blocking drugs, like propranolol and acebutolol,
act to reduce sympathetic effects on the heart.
Class III drugs, used for life-threatening ventricular arrhythmias, include bretylium and amioda-
rone. Class IV drugs include the calcium channel
blocking drugs, verapamil and diltiazem. Digitalis
is also used to treat atrial arrhythmias but it is not
given a class number. Only quinidine and lidocaine are discussed here; the pharmacology of
other antiarrhythmics are presented elsewhere in
this chapter.

Quinidine

Quinidine is a general myocardial depressant that
has both direct and indirect actions on the heart.
Its direct actions include a decrease in myocardial
excitability, conduction velocity, and automatic-
ity. It slows the cardiac rhythm by increasing the
time of the refractory period. The indirect effect
of quinidine is atropine-like; that is, it reduces the
vagal influence on the myocardium. Clinically,
quinidine is used for the treatment and prevention of supraventricular tachyarrhythmias and
ventricular tachycardia.

Oral doses of quinidine can cause nausea and
vomiting. Larger oral doses cause tinnitus, transient deafness, and headache described by the
term "cinchonism." This latter term is derived
from the botanical name for the source of quinidine. The most serious hypersensitivity reaction
associated with the use of quinidine is thrombocytopenia purpura. Given parenterally, quinidine
can produce severe hypotension.

Lidocaine

Lidocaine is a common dental local anesthetic
that is useful parenterally in the treatment of ventricular premature beats and tachycardia. It is
commonly employed in emergency situations
such as myocardial infarction or to control arrhythmias in patients recovering from cardiac surgery. Its short duration of action and lack of hypotensive complications are advantages over other

antiarrhythmic drugs. Doses of lidocaine are
given by intravenous (IV) infusion and adjusted to
control the arrhythmia without the production of
objectionable side effects. Cardiac lidocaine solutions should not be confused with the dental local
anesthetic solution. Additional pharmacology concerning lidocaine is included in Chapter 9 on local
anesthetic drugs.

ANTIANGINAL DRUGS
Angina pectoris

Angina pectoris is a common cardiovascular disease characterized by pain or discomfort in the
chest radiating to the left arm and shoulder. Pain
may also be reported in the neck, back, and lower
jaw. Lower jaw pain can be of such intensity that
it may be confused with a toothache. The cause
of angina is related to a failure of the coronary
arteries to supply a sufficient amount of oxygen to
the myocardium on demand. Anginal pain can be
precipitated by the stress induced by physical exercise and emotional states such as the anxiety
and apprehension generated by a dental appointment.

Major drugs

At one time the nitrites and nitrates were about
the only class of drugs that could effectively relieve the symptoms of angina. More recently, the
β-adrenergic blocking agents and the calcium
channel blocking drugs have added a new dimension to drug therapy for angina. The basic pharmacologic effect of these drugs is to reduce the
workload of the heart, thereby lowering the oxygen requirements of the myocardium that in turn
relieves the painful symptoms of angina. It is important, however, to keep in mind that these
drugs are not curative and the dental hygienist
should be alert to the fact that an angina episode
could occur at any given time. Table 15-2 lists the
major antianginal drugs and some of their more
pertinent characteristics.

Nitrates

Nitroglycerin (glyceryl trinitrate, NTG) is by far
the most frequently used nitrate for the manage-

Table 15-2. Antianginal preparations

Drugs	Route(s)	Onset (min)	Duration (hr)	Comments
Nitrites				
Amyl nitrite	Inhalation	1/2	3–5	To treat acute anginal attacks
Nitrates				
Short acting				
Nitroglycerin (NTG) (Nitrostat) (Nitrolingual)	Sublingual Oral spray	3	10–30	To treat acute anginal attacks
Isosorbide dinitrate	Sublingual	2–5	10–60	To treat acute anginal attacks
Long acting				
Nitroglycerin (Nitro-Bid)	Sustained-release oral tablets	Slow	6–8	Prophylactically
	Ointment		6–8	Prophylactically
	Transdermal patches		12–24	Prophylactically
Isosorbide dinitrate (Isordil, Sorbitrate)	Oral	15–30	4–6	Prophylactically
Pentaerythritol tetranitrate (Peritrate)	Oral	Slow	6–8	Prophylactically
Erythrityl tetranitrate (Cardilate)	Oral	Slow	6–8	Prophylactically
β-blockers				
Propranolol (Inderal)	Oral	30	6–8	Chronic angina
Calcium channel blockers				
Verapamil	Oral	30	6–8	Acute and chronic angina
(Calan, Isoptin)	IV	2		Acute anginal attack

ment of acute anginal episodes and to prevent anginal attacks induced by stress or exercise. Nitroglycerin is thought to relax vascular smooth muscle throughout the body reducing the resistance against which the heart must pump. The reduced workload on the heart is believed to result in a decreased oxygen demand with a relief or reduction of angina pain. Other nitrates are presumed to act in a similar manner. Amyl nitrite, a volatile agent, can be used by inhalation to treat anginal emergency situations.

Nitroglycerin can be used sublingually to treat acute angina attacks. It has a rapid onset by this route, and its effect can last up to 30 minutes. It is available as a sublingual tablet (Nitrostat) or spray (Nitrolingual). The dental office emergency kit should contain one of these. For prophylaxis of anginal attacks, nitroglycerin is available for oral administration in tablet form and for topical administration in ointment and patch form. Patients should be encouraged to bring their own medication to each dental appointment.

An adverse reaction associated with nitroglycerin occurs because it produces vascular relaxation resulting in hypotension and fainting. Hypotension is enhanced by alcohol or hot weather. Severe headaches are also frequently reported. With long-term use, tolerance develops to this effect.

Dental implications

1. Treatment of an acute anginal attack. The patient's own supply of nitroglycerin tablets should be available in case an acute attack occurs.

2. Prevention of anginal attack

a. Sedation. A benzodiazepine may be prescribed to allay anxiety and prevent an acute attack in an anxious patient.

b. Nitroglycerin. Nitroglycerin can be administered before any anxiety-provoking procedure to prevent an anginal attack. For example, the patient can be given nitroglycerin before an injection of local anesthetic.

3. Myocardial infarct. A patient with acute chest pain may be experiencing an anginal attack or a myocardial infarct. If the patient has not been previously diagnosed as having angina, he should be taken to an emergency room for diagnosis.

4. Storage. Since nitroglycerin breaks down easily during storage, it should be stored in its original container out of the reach of heat and moisture. If the bottle is unopened, it is active until the expiration date printed on the bottle. If opened, it should be discarded after 3 months (note the date the bottle is opened on the container).

5. Dosage forms. Since the activity of the nitrates is reduced by stomach acid, routes other than oral are commonly used. When administered sublingually, they cause a burning sensation under the tongue. If used topically, they should be applied with the applicator provided.

Calcium channel blocking agents

The newest drugs approved for use in angina pectoris are termed the calcium channel or slow channel blocking agents. The currently marketed products are verapamil (Calan, Isoptin), diltiazem (Cardiazem) and nifedipine (Procardia, Adalat). Their mechanism of action is related to the inhibition of calcium movement during the contraction of cardiac and vascular smooth muscle. In addition to their use in angina, these drugs are also used in the treatment of cardiac arrhythmias and hypertension. Adverse effects include dizziness, weakness, constipation and hypotension. Nifedipine has been associated with gingival hyperplasia and dysgeusia. The hyperplasia is similar to that produced by phenytoin and it too is amendable to scrupulous oral hygiene. Dental patients receiving these drugs should be managed like other anginal patients. Additional attention to oral hygiene is also indicated.

β-adrenergic blockers

Three marketed β-adrenergic blocking drugs, propranolol (Inderal), nadolol (Corgard), and atenolol (Tenormin) are used in the treatment of angina pectoris. These drugs block the β-response to catecholamine stimulation thereby reducing both the chronotropic and inotropic effects. The net result is a reduced myocardial oxygen demand. β-adrenergic blockers are effective in reducing both exercise- and stress-induced anginal episodes. Dosage is adjusted to the patient's requirements with nadolol given on a once-a-day basis. Adverse effects include bradycardia, congestive heart failure, headache, dry mouth, blurred vision, and unpleasant dreams.

ANTIHYPERTENSIVE AGENTS
Hypertension

Hypertension is the most common of all cardiovascular diseases, affecting some 60 million Americans. It is usually defined as a blood pressure greater than 140/90 mm Hg, although this figure is arbitrary. It produces few if any symptoms until some damage has occurred to the "target organs" such as the heart, kidney, brain, or retina. A sustained elevated blood pressure eventually damages the body's organs, so that untreated hypertensive patients are more likely to have kidney and heart disease and cerebrovascular accidents. Fortunately, early detection and treatment with drug therapy reduces the possibility of damage to vital organs and extends the patient's lifetime.

Hypertensive disease is generally divided into the following categories based on the cause or progression of the disease:

1. Essential hypertension. Approximately 90% of the diagnosed hypertensive patients have essential or primary hypertension. In this case the cause is unknown. Antihypertensive agents are used to control the elevated blood pressure in this group of patients.

2. Secondary hypertension. In approximately 10% of hypertensive patients, the cause can be associated with a specific disease process involving the endocrine or renal systems. For example, renal hypertension can result from a narrowed renal artery. This category is termed secondary hypertension. The hypertension in this case can be eliminated by removing the cause, for example, surgically correcting the narrowing in the renal artery.

3. Malignant hypertension. The third group of hypertensive patients are those with malignant hypertension. Blood pressures are very high or rapidly rising, and there is usually evidence of retinal and renal damage. The small number of patients in this group must be treated aggressively with antihypertensive agents. Malignant hypertension can develop in about 5% of patients with primary or secondary hypertension.

Pharmacologic management of hypertension involves a stepped-care approach as diastolic pressures range above 90 mm Hg. In step 1, therapy is initiated with the smallest effective dose of either a thiazide diuretic or a β-blocking drug. Diuretics are usually preferred in the over 50-age group and in patients with complicating periph-

eral vascular disease or pulmonary disorders. β-blockers are used frequently for those under age 50 and in patients with ischemic heart disease. Step 2 therapy is used when maximal doses of the step 1 drugs fail to control hypertension. Step 2 drugs can be either a thiazide or β-adrenergic blocker depending on which of these drugs was initially selected in step 1. Angiotensin-converting enzyme inhibitors may be substituted as required. Step 3 drugs include a direct-acting vasodilator like hydralazine or minoxidil, if additional drugs are required to control the hypertension. Step 4 care includes the addition of a neuronal blocker such as guanethidine. Calcium channel blocking drugs have been used as step 2 or step 3 drugs, but can be the only drug used for a hypertensive patient. Some have suggested that an α-antagonist such as prazosin or a centrally acting agent like clonidine may be suitable alternatives to step 1 drugs. The exact combination of drugs selected depends not only on the control of hypertension, but also on the patient's tolerance to the side effects. It may not be unusual to see a hypertensive patient taking several drugs for adequate management.

The control of blood pressure is an interplay of many factors and treatment of hypertension is directed at some of the forces that alter blood pressure. Fig. 15-1 illustrates these factors. Both the cardiac output and the peripheral resistance determine blood pressure. Since the sympathetic nervous system can affect the peripheral resistance, agents that block the sympathetic nervous system reduce blood pressure through their effect on peripheral resistance.

The blood pressure of each hypertensive patient seen in the dental office should be measured and recorded. Only with a serial record can the degree of control be evaluated. Also, because control is so important to patient health, patients should be questioned about their compliance. It is of little use for a patient to have clean teeth and a restored mouth if that patient has a fatal myocardial infarction resulting from untreated hypertension.

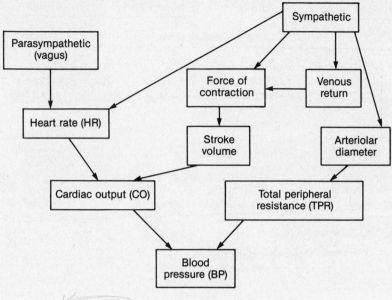

Fig. 15-1. Factors controlling blood pressure.

Major drugs

Table 15-3 lists the antihypertensive agents and their various sites of action and side effects. The agents marked with an asterisk are discussed in the text. Antihypertensive drugs may contain one or more than one constituent.

Diuretic agents

Thiazide diuretics. The thiazide diuretics are among the most commonly used agents for the treatment of hypertension. Many patients with mild hypertension may be treated solely with these agents. Even when other antihypertensives are used, they are frequently used in combination with the thiazides. Although a large number of thiazide and thiazide-like diuretics are currently available, these agents all have essentially the same pharmacologic effects. Their major pharmacologic effect is diuresis produced by the inhibition of sodium reabsorption in the distal tubule of the kidney. Since chloride ion and water accompany the sodium, diuresis results. Because an in-

creased amount of sodium is present at the site of sodium-potassium exchange, there is also an increase in potassium excretion.

The antihypertensive effect of the thiazide diuretics is believed to be related to the reduction in extracellular fluid volume because of its natriuretic action. Volume reduction is associated with a reduction in cardiac output, and peripheral resistance is lowered in response.

The adverse reactions most commonly associated with the thiazides include hypokalemia, anorexia, hyperuricemia, and hyperglycemia. Rarely, they have been associated with oral lichenoid eruptions indistinguishable from lichen planus. This condition is reversible on discontinuation (at least 1 month).

Because the thiazides can cause hypokalemia, they can sensitize the myocardium to the development of arrhythmias. This is a problem especially in patients taking digitalis or epinephrine, which may also cause arrhythmias. The thiazide diuretics also potentiate the action

Table 15-3. Mechanism of action and adverse effects of antihypertensive drugs

Drug	Mechanism of action	Frequent adverse effects
Diuretics		
Thiazides	Sodium excretion and volume reduction	Hyperuricemia, hypokalemia, hyperglycemia
Hydrochlorothiazide (Dyazide)		
Loop diuretics		
Furosemide (Lasix)		Like thiazides and profound diuresis and electrolyte imbalance
Potassium-conserving diuretics		
Spironolactone (Aldactone)	Antagonizes aldosterone	Gastrointestinal disturbances, dry mouth
Sympatholytics		
Centrally acting	Act in the CNS to reduce sympathetic tone	
Clonidine (Catapres)		Sedation, dizziness, constipation, dry mouth, parotid gland swelling and pain
Methyldopa (Aldomet)		Like clonidine plus positive Coombs test (hemolytic anemia)
Adrenergic receptor blockers		
Prazosin (Minipress)	α-receptor blocker	Sudden syncope, dizziness and vertigo, palpitation, edema, dyspnea, headache and depression, drowsiness, weakness, anticholinergic effects
Propranolol (Inderal)	β-receptor blocker	Bradycardia, reduced exercise tolerance, congestive heart failure, gastrointestinal disturbances, increased airway resistance, rare blood dyscrasias and other allergic disorders
Labetalol (Trandate)	α- and β-receptor blocker	Similar to other adrenergic blockers
Neuronal blockers	Block release of norepinephrine from sympathetic nerve ending; reduced amount of norepinephrine stored in synaptic vesicles	
Guanethidine (Ismelin)		Orthostatic hypotension, diarrhea, may aggravate bronchial asthma, bradycardia, inhibition of ejaculation, sodium and water retention

Table 15-3. Mechanism of action and adverse effects of antihypertensive drugs—cont'd

Drug	Mechanism of action	Frequent adverse effects
Reserpine (Serpasil)		Psychic depression, nightmares, nasal stuffiness, drowsiness, gastrointestinal disturbances, bradycardia, impotence
Ganglionic blockers Mecamylamine (Inversine) Trimethaphan (Arfonad)	Block sympathetic ganglia	Tachycardia, xerostomia, severe postural hypotension, constipation, urinary retention, paralytic ileus
Direct-acting vasodilators Hydralazine (Apresoline)	Produce arteriole dilation by a direct effect	Gastrointestinal disturbances, tachycardia, aggravation of angina, headache and dizziness, fluid retention, nasal congestion, rashes and other allergic disorders, lupuslike syndrome
Diazoxide (Hyperstat)		Sodium and water retention, hypotension, arrhythmias
Sodium nitroprusside (Nipride)		Nausea, retching, diaphoresis, headache, palpitations, dizziness
Calcium channel blockers Nifedipine (Procardia)	Blocks calcium ion movement	Edema, hypotension, dizziness, nausea, flushing, impotence, headache, congestive heart failure
Angiotensin-converting enzyme (ACE) inhibitors Captopril (Capoten) Enalapril (Vasotec)	Antagonizes renin-angiotensin system	Polyuria, neutropenia, pruritus, tachycardia, gastric irritation, dysgeusia, aphthous ulcers and dry mouth

of the other antihypertensives, leading to hypotension.

Loop diuretics. The loop diuretics include furosemide (Lasix), ethacrynic acid (Edecrin), and bumetanide (Bumex). These are high-potency diuretics that can be used when rapid diuresis is required, as in an emergency. Furosemide is also used in the management of the hypertensive patient. The principal site of action of the loop diuretics is on the ascending limb of Henle's loop with some effect on the distal tubule as well. As is the case with the thiazides, the main effect is to inhibit the reabsorption of sodium with a con-

current loss of fluids. As with use of the thiazide diuretics, excessive loss of potassium can occur. Side effects and drug interactions are similar to the thiazide diuretics also.

Potassium-conserving diuretics. The renin-angiotensin system is a complex but important homeostatic mechanism involved with sodium ion and circulatory volume regulation. Renin catalyzes the conversion of angiotensinogen to angiotensin I (Fig. 15-2). A second enzyme, angiotensin-converting enzyme, converts angiotensin I to angiotensin II, which then acts to increase peripheral resistance. In addition, angiotensin II

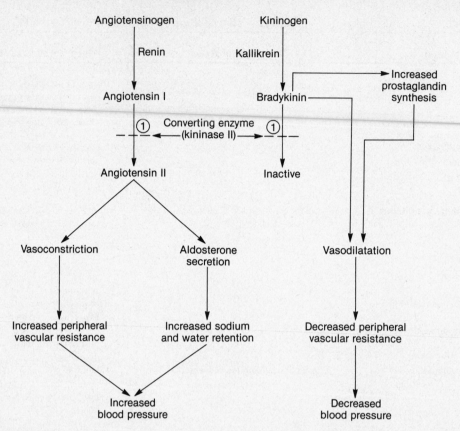

Fig. 15-2. Site of action of angiotensin-converting enzyme (ACE) inhibitors *(1)*. (Adapted from Katsung, B.G.: Basic and clinical pharmacology, ed. 2, Los Altos, Calif., 1984, Lange Medical Publications.)

stimulates the adrenal cortex to release aldosterone, which also increases water retention. All of these events serve to increase sodium and fluid volume retention and hence blood pressure.

Spironolactone (Aldactone) is a diuretic that is chemically similar to and competitively antagonizes the action of aldosterone. The result is sodium excretion and loss of fluid volume through the attendant diuresis. However, potassium ion is conserved as some of the potassium is reabsorbed at the expense of sodium in the sodium-potassium exchange system in the distal tubule. Triamterene (Dyrenium) is also a potassium-conserving diuretic that acts by a direct effect on the kidney tubule rather than as an aldosterone antagonist.

The diuresis and potassium conservation that occurs resembles that of spironolactone. Because these diuretics have a different site and mechanism of action, they can logically be combined with the thiazides in the hypertensive patient. This combination is designed to reduce the amount of potassium lost and prevent hypokalemia. The combination of triamterene and hydrochlorothiazide (Dyazide) is one of the most frequently used preparations.

Potassium (K) salts

Potassium is involved in many important physiologic processes, such as nerve impulses, contraction of smooth, cardiac, and skeletal muscles, and maintenance of normal renal function, to name a few. It is indicated in the treatment of hypokalemia, either from inadequate dietary intake or that produced by diuretics. It is contraindicated in patients with severe renal impairment or those receiving potassium-sparing diuretics. Its most common adverse reactions are nausea and abdominal discomfort caused by gastrointestinal irritation. It can produce gastrointestinal lesions from the esophagus to the lower gastrointestinal tract. Liquid preparations, although less palatable than the solid dosage forms, are less likely to produce gastrointestinal problems. Diluting the liquid potassium or taking the solid dosage forms with water and food can also reduce symptoms. Patients taking potassium supplements, such as Slo-K or Micro-K, should be questioned about diuretic use and the possibility of cardiovascular diseases when the hygienist takes a drug history.

Centrally acting drugs

Clonidine (Catapres) is a commonly encountered central nervous system (CNS)–mediated antihypertensive drug. Clonidine reduces peripheral resistance through a CNS-mediated action on the α-receptor. Stimulation of postsynaptic α_1-receptors (Fig. 15-3) in the vasomotor center and of the hypothalamic presynaptic α_2-receptor results in a decrease of sympathetic outflow. Thus clonidine reduces heart rate, cardiac output, and total peripheral resistance. It is indicated for the management of essential hypertension and can be administered orally or by a transdermal patch.

Adverse effects include a rather high incidence of sedation, dizziness, and xerostomia (40%). Parotid gland swelling and pain have been noted in a small number of patients. Other side effects include an unpleasant taste, possibly related to the xerostomia. Rapid elevation of blood pressure has occurred with abrupt discontinuation. CNS depressants employed in dental conscious-sedation techniques may contribute to postural hypotension when used in a patient taking clonidine.

Two other centrally acting antihypertensive drugs, methyldopa (Aldomet) and guanabenz (Wytensin), are also available for use. Adverse ef-

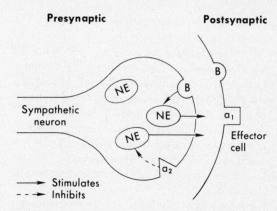

Fig. 15-3. Simplified schematic view of the adrenergic nerve ending showing that norepinephrine (NE) is released from its storage granules when the nerve is stimulated and enters the synaptic cleft to bind to α_1- and β-receptors on the effector cell (postsynaptic). In addition, a short feedback loop exists, in which NE binds to α_2- and β-receptors on the neuron (presynaptic), either to inhibit or to stimulate further release. (From Kaplan, N.M.: Systemic hypertension: therapy. In Braunwald, E., editor: Heart disease: a textbook of cardiovascular medicine, vol. 1, Philadelphia, 1980, W.B. Saunders Co.)

fects and indications for use are similar to clonidine. The centrally acting antihypertensive drugs may be combined with a diuretic in essential hypertension management.

Adrenergic blocking drugs

A large number of drugs with antagonist actions for the peripheral α- and β-adrenergic receptors have been developed for the management of hypertension as well as other cardiovascular diseases. In fact, these drugs have had a significant impact on the control of hypertension. Two subtypes of α-receptors, α_1 and α_2, have been identified (Fig. 15-3). The α_1-receptors, located on postsynaptic receptor tissues, are responsible for producing vasoconstriction and increasing peripheral resistance. α_2-receptors are located on the presynaptic tissue sites and their stimulation inhibits the feedback release of norepinephrine. This latter action is necessary to maintain sympathetic tone and blood pressure.

β-receptors are subtyped into β_1 and β_2

Read p. 183 184

groups. β_1-receptor stimulation is associated with an increase in heart rate, cardiac contractility, and AV conduction. β_2-receptors are responsible for vasodilation in skeletal muscles and bronchodilation in the pulmonary tissues. Stimulation of a presynaptic β-receptor is believed to cause release of the neurotransmitter norepinephrine. Thus drugs with adrenergic receptor blocking activity can influence many cardiovascular parameters involved with blood pressure regulation. These receptors are initially discussed in Chapter 5.

α-Adrenergic blockers. The most commonly encountered α-adrenergic receptor blocking drug is prazosin (Minipress). It lowers blood pressure by a peripheral blocking action on the α_1-receptor. Since prazosin does not affect the α_2-receptor, the normal feedback system remains functional thereby avoiding the reflex tachycardia often associated with the older types of α-adrenergic blocking drugs. Prazosin is used for moderate to severe hypertension but is seldom used as a single agent because of fluid retention. For this reason, it is often used in combination with a thiazide diuretic. A similar-type drug, terazosin (Hytrin) is also available for use.

The first dose of prazosin can produce orthostatic hypertension with syncope. Common side effects include dizziness, headache, weakness, and nausea. Dry mouth, orthostatic hypotension, and fluid retention can also occur. As with other antihypertensive drugs, drugs used in conscious sedation techniques in dentistry may contribute to the incidence of orthostatic hypotension.

β-Adrenergic blockers. Presently there are nine β-adrenergic blocking drugs approved for use in the management of hypertension (Table 15-4). The nonselective β-adrenergic receptor blocking drugs, like propranolol, block both types of β-receptors. The selective β-adrenergic receptor blocking drugs, like metoprolol, selectively block the β_1-receptor in usual doses. At larger doses, receptor selectivity disappears. Pindolol and acebutolol have partial agonist activity and cause some β-stimulation while blocking catecholamine action. The selective blockers have some advantages in patients who may have preexisting bronchospastic disease. Labetalol has both β- and α-blocking action.

The exact mechanism of the antihypertensive effects of the β-adrenergic blockers is still somewhat unclear because of their wide-ranging pharmacologic activities. Possible explanations for their hypotensive action include (1) a decrease in cardiac output, (2) a lowering of plasma renin levels, (3) a reduction in plasma volume and venous return, (4) a CNS effect, and (5) a reduction in peripheral resistance. These drugs are often used as step 1 drugs either as a single drug or in combination with other antihypertensive drugs. Doses must be individualized for each patient.

α- and β-Adrenergic blocking drug (labetalol). Labetalol (Trandate, Normodyne) is a nonselective β-adrenergic receptor blocking drug that also has α-receptor blocking activity. In addition to the typical β-adrenoceptor blocking effects, labetalol also reduces peripheral resistance through its α-blocking action. Labetalol is used either alone or in combinations with the diuretics. Side effects and drug interactions are similar to the β- and α-adrenergic blockers.

Neuronal blockers

Guanethidine. Guanethidine (Ismelin) acts by blocking the release of norepinephrine from the sympathetic nerve endings. It also depletes the amount of norepinephrine stored in synaptic ves-

Table 15-4. β-Adrenergic receptor blocking drugs

Nonselective β-blockers	Selective (β_1) β-blockers
propranolol (Inderal)	metoprolol (Lopressor)
timolol (Blocadren)	atenolol (Tenormin)
nadolol (Corgard)	acebutolol (Tenormin)
pindolol (Visken)	esmolol (Brevibloc)

α- and β-blocker
labetalol (Normodyne, Trandate)

icles. Both actions decrease the amount of norepinephrine that can be released with sympathetic stimulation, thereby reducing sympathetic
nervous system tone and decreasing blood pressure (see Fig. 15-1). Guanethidine has a delayed
onset of action, and its effects can persist for at
least 2 weeks after it is discontinued.

Guanethidine causes severe postural and exer-
tional hypotension, which is exacerbated by any-
thing that causes vasodilation, such as warm
weather, ingestion of alcohol, or exercise. Hypotension is most severe after the patient has spent
several hours in a supine position, for example, in
the dental chair. Other adverse reactions include
diarrhea, interference with ejaculation, and cardiac problems. Muscle weakness has also been reported.

Reserpine. Originally employed as a tranquilizer, reserpine currently is used in low doses as
an antihypertensive agent. Like guanethidine, reserpine depletes norepinephrine from the sym-
pathic nerve endings and can accumulate in the
body. Adverse reactions include diarrhea, bad
dreams, sedation, and even psychic depression
leading to suicide. Reserpine increases the production of stomach acid and aggravates peptic ulcer. It can also produce glactorrhea, breast en-
gorgement, and gynecomastia.

Vasodilators

Hydralazine. Hydralazine (Apresoline) exerts
its antihypertensive effect by acting directly on
the arterioles to reduce peripheral resistance. At
the same time a rise in heart rate and output occurs. Propranolol is often administered concurrently to reduce the reflex tachycardia and increased cardiac output. Hydralazine is often used
in combination with the thiazides or other antihypertensive agents. Both diastolic and systolic
blood pressures are reduced proportionately, and
there is little orthostatic hypotension. The most
commonly reported side effects associated with
hydralazine are cardiac arrhythmias, angina,
headache, and dizziness. A serious toxic reaction
produces symptoms like those of systemic lupus
erythematosus (lupuslike reaction).

Calcium channel blocking drugs

The calcium channel blocking drugs, verapamil
(Isoptin, Calan), nifedipine (Procardia, Adalat),
and diltiazem (Cardiazem) have all been used in
the treatment of hypertension. These drugs block
the movement of calcium ion across vascular
smooth muscle membrane at the "slow channel"
entry site for calcium. The net result is a relaxation of vascular smooth muscle and a decrease in
peripheral resistance. They also affect calcium ion
movement in cardiac muscle, which accounts for
their use in angina. Nifedipine, however, has its
action on vascular smooth muscle and is the primary choice for hypertension for this particular
group of drugs. The other two drugs, verapamil
and diltiazem, have been used in certain cases of
hypertension but only nifedipine is approved for
this indication. Side effects associated with nifedipine include dizziness, lightheadedness, nausea,
weakness, flushing, hypotension, headache, and
peripheral edema. Gingival hyperplasia and dysgeusia have been reported with the use of nifedipine.

Nifedipine has been used as a step 3 drug in
combination with a β-adrenergic blocking drug, a
thiazide diuretic, or one of the centrally acting
agents.

Angiotensin-converting enzyme (ACE) inhibitors

The latest group of drugs to be added to the antihypertensive category are the angiotensin-converting enzyme (ACE) inhibitors, captopril (Ca-
poten), enalapril (Vasotec), and lisinopril (Prinivil,
Zestril). Their mechanism involves inhibition of
the conversion of angiotensin I to angiotensin II
(see Fig. 15-2). Angiotensin II increases blood
pressure by producing vasoconstriction leading to
an increase in resistance, and by increasing aldosterone secretion leading to sodium and water retention. ACE inhibitors, by blocking the conversion of angiotensin I to angiotensin II, reduce
blood pressure. Cardiac output and heart rate are
relatively unaffected. Side effects reported with
the ACE inhibitors include neutropenia, pancytopenia, proteinuria, altered sense of taste, al-

lergic skin reactions, drug fever, and hypotension. The ACE inhibitors may be used alone as a step 1 drug or in combination with a β-blocker or thiazide diuretic. These drugs are becoming very popular and the dental hygienist will treat many patients taking these agents.

Dental implications

Although the antihypertensives cause a variety of adverse reactions, many of them exert similar actions that can alter dental treatment. Since antihypertensive medications can cause hypotension or be unable to control a patient's hypertension, the blood pressure of each patient should be measured on each visit to the dental office. Not uncommonly, a patient whose blood pressure is "normal" on one visit might be found to be severely hypertensive on a subsequent visit. Each of the following adverse effects can alter a patient's dental treatment:

1. Xerostomia. A dry mouth is an adverse reaction frequently associated with several of the antihypertensives. If the dental hygienist notices this effect, it is imperative to question the patient about methods used to alleviate this discomfort.

2. Dysgeusia. An altered sense of taste may or may not be related to xerostomia.

3. Gingival hyperplasia. When a drug, such as nifedipine, produces hyperplasia, meticulous oral hygiene and frequent recall appointments are necessary.

4. Orthostatic hypotension. When a patient has been in a supine position and is suddenly raised to an upright position, there can be a sudden fall in blood pressure. This is termed orthostatic hypotension. Patients taking antihypertensive agents who have been lying down for some time should be raised from that position slowly. Guanethidine causes this problem frequently; other agents produce variable amounts of orthostatic hypotension.

5. Constipation. Opioids can produce additive constipating effects with the antihypertensives, which cause constipation. A stool softener or laxative may be considered if an opioid is prescribed for a patient receiving antihypertensive medication.

6. CNS sedation. Additive sedation with other CNS depressants such as opioids or benzodiazepines can occur. Also the psychic depression caused by the antihypertensive agents can lead to suicide attempts, so the dosage of potentially lethal medication prescribed in the dental office should be limited if depression is evident.

ANTIHYPERLIPIDEMICS
Drugs for hyperlipoproteinemia

Elevation of plasma lipid concentrations above accepted normal values has been identified as a significant risk factor in the development of arteriosclerosis. Cholesterol and other plasma lipids are transported in the blood in the form of protein complexes (lipoproteins) to make them more soluble in the plasma. Low density lipoproteins (LDL) carry the greatest concentration of cholesterol, whereas high density lipoproteins (HDL) have the lowest cholesterol content. Therapy of hyperlipoproteinemia is directed at lowering the level of LDL cholesterol in those patients who have not responded to other forms of treatment and are still at high risk for the complications of arteriosclerosis. Drugs are available that may provide some benefit in reducing hyperlipoproteinemia, but the long-term benefits remain to be established. The specific type of hyperlipoproteinemia must be identified before starting drug treatment.

Among the drugs used in the treatment of hyperlipoproteinemia are the bile acid binding resins, cholestyramine (Questran) and colestipol (Colestid). The bound bile acids are made insoluble and are lost through the gastrointestinal tract. These drugs lower cholesterol concentrations because cholesterol is required for the synthesis of the new bile acids. Gemfibrozil (Lopid) is frequently used to lower cholesterol levels but an exact mechanism of action remains to be determined. This drug causes fewer gastrointestinal complaints than the bile acid binding drugs, but it can promote gallstone formation. It has been suggested that niacin (nicotinic acid) in therapeutic doses—as opposed to nutritional doses—lowers cholesterol levels by reducing LDL synthesis. At these larger doses, niacin commonly produces flushing and dry skin. Lovastatin (Mevacor) is the most recent drug approved for treatment of hyperlipoproteinemia. Lovastatin reduces cholesterol synthesis by inhibition of HMG-CoA reductase, the rate-limiting enzyme in cholesterol synthesis. Adverse effects include gastrointestinal complaints, myositis, some hepatotoxicity, and lens opacities. Other drugs have also been used in an effort to lower plasma lipid levels; these include neomycin, probucol (Lorelco), clofibrate (Atromid S), and dextrothyroxine (Choloxin).

ANTICOAGULANTS

Hemostasis is a mechanism designed to prevent the loss of blood after injury to the blood vessel.

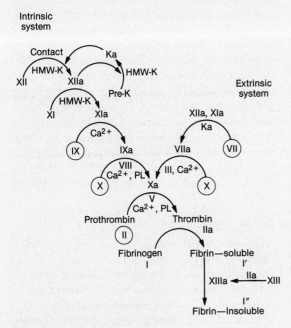

Fig. 15-4. Intrinsic and extrinsic systems of blood coagulation. The circled clotting factors (II [prothrombin], VII [extrinsic], IX [intrinsic], and X) are dependent on vitamin K for their synthesis. (Reproduced, with permission, from O'Reilly, R.A.: Anticoagulant, antithrombotic, and thrombolytic drugs. In Gilman, A.G., et al., editors: Goodman and Gilman's The Pharmacological Basis of Therapeutics, ed. 7, New York, 1985, Macmillan, Inc.)

The leaking vessel is plugged by a complicated process of clot formation. In the presence of a vascular injury the entire clotting mechanism is initiated. Thromboplastin, factors V, VII, and X, and calcium ions form prothrombin, thrombin, and finally fibrinogen and fibrin. The fibrin, along with vascular spasms, platelets, and red blood cells, quickly forms the clot.

If the blood vessel's interior remains smooth, circulating blood does not clot. However, if internal injury to the vessel occurs and a roughened surface develops, intravascular clotting will take place. This process involves an intrinsic prothrombin activator that includes a platelet factor, factors V and factors VIII through XII, and calcium ions. The prothrombin activator formerly called thromboplastin converts prothrombin to thrombin. Thrombin then converts fibrinogen to fibrin, and there is clot formation (Fig. 15-4).

Many of the factors required in the clotting process are synthesized by normal metabolic processes. Factors VIII, IX, and X and prothrombin require vitamin K for synthesis. One mechanism for producing an anticoagulant effect is by interference with vitamin K.

Uses

In certain disease processes intravascular clots occur. These clots or thrombi may break loose, forming emboli that lodge in the smaller vessels to the major organs such as the heart, brain, and lungs, producing severe and even fatal thromboembolic diseases. Anticoagulant therapy attempts to reduce the incidence of intravascular clotting and prevent life-threatening situations. Each person's anticoagulant therapy must be adjusted to suit that patient's needs. If the dose of the anticoagulant is too large, hemorrhage may occur. If the dose is too small, the danger of embolism remains.

Major drugs
Heparin

Heparin is one of the most commonly employed anticoagulant agents. Because it must be given by injection and cannot be used orally, its use is limited to hospitalized patients. It is the first anticoagulant given to hospitalized patients with clotting problems. Patients who might receive heparin are those with myocardial infarction or thrombophlebitis. Patients who have an overdose of heparin are treated with protamine sulfate, which immediately reverses its anticoagulant effects.

Coumarins

The coumarins, most commonly warfarin (Coumadin), are also referred to as the oral anticoagulants. These agents act as vitamin K antimetabolites and therefore interfere with the synthesis of factors VII, IX, and X and prothrombin (II) (Fig. 15-4, circled). There is a delay in the onset of action until the blood level of these agents builds up and the usual plasma stores of the clotting factors are depleted. Because the coumarins are orally effective and less expensive than heparin, they are used in long-term treatment of thromboembolic diseases such as thrombophlebitis and myocardial infarction.

The most common adverse effect associated with the oral anticoagulants is hemorrhage. Because of the narrow therapeutic index, serious reactions can easily occur. Another problem with these agents is drug interactions. Their most serious drug interaction is with the salicylates such as aspirin. Patients taking warfarin should not be given salicylates because bleeding episodes or fatal hemorrhages can result.

Aspirin interacts with warfarin in several ways. First, aspirin causes hypoprothrombinemia and alters platelet adhesiveness (see Chapter 6). These effects in themselves reduce clotting ability. Also, warfarin is more than 99% bound to plasma proteins and therefore is largely inactive. Only free drug (less than 1%) possesses the pharmacologic effect of decreased clotting. Warfarin and aspirin compete for the same plasma protein binding site. Aspirin displaces the bound warfarin on the plasma protein, thereby increasing the proportion of free (unbound) warfarin and so its activity. Even a small increase in free warfarin can lead to dire consequences—including hemorrhage.

The antibiotics can also potentiate the effect of the coumarins. The antibiotics reduce the flora in the gastrointestinal tract, which normally synthesize vitamin K. This results in a decrease in vitamin K absorption. Since warfarin also inhibits vitamin K, there can be an added anticoagulant effect.

The effect of the coumarins may be reduced by the barbiturates, especially phenobarbital, because phenobarbital induces the liver microsomal enzymes that would normally destroy the anticoagulant.

Other anticoagulants

Enzymes are sometimes used in the therapy of deep vein thrombosis, arterial thrombosis, pulmonary embolism, and acute coronary artery thrombosis associated with myocardial infarction. Examples would include streptokinase (Streptase, Kabikinase), urokinase (Abokinase), and the recombinant tissue-type plasminogen activator, alteplase (tPA, Activase). These may appropriately be termed thrombolytic drugs because they promote the conversion of plasminogen to plasmin, the natural clot resolving enzyme. They are usually administered by direct vessel perfusion to the clot site. Considerable technical skill and immediate treatment of the thrombus is required for satisfactory results. Since streptokinase is a protein, allergic reactions can occur: hemorrhage may result from the use of any of these drugs and they are contraindicated in patients at risk for hemorrhage.

Dental implications

1. Bleeding. Although many surgical procedures can be carried out on a patient receiving therapeutic doses of anticoagulants, it is wise to check with the prescribing physician concerning special considerations or contraindications.

2. Analgesics. Aspirin and aspirin-containing products are absolutely contraindicated in patients taking warfarin. Acetaminophen or any opiod alone or together, may be substituted if analgesia is desired.

PENTOXIFYLLINE (TRENTAL) Skip

Pentoxifylline is a dimethylxanthine that improves blood flow by its hemorrheologic effects, which include lowering blood viscosity and improving the flexibility of red blood cells. It is indicated for intermittent claudication produced by chronic occlusive artery disease of the limbs. Side effects associated with pentoxifylline include cardiovascular and gastric symptoms. Dry mouth, bad taste, excessive salivation, and swollen neck glands have infrequently been reported.

REVIEW QUESTIONS

1. Describe some contraindications to dental treatment that are associated with the cardiovascular system.
2. Describe the major pharmacologic effect associated with digoxin.
3. Describe the adverse effect associated with the digitalis glycosides that can be additive with epinephrine. Name another agent that would exacerbate this side effect.
4. Explain the rationale for determining the location of a patient's angina medication before rendering dental treatment. Tell what other measures might be taken in ambulatory patients to minimize the chance for problems.

5. For each of the following drugs state their mechanism of action and two major side effects:
   a. Hydrochlorothiazide
   b. Clonidine
   c. Propranolol
   d. Prazosin
   e. Captopril
6. Describe the alterations in dental treatment required for each of the following adverse reactions:
   a. Orthostatic hypotension
   b. Xerostomia
   c. Psychic depression
   d. Gingival hyperplasia
7. Explain the procedures that must be followed when treating a patient taking warfarin. Name one drug that should not be administered to such a patient for pain relief. State the laboratory test used to follow warfarin therapy.
8. Explain the use of diuretics for the cardiovascular patient. Name their major side effect and state a management strategy.

Anticonvulsants

EPILEPSY   Neurological disorder

The epilepsies are a group of disorders that involves a chronic stereotyped recurrent attack of involuntary behavior or experience or changes in neurologic function. Each episode is termed a seizure. The seizure may be accompanied by motor activity such as convulsions or by other neurologic changes (e.g., sensory or emotional). Since seizure disorders are estimated to affect between 0.5% and 2% of the population, the dental hygienist is likely to encounter a patient with a history of epilepsy. Because these agents are administered chronically, their adverse reactions must be considered when these patients are receiving dental treatment.

Epilepsy has many etiologies including infection, trauma, toxicity to exogenous agents, genetic or birth influences, circulatory disturbances, metabolic or nutritional alterations, neoplasms, hereditary factors, fevers, and degenerative diseases. The majority of epileptic patients have idiopathic epilepsy, a term used when the cause is unknown.

Epilepsy has been classified based on causes, symptoms, duration, precipitating factors, postictal state, and aura. Currently, the most useful method of classification uses the clinical symptoms as its basis. The classification of seizures developed by the International League Against Epilepsy and the World Health Organization divides seizure types into primary generalized, partial, secondary generalized, and unclassified epilepsies. The more common seizure types are briefly discussed. The treatable epilepsies, their symptoms and drug treatment, have been reviewed[1,2] in 1983.

Primary generalized seizures

The primary generalized seizures are divided into two large groups: absence and tonic-clonic types. Consciousness is lost in both types. In absence seizures there are very short periods of unconsciousness with little movement, whereas in tonic-clonic seizures longer periods of unconsciousness with major movement of large muscle groups of the entire body occur. Management of seizures are discussed at the end of this chapter.

Absence seizures (petit mal). The symptoms of absence seizures include a brief (few seconds) loss of consciousness with characteristic electroencephalographic (EEG) waves. Absence seizures usually begin during childhood and disappear in middle age. The patient is usually unaware that these seizures are occurring and body tone is not lost. There is no aura or postictal state, and the patient quickly returns to normal activity. The drug of choice in the treatment of typical absence seizures is either ethosuximide or valproic acid (Table 16-1).

Absence seizures pose no management problems for the dental hygienist. The hygienist's main concern when treating patients with absence seizures is the adverse reactions that can occur from long-term administration of the drugs used to treat the disease.

Tonic-clonic (grand mal). Generalized tonic-clonic seizures include loss of consciousness and major motor activity. The seizure begins by the body becoming rigid and the patient falling to the floor. Urination, apnea, and a cry may be present. Tonic rigidity is followed by clonic jerking of the face, limbs, and body. Finally the patient becomes limp and comatose. Consciousness is grad-

Table 16-1. Anticonvulsant drugs of choice

Seizure disorder	Drugs	
	First choice	Alternatives
Tonic-clonic (grand mal)	Phenytoin (Dilantin) Carbamazepine (Tegretol) Valproic acid (Depakene)	Phenobarbital (Luminal) Primidone (Mysoline)
Partial, including secondary generalized	Carbamazepine (Tegretol) Phenytoin (Dilantin)	Phenobarbital (Luminal) Primidone (Mysoline)
Absence (petit mal)	Ethosuximide (Zarontin) Valproic acid (Depakote)	Clonazepam (Clonopin)
Atypical absence, myoclonic, atonic	Valproic acid (Depakote)	Clonazepam (Clonopin)
Status epilepticus	Diazepam (Valium)	Phenytoin (Dilantin) Phenobarbital (Luminal)

ually returned, with postictal confusion, headache, and drowsiness. Some patients experience prodromal periods of varying durations, but a true aura does not occur. Because this seizure type involves the violent movement of major muscle groups, it is more likely to result in serious injury to the patient. Phenytoin, phenobarbital, and carbamazepine are used to treat grand mal seizures.

Continuous tonic-clonic seizures, also termed status epilepticus seizures, are seizures that last 30 minutes or longer or reoccur before the end of the postictal period of the previous seizure. Since this is an emergency situation, rapid therapy is required especially if the seizure activity has produced hypoxia. Parenteral benzodiazepines are the drugs of choice to control this seizure type (see Chapter 10).

Partial (focal) epilepsies

Partial epilepsies involve activation of only part of the brain and the location of the activity determines the clinical manifestation. When consciousness is not impaired, the attack is called an elementary (simple) partial attack. When consciousness is impaired, the attack is termed a complex partial attack. The complex seizures are also called psychomotor, temporal-lobe seizures, fugues epileptiques, and Dammer attacken. In contrast to absence seizures that last a few seconds, these complex partial seizures last several minutes. Some patients with complex partial seizures have an aura and full consciousness is slow to return. For the partial epilepsies carbamazepine, phenytoin, phenobarbital, and primidone are used.

DRUG THERAPY OF EPILEPTIC PATIENTS

Drug therapy of the epileptic patient can also produce problems. Anticonvulsant agents are central nervous system (CNS) depressants that attempt to prevent epileptic seizures without causing excessive drowsiness. Although their exact mechanisms of action are unknown, these agents prevent the spread of abnormal electric discharges in the brain.

The anticonvulsant drug used to treat a specific patient depends on the type of seizures the patient has. Since these agents are taken for life, their chronic toxicity becomes an important consideration in choosing a particular anticonvulsant agent and determining their dental implications. The drugs of choice and their alternatives for traditional grand mal (clonic-tonic-clonic or tonic-clonic) seizures, absence seizures, status epilepticus, and other seizure types are listed in Table 16-1.

General adverse reactions

The dental hygienist needs to be aware of the side effects of the anticonvulsant agents that might influence dental treatment. The anticonvulsant drugs possess a unique set of adverse reactions. The adverse reactions that the anticonvulsants have in common are discussed first.

Altered CNS function is a common side effect of the anticonvulsant agents. Impaired learning and cognitive abilities occur in some patients. Behavior alterations reported include both hyperactivity and sedation. Another CNS side effect is exacerbation of a seizure type that is not being treated.

A wide range of idiosyncratic reactions occur with the anticonvulsants. Dermatologic side effects include rash, Stevens-Johnson syndrome, exfoliative dermatitis, and erythema multiforme. Drug-induced systemic lupus erythematosus and hematologic effects have also been reported with most of these agents.

Many drug interactions can occur with the anticonvulsants. They may interact not only with each other but also with other drugs. The mechanisms of drug interactions include altering absorption or renal excretion and inducing or inhibiting metabolism. The outcome may alter the levels of the inducing drug itself, another concomitant anticonvulsant, or some other drug that is extensively metabolized by the liver microsomal enzymes. Drug interactions are more significant with the anticonvulsants than with other drug groups because their therapeutic index is narrow. If the level of an anticonvulsant is altered sufficiently by a drug interaction, either toxicity (level too high) or loss of seizure control (level too low) can result. Before any changes or additions are made to a patient's therapy, the possibility of a drug interaction should be considered.

A variety of reports have associated the anticonvulsant agents with alteration in growth, as well as teratogenic potential. Thickening of the facial structures secondary to a thickening of the calvarium and facial subcutaneous tissues has been associated with anticonvulsant medication. In addition, a coarseness of the facial features including enlargement of the nose and lips has been noted. These effects have the most profound effect on children receiving anticonvulsant medications during growth and development. Several of the anticonvulsant medications have been implicated in the production of fetal anomalies.

Abrupt withdrawal of any convulsant medication can precipitate seizures. Although many patients require medication for life, certain seizure types tend to disappear as the patient grows older. In these patients, gradual withdrawal of their seizure medication under controlled conditions can be undertaken after an appropriate interval of drug use.

Barbiturates (phenobarbital)

The barbiturates used in the treatment of epilepsy include phenobarbital (most common), mephobarbital, and metharbital (see Table 16-2). Both mephobarbital and primidone are metabolized to phenobarbital in the body. Since these three agents are very similar in their action, phenobarbital is discussed as the prototype.

Phenobarbital is used both alone and in combination with other anticonvulsants such as phenytoin. It is used to treat tonic-clonic and partial seizure types. Because of its relative safety compared with other anticonvulsants, it is often used first.

The most common side effect associated with phenobarbital is sedation. With continued use, tolerance to the drowsiness, but not the anticonvulsant effect, often develops. This CNS depression is additive with that produced by other CNS depressants. If another CNS depressant is given to the patient, such as an opioid analgesic agent or a benzodiazepine, the dose of these agents should be reduced. In children, excitement and hyperactivity are often produced. The elderly sometimes exhibit confusion, excitement, or depression.

Skin reactions occur in 1% to 3% of patients. Rarely exfoliative dermatitis, erythema multi-

Table 16-2. Anticonvulsants by chemical group

Drug	Indications*
Barbiturates	
Phenobarbital (Luminal)	TC,SE,F
Mephobarbital (Mebaral)	TC
Metharbital (Gemonil)	TC,MX
Hydantoins	
Phenytoin (Dilantin)	SE,TC,P
Mephenytoin (Mesantoin)	TC,P,F,J
Ethotoin (Peganone)	TC,P
Succinimides	
Ethosuximide (Zarontin)	A
Methsuximide (Celontin)	A
Phensuximide (Milontin)	A
Oxazolidinediones	
Trimethadione (Tridione)	A
Paramethadione (Paradione)	A
Benzodiazepines	
Clonazepam (Clonopin)	A,M,AK
Diazepam (Valium)	SE
Chlorazepate (Tranxene)	P-Ad
Other agents	
Carbamazepine (Tegretol)	TC,MX,P
Valproic acid (Depakene, Depakote)	A
Primidone (Mysoline)	TC,P,F
Phenacemide (Phenurone)	Severe: MX,P

*A, absence; AK, akinetic; F, focal; J, jacksonian; M, myoclonic; MX, mixed; P, psychomotor; P-Ad, partial, adjunct; SE, status epilepticus; TC, tonic-clonic.

forme, or Stevens-Johnson syndrome have been reported. Stomatitis may herald the onset of cutaneous reactions, some of which have been fatal. The barbiturates should be discontinued if any skin reactions occur. Other rare adverse reactions of phenobarbital include blood dyscrasias, exacerbation of acute intermittent porphyria, and respiratory depression. The barbiturates are discussed in more detail in Chapter 10.

Hydantoins (Phenytoin)

Since phenytoin (dilantin), formerly called diphenylhydantoin (DPH), is the most commonly used hydantoin, it is discussed as the prototype for the hydantoin group. Because phenytoin is associated with gingival hyperplasia, patients taking it require thorough dental education, monitoring, and appropriate dental treatment to maintain optimal oral health. The dental hygienist plays an integral role in the management of these patients.

Phenytoin is used to treat both tonic-clonic and partial seizures with complex symptomatology. It is not useful in the treatment of pure absence seizures, but may be used in combination with other agents indicated for absence seizures to control combined seizure types. It has also been used to treat trigeminal neuralgia. In addition to its anticonvulsant properties, phenytoin has quinidine-like antiarrhythmic properties.

Adverse reactions

The adverse reactions associated with phenytoin are frequent, affect many body systems, and may rarely be serious. Because of phenytoin's narrow therapeutic index, adverse reactions associated with elevated blood levels can occur. The chance for toxicity is also increased because phenytoin's metabolism is a saturable process. This means that very small changes in the dose can result in large changes in the blood level. Another problem with phenytoin is its propensity for drug interactions.

1. Gastrointestinal. Gastrointestinal adverse reactions including nausea, vomiting, loss of taste, and anorexia are not uncommon. Taking the medication with food can reduce these side effects. Prescribing other drugs with the potential for adverse gastrointestinal effects, such as opioids, should be minimized.

2. Central nervous system (CNS). The CNS effects that can occur with phenytoin include mental confusion, nystagmus, ataxia, slurred speech, blurred vision, diplopia, amblyopia, dizziness, and insomnia. Because some of these effects are

dose related, they can often be controlled by reducing the dose of phenytoin. Long-term administration has been associated with a sensory peripheral neuropathy.

3. Dermatologic effects. Skin reactions to phenytoin range from rash, to rarely exfoliative dermatitis, lupus erythematosus, or Stevens-Johnson syndrome. Some patients experience irreversible hypertrichosis, or excessive hairiness, on their trunk and face. This is one reason why alternative drugs are often selected, especially in the young female patient.

4. Vitamin deficiency. Vitamin deficiency states produced by phenytoin may involve both vitamin D and folate. Osteomalacia may result from phenytoin's interference with vitamin D metabolism. Rarely patients on long-term phenytoin may show the symptoms of adult rickets. The first symptoms of folate deficiency may be oral mucosal changes such as ulcerations or glossitis. Treatment involves the administering of folic acid.

5. Other adverse effects. Other adverse reactions include a mononucleosis syndrome, lymphadenopathy, lymphoma, and toxic hepatitis.

6. Gingival hyperplasia. The incidence of gingival hyperplasia quoted in the literature varies greatly; it occurs in approximately 50% of all chronic phenytoin users. Hyperplasia severe enough to require surgical intervention occurs in about 30% of affected patients.

The clinical symptoms of gingival hyperplasia may appear a few weeks or as long as a few years after initial drug therapy. It often begins as a painless enlargement of the gingival margin. The gingiva is pink and does not bleed easily unless other factors are present. With time, the interproximal papillae become involved finally coalescing to cover even the occlusal surfaces of the teeth. The hyperplasia is more commonly located in the anterior rather than the posterior surfaces, and the buccal rather than the lingual surfaces. Most agree that, in order of severity, the affected areas of the mouth are the maxillary anterior facial, mandibular anterior facial, maxillary posterior facial, and the mandibular posterior facial. In the affected patient both normal and abnormal

tissue may be found. Edentulous areas are rarely involved.

Although the relationship between dental plaque and gingival hyperplasia has been repeatedly debated, the better the patient's oral hygiene is the less likely the lesions are to occur, or the less severe they will be if they do occur. Younger patients are more likely to experience this adverse reaction. Controversy exists on the contribution of dose and duration of therapy to the risk for the development of gingival hyperplasia.

The cause of phenytoin gingival hyperplasia is unknown. Many causes have been investigated including alteration in the function of the adrenal gland, hypersensitivity or allergic reaction, and vitamin C or folate deficiency. Since it is known that phenytoin occurs in the saliva, some investigators suggest a local etiology. Dahllof and co-workers[3] suggest that T-cell-mediated immunologic reactions may play a part in the lesions.

The management of phenytoin-induced gingival hyperplasia requires consultation between dental personnel and the patient's physician. Some of the alternatives are as follows:

• Alter drug. Choosing another effective antiepileptic drug is one method of handling the gingival hyperplasia produced by phenytoin. Often the alternatives available have as many, and often more potential for, adverse effects than phenytoin.

Ethotoin, another hydantoin, has traditionally been said to have less seizure control efficacy, but other authors attribute this reduced efficacy to inadequate doses. Some patients with gingival hyperplasia from phenytoin have experienced a regression in the gum hypertrophy when ethotoin was substituted for phenytoin.

Patients who have phenytoin discontinued will experience a decrease in gingival hyperplasia over a 1-year period. Surgical intervention should wait until at least 18 months after cessation of therapy because some patients experience additional reduction in the hyperplasia after the 1-year period.

- Improve oral hygiene. Scrupulous oral hygiene may reduce the rate of formation of hyperplasia. Avoiding irritating restorations may also reduce hyperplasia. Even with ideal oral hygiene, hyperplasia is not always totally preventable and once it has formed is not easily reversed.
- Gingivectomy. When gingival hyperplasia interferes with plaque control, esthetics, or mastication and when oral hygiene has not been successful in controlling hyperplasia, surgical elimination is indicated. It is not a final or permanent solution since hyperplasia quickly returns in most cases and can progress to the presurgical level in a short period of time if the patient continues on phenytoin.
- Other drugs. Although many types of drugs have been tried in the treatment of this condition, such as diuretics, corticosteroids, mouthwashes, vitamin C, folic acid, and antihistamines, none have been shown to be effective in controlled trials.

7. Teratogenicity. Fetal hydantoin syndrome is the term given to the congenital abnormality associated with maternal ingestion of phenytoin. It includes craniofacial anomalies, limb defects, growth deficiency, and mental retardation. Its existence as a direct consequence of exposure to phenytoin is controversial.

Phenytoin dental implications

1. Review emergency management of epileptic patients.
2. Take a thorough medical and drug history.
3. Use CNS depressants cautiously.
4. Avoid drugs that are gastric irritants, for example, nonsteroidal antiinflammatory agents (NSAIAs).
5. Monitor gingival hyperplasia.
6. Perform frequent prophylaxis; give instructions.

Valproic sodium/acid (Depakene) and divalproex sodium (Depakote)

Valproic acid, valproate sodium, and divalproex sodium are structurally unrelated to other anti-convulsants. Divalproex sodium is a 1:1 ratio of valproic acid and valproate sodium. The mechanism of action of valproic acid may be due to an increase in the inhibitory neurotransmitter, γ-aminobutyric acid (GABA).

Adverse effects

1. Gastrointestinal. Indigestion, nausea, and vomiting are the most frequent adverse effects associated with valproic acid. These can be minimized by giving the drug with meals or increasing the dose very gradually. Divalproex sodium may have fewer adverse gastrointestinal effects than its components. Other gastrointestinal side effects include hypersalivation, anorexia, increased appetite, cramping, diarrhea, and constipation.

2. CNS effects. Sedation and drowsiness have been reported with valproic acid. Rarely ataxia, headache, and nystagmus have been noted. Some children exhibit hyperactivity, aggression, and other behavioral disturbances.

3. Hepatotoxicity. Dose-related changes in liver enzymes frequently occur in these patients. Deaths caused by hepatic failure have also been reported. Because valproic acid can produce serious hepatotoxicity, hepatic function tests should be performed at frequent intervals, especially at the beginning of therapy.

4. Bleeding. Because valproic acid inhibits the second phase of platelet aggregation, bleeding time may be prolonged. Thrombocytopenia, petechiae, bruising, and hematoma have been reported. Platelet counts, bleeding time, and coagulation studies should be performed before surgical procedures.

5. Teratogenicity. Several reports suggest an association between the use of valproic acid in pregnant women and an increase in birth defects (particularly neural tube defects). The risk to the fetus for seizures must be weighed against this drug's potential for teratogenicity.

6. Drug interactions. Other drugs that are CNS depressants can have an additive CNS depressant effect when used in conjunction with valproic acid. When valproic acid is combined with phenobarbital, excessive sedation has been reported.

Valproic acid has also been associated with drug interactions with phenytoin—either decreased or increased phenytoin levels. Because valproic acid can affect bleeding, other drugs that affect bleeding should be used cautiously.

Valproic acid dental implications

1. Review emergency management of epileptic patients.
2. Take a thorough medical and drug history.
3. Use drugs that can alter coagulation cautiously.
4. Use CNS depressants cautiously.
5. Avoid drugs that are gastric irritants, for example, NSAIAs.
6. Look for signs of hepatotoxicity.

Carbamazepine (Tegretol)

Carbamazepine is structurally related to the tricyclic antidepressants. Although it is used to treat convulsions, it is of special interest in dentistry because of its use in the treatment of trigeminal neuralgia (tic douloureux). Carbamazepine's anticonvulsant action involves limiting the seizure propagation by reducing posttetanic potentiation of synaptic transmission. In the treatment of trigeminal neuralgia, carbamazepine appears to reduce synaptic transmission within the trigeminal nucleus.

Pharmacologic effects

Carbamazepine has anticonvulsant, anticholinergic, antidepressant, sedative, and muscle relaxant properties. It also has antiarrhythmic, antidiuretic, and neuromuscular transmission-inhibitory actions.

Adverse reactions

Carbamazepine can have serious adverse effects on a variety of organs including the hematopoietic, cardiovascular, hepatic, and renal systems. Its use should not be undertaken lightly.

1. Hematologic. Aplastic anemia secondary to carbamazepine therapy has been fatal. Agranulocytosis, thrombocytopenia, and leukopenia have also been reported. Because of the hematologic adverse effects, laboratory tests are necessary to follow these patients. Patients should be made aware of the symptoms of these blood dyscrasias and warned to stop the drug and report any of the symptoms immediately. The dental hygienist should observe the oral cavity of patients taking carbamazepine with these side effects in mind.

2. Nervous system. Carbamazepine has been known to cause dizziness, vertigo, drowsiness, fatigue, ataxia, confusion, headache, nystagmus, and visual and speech disturbances. Activation of a latent psychosis, abnormal involuntary movements, depression, and peripheral neuritis occur rarely.

3. Gastrointestinal. Gastrointestinal side effects include nausea, vomiting, and gastric distress. Abdominal pain, diarrhea, constipation, and anorexia have also been noted. Dry mouth, glossitis, and stomatitis can sometimes be seen in patients taking carbamazepine.

4. Dermatologic. Rashes, urticaria, photosensitivity reactions, and altered skin pigmentation can occur. Erythema multiforme, erythema nodosum, and aggravation of systemic lupus erythematosus have been reported. Alopecia can also occur.

5. Dental. The pediatric dosage form of carbamazepine contains 63% sugar in its chewable tablet. It is usually indicated to be chewed four times daily. When the dental hygienist is questioning the mother about a child's medication usage, the topic of the particular dosage form and its sugar content should be explored.

6. Other effects. Cardiovascular side effects include congestive heart failure and alterations in blood pressure. Abnormal liver function tests and cholestatic jaundice have been reported. Urinary frequency and retention, oliguria, and impotence have been reported with carbamazepine use. Elevated blood urea nitrogen (BUN) levels, albuminuria, and glycosuria have been seen. Lymphadenopathy, aching joints, and punctate lens opacities have occurred rarely.

7. Drug interactions. Carbamazepine possesses many drug interactions. Since it can induce liver microsomal enzymes, the metabolism of many drugs, including carbamazepine itself, may be increased. Carbamazepine can decrease the effect

of doxycycline, warfarin, theophylline, and oral contraceptives. Carbamazepine's effect may be increased by erythromycin, isoniazid, propoxyphene, and calcium channel blockers.

Carbamazepine dental implications

1. Check for dry mouth, glossitis, and stomatitis.
2. Look for symptoms of blood dyscrasias.
3. Perform appropriate laboratory testing (if being prescribed by the dentist for trigeminal neuralgia):
   a. Hematologic tests
   b. Ophthalmologic examination
   c. Complete urinalysis
   d. Liver function tests

Miscellaneous anticonvulsant agents

Ethosuximide. Ethosuximide (Zarontin) is the drug of choice for the treatment of absence seizures. It is ineffective in partial seizures with complex symptoms or in tonic-clonic seizures. In the treatment of mixed seizures, agents effective against tonic-clonic seizures must be used in addition to ethosuximide.

Gastrointestinal adverse effects include anorexia, gastric upset, cramps, pain, diarrhea, and nausea and vomiting. CNS adverse effects include drowsiness, hyperactivity, headache, and hiccups. Adverse psychiatric and psychologic manifestations include sleep disturbances and aggressiveness or rarely even paranoia or suicidal attempts. Ethosuximide has been associated with blood dyscrasias, positive direct Coombs test, systemic lupus erythematosus, and Stevens-Johnson syndrome. Gum hypertrophy, hirsutism, and swelling of the tongue have also occurred.

Trimethadione. Because of the potential for severe toxicity, trimethadione (Tridione) is used only to manage absence seizures that are refractory to other anticonvulsant agents. It is used in combination with other anticonvulsants to treat combination seizure disorders. The most frequent adverse effects are drowsiness and visual disturbances. Severe side effects include aplastic anemia, fetal malformations, exfoliative dermatitis, erythema multiforme, nephrotic syndrome, hepatitis, systemic lupus erythematosus, malignant lymphoma syndrome, and myasthenia gravis.

Benzodiazepines (Clonazepam). The benzodiazepines clonazepam (Clonopin) and chlorazepate (Tranxene) are used orally as anticonvulsants. Diazepam (Valium) and lorazepam (Ativan) are used parenterally to treat recurrent tonic-clonic seizures. The antianxiety use of the benzodiazepines is discussed in Chapter 10. Clonazepam, the oral benzodiazepine anticonvulsant prototype, is discussed here.

Clonazepam is used as an adjunct to treat certain seizure types not responsive to ethosuximide. Drowsiness and ataxia occur frequently. Behavioral disturbances as well as adverse neurologic effects can occur. Other side effects reported relate to the gastrointestinal tract, and dermatologic and hematologic systems. Increased salivation and hypersecretion in the upper respiratory passages may occur. Other oral manifestations of clonazepam include coated tongue, dry mouth, encopresis, abnormal thirst, and sore gums.

Primidone (Mysoline). Primidone, a structural analogue of phenobarbital, shares many of phenobarbital's actions. It is used to treat seizures that are refractory to other anticonvulsants and it is often used in combination with other anticonvulsants. Like phenobarbital, primidone can cause hyperkinetic behavior in children. It has also been associated with diplopia, nystagmus, rash, alopecia, edema, lymphoma-like syndrome, and lupus erythematosus–like syndrome. Megaloblastic anemia responsive to folic acid has been reported.

DENTAL TREATMENT OF THE EPILEPTIC PATIENT

The dental hygienist should not treat a patient who has a history of seizure disorders without reviewing the management of the epileptic patient, including the procedures for handling a patient experiencing tonic-clonic seizures. Preventive measures include a detailed seizure history, treatment planning to avoid excessive stress and missed medications, and education of the entire dental office staff. The management of the patient experiencing tonic-clonic seizures should include moving the patient to the floor if possible, tilting the patient's head to one side to prevent aspiration, removing objects from the patient's mouth before the seizure to prevent fractured teeth. Tongue blades are not recommended because they may split and produce additional trauma.

REVIEW QUESTIONS

1. Briefly describe the most common seizure types, including the following:
   a. Grand mal (tonic–clonic)
   b. Absence (petit mal)
   c. Status epilepticus
2. State the general measures with which the dental hygienist should be familiar before treating an epileptic patient.
3. Explain the major adverse reactions associated with these anticonvulsants:
   a. Phenytoin
   b. Phenobarbital
   c. Carbamazepine
   d. Depakote
4. Describe a few major adverse reactions caused by the less frequently used anticonvulsants.
5. Discuss the gingival hyperplasia associated with phenytoin, including its incidence, cause, minimization, and treatment. Explain the dental hygienist's essential role in preventing and treating this condition.
6. Describe a dentally related use of carbamazepine and name what laboratory test monitoring is involved.
7. Enumerate the adverse reactions associated with epileptic patients who are taking several medications.

REFERENCES

1. Delgado-Escueta, A.V., et al.: Treatable epilepsies, N. Engl. J. Med. **308:**1508-1514, 1983.
2. Delgado-Escueta, A.V., et al.: Treatable epilepsies, N. Engl. J. Med. **308:**1576-1584, 1983.
3. Dahllof, G., et al.: Subpopulations of lymphocytes in connective tissue from phenytoin-induced gingival overgrowth, Scand. J. Dent. Res. **93:**507-512, 1985.

Chapter 17

10/27/93

Psychotherapeutic agents

Many drugs have the ability to affect mental activity. Some of these drugs are used in the treatment of psychiatric disorders. The dental hygienist is most likely to encounter the use of these agents in dental patients who have had them prescribed by psychiatrists or other physicians. Because these agents are so widely prescribed and they can alter the patient's dental treatment, the dental hygienist must understand their pharmacologic effects, adverse reactions, and dental implications.

The agents used in the treatment of the major psychiatric disorders will be discussed in this chapter. Those used to treat anxiety are discussed in Chapter 10. Because the psychotherapeutic drugs are classified by their therapeutic use, a brief discussion of the common psychiatric illnesses follows.

PSYCHIATRIC DISORDERS

There are many psychiatric disorders. They may be divided into two types, organic and functional, depending on their suspected cause. Organic illness is congenital or caused by an injury or disease. Functional disorders are partially of psychogenic origin, without any evidence of structural or biochemical abnormality. Functional disorders include the following categories:

1. Psychoses, the most violent type of psychiatric disorder, are divided into schizophrenia and the affective disorders.
   a. Schizophrenia is an extensive disturbance of the patient's personality function with a loss of perception of reality.
   b. Affective disorders include endogenous, exogenous, and manic depression. Endogenous (involutional) depression seems to be unrelated to external events, whereas exogenous (reactive) depression appears to be related to specific external events. Manic depressive illness is characterized by alternating periods of mania (elation) and depression.

2. Neuroses, less severe than psychoses, can also be helped by drug therapy. Examples include anxiety, phobias, and compulsiveness.

3. Psychophysiologic (somatic) disorders are those that have an emotional origin but are manifested by physiologic symptoms.

4. Personality disorders include sexual deviation, alcoholism, and drug dependence.

This presentation is an oversimplification of the classifications of psychiatric disorders. The drug groups to be discussed in this chapter include the antipsychotic agents, used in the treatment of psychoses, and the antidepressants, used in the treatment of affective disorders. Lithium, used in the treatment of manic depression, is also mentioned. The minor tranquilizers, used to manage various neuroses, are discussed in Chapter 10.

Before the antipsychotic drugs were introduced into the management of psychiatric disorders, many physical methods were employed to treat patients. Only electroconvulsive therapy (ECT, shock therapy) is still used.

When treating patients with mental disorders, the following cautions should be observed:

1. Patients with various mental disorders may perceive comments from the dental hygienist as threatening, and office discussion should be carefully monitored.

2. Patients undergoing drug therapy for the treatment of psychoses often do not take their medication. A thorough health history including

199

the patient's medication and its dosage should be obtained.

3. Depressed patients may attempt suicide. Therefore the amount of any drug prescribed at one time should not exceed a lethal dose. In a suicide attempt drugs are often combined. For example, a patient may mix an opioid analgesic given for the relief of a toothache, a sedative-hypnotic prescribed for dental anxiety, and an antidepressant medication prescribed by the patient's physician.

ANTIPSYCHOTIC AGENTS

The phenothiazines are the most frequently used group in the treatment of psychoses. Table 17-1 lists the common phenothiazines and other groups with antipsychotic action and their usual adult daily dose for outpatient treatment.

The actions of the antipsychotic agents are diverse. No single agent is clearly superior in its antipsychotic action. Clinical judgment and the drug's side effect profile in a particular patient determine which agent is used. In general, the lower potency agents like chlorpromazine have more sedation, more peripheral side effects, and more autonomic effects (e.g., dry mouth), while the higher potency agents like haloperidol have more extrapyramidal effects and less sedation. The phenothiazines, because they are the most frequently used antipsychotic agents, are discussed as the prototype.

Pharmacologic effects and adverse reactions

When the phenothiazines are used for the treatment of psychoses, any effect other than the antipsychotic effect could be considered an adverse reaction. Therefore the pharmacologic effects and the adverse reactions will be considered simultaneously.

1. Antipsychotic effects. All phenothiazines possess antipsychotic effects associated with slowing of the psychomotor activity in an agitated patient and calming of emotion with suppression of hallucinations and delusions. There is also a lack of response without a loss of intellectual function.

Table 17-1. Antipsychotic agents

Drug	Daily dose (mg)*
Phenothiazines	
Aliphatic	
Chlorpromazine (Thorazine)	100–400
Promazine (Sparine)	500–1000
Piperazine	
Fluphenazine (Prolixin)	1–5
Trifluoperazine (Sterlazine)	4–10
Prochlorperazine (Compazine)	20–60
Piperidine	
Thioridazine (Mellaril)	100–400
Butyrophenones	
Haloperidol (Haldol)	2–6
Droperidol (Inapsine)	IV
Thioxanthenes	
Thiothixene (Navane)	6–30
Chlorprothixene (Taractan)	50–400
Dihydroindolones	
Molindone (Moban)	15–60
Dibenzoxazepines	
Loxapine (Loxitane)	15–40

*Usual oral dosage range for outpatient treatment in milligrams; inpatient treatment uses higher doses.
IV, Intravenous.

2. Sedation. Although the phenothiazines differ in the degree of sedation and drowsiness they produce, many patients are sedated by these agents. In contrast to the sedative-hypnotic agents, with higher doses the phenothiazines do not produce anesthesia and the patient is easily aroused. Tolerance develops to the sedative effect but not to the antipsychotic effect.

3. Antiemetic effect. The phenothiazines antiemetic effect is due to depression of the chemoreceptor trigger zone (CTZ). These agents are useful in the symptomatic treatment of certain types of nausea and vomiting.

4. Orthostatic hypotension. Because these

agents depress the central sympathetic outflow and block the peripheral adrenergic receptors (α-sympathetic blockers) they can produce orthostatic hypotension that is additive. When a patient is elevated rapidly from the supine position, a compensatory tachycardia can accompany the orthostatic hypotension.

5. Extrapyramidal effects. The most common type of adverse reaction associated with these agents is due to stimulation of the extrapyramidal system. All phenothiazines produce this effect, although the incidence of the reaction varies. The following types of extrapyramidal effects can occur:

a. Acute dystonia consisting of muscle spasms of the face, tongue, neck, and back.

b. Parkinsonism with symptoms of resting tremor, rigidity, and akinesia

c. Akathisia or increased, compulsive motor activity

d. Tardive dyskinesia, an irreversible dyskinesia involving the tongue, lips, face, and jaw. Tardive dyskinesia is typically seen in patients who are over 40 years old and have been taking large doses of the phenothiazines for a minimum of 6 months to 2 years. The onset is gradual and the movements are coordinated and rhythmic. This effect is exacerbated by drug withdrawal. The involuntary movements, especially those involving the face, jaw, and tongue, can make home care difficult if not impossible. Performing an oral prophylaxis is difficult because of the strength of the oral facial muscles. Since it cannot be determined whether these abnormal movements are irreversible tardive dyskinesia, the dental hygienist should discuss the patient's condition with the patient's physician.

e. Temporomandibular joint (TMJ) pain. The extrapyramidal effects of the phenothiazines can cause severe intermittent pain in the region of the TMJ, produced by a spasm of the muscles of mastication. In an acute attack it becomes difficult or impossible to open or close the jaw. Dislocations of the mandible can occur. Should muscle spasm be present, force should not be exerted to open the patient's mouth for dental treatment. Treatment of the acute spasm of the mandible must be undertaken after consultation with the patient's prescribing physician. Alternatives may include decreasing the patient's dose of medication, adding an anticholinergic medication to counteract the spasm, or changing the patient's antipsychotic medication to one which produces fewer extrapyramidal effects.

6. Seizures. Since the phenothiazines lower the convulsion threshold, seizures may be more easily precipitated in a patient taking these agents, especially if a previous history of epilepsy exists.

7. Anticholinergic effects. The anticholinergic effects of the phenothiazines produce blurred vision, xerostomia, and constipation. This is especially significant because the anticholinergic effects of other medications the patient may be taking are additive. The dental hygienist should be aware of the presence of xerostomia and should question patients regarding their self-treatment.

8. Other effects. As previously mentioned, phenothiazines have many adverse effects including blood dyscrasias, cholestatic jaundice, skin eruptions, and photosensitivity reactions that are exaggerated by sunlight or even by the light from the dental unit.

Drug interactions

1. Central nervous system (CNS) depressants. The phenothiazines interact in an additive or even potentiating fashion with all CNS depressants including the barbiturates, alcohol, the general anesthetics, and the opioid analgesics. Sedation, as well as respiratory depression can occur.

2. Epinephrine. Because the phenothiazine agents are α-adrenergic blockers, epinephrine should not be used to treat vasomotor collapse (acute drop in blood pressure), since it could cause a further decrease in blood pressure. This occurs because of the predominant β (vasodilating) activity of epinephrine in the presence of the

phenothiazines (α-blockers). Epinephrine, as a vasoconstrictor in local anesthetic solutions, can be safely used in patients taking phenothiazines.

3. Anticholinergic agents. To control excessive extrapyramidal stimulation, phenothiazine therapy often has to be combined with antiparkinsonian medication of the anticholinergic type, for example, benztropine (Cogentin). This combination is bound to exacerbate antimuscarinic peripheral effects such as xerostomia, urinary retention, bowel paralysis, and inhibition of sweating.

Uses

1. Antipsychotic effects. Phenothiazines are the drugs of choice for the treatment of schizophrenia. Long-acting injectable phenothiazines are available for schizophrenic patients who fail to take their oral medication.

2. Antiemetic effects. Because the phenothiazines prevent or inhibit vomiting, they are useful in the treatment of some types of nausea and vomiting. Prochlorperazine has traditionally been used.

3. Treatment of hiccoughs. Intractable hiccoughs have been successfully treated with the phenothiazines.

Dental implications

1. Sedation. Sedation, an adverse reaction of the phenothiazines, is additive with that of other sedating agents.

2. Anticholinergic effects. The phenothiazines are additive with other agents with atropine-like effects; this combination can lead to toxic reactions including tachycardia, urinary retention, blurred vision, constipation, and xerostomia. The hygienist should be aware that patients may use sugar-containing candy to counteract xerostomia. Use of sugarless products or artificial saliva (Orex, Xero-Lube, Moi-Stir) should be encouraged.

3. Orthostatic hypotension. This effect can be minimized by raising the dental chair slowly.

4. Epinephrine. Epinephrine's use should be avoided in acute hypotensive crisis. It may be used in local anesthetic solutions.

5. Temporomandibular joint pain. As a result of the phenothiazine's extrapyramidal effects, the muscles of mastication may be in spasm.

6. Tardive dyskinesia. Since this effect is irreversible, it should be reported to the patient's physician.

The other antipsychotic drugs have essentially the same pharmacologic effects, adverse reactions, and dental implications as the phenothiazines. They differ only in the relative degree of these effects. For example, haloperidol has more extrapyridamal side effects but less sedation than chlorpromazine.

ANTIDEPRESSANTS
Depression

Until the late 1950s, there was no widely accepted pharmacologic treatment for depression. Forms of mild depression were treated with psychotherapy, and severe depression was treated with electroconvulsive therapy (ECT). Several classes of antidepressants are presently available, and they are discussed separately. Nevertheless, ECT is still used in the treatment of severely suicidal patients as well as those resistant to antidepressants.

Tricyclic antidepressants

The tricyclic antidepressants (TCAs) are structurally similar to the phenothiazines. Table 17-2 lists the antidepressants with their usual adult outpatient daily dose in milligrams. All TCAs are similar in their antidepressant effectiveness, differing only in their side effect profile.

Pharmacologic effects

The action of TCAs on normal and depressed patients is somewhat different. In the normal patient an undesirable sedation and fatigue with strong atropine-like side effects are noted. In the depressed patient, a feeling of well-being, elevation of mood, and a dulling of depressive ideation are noted. Sedation occurs frequently, but toler-

Table 17-2. Antidepressants

Drug	Daily dose (mg)*
Tricyclic antidepressants	
Imipramine (Tofranil)	50–150
Amitriptyline (Elavil)	50–150
Protriptyline (Vivactil)	10–40
Nortriptyline (Pamelor, Aventyl)	50–150
Doxepin (Sinequan, Adapin)	75–150
Desipramine (Norpramine)	75–150
Monoamine oxidase inhibitors	
Isocarboxazid (Marplan)	10–30
Tranylcypromine (Parnate)	20–30
Phenelzine (Nardil)	15–45
Second-generation antidepressants	
Amoxapine (Asendin)	100–200
Maprotiline (Ludiomil)	75–200
Trazodone (Desyrel)	100–300
Fluoxetine (Prozac)	20

*Usual oral dosage range for outpatient treatment in milligrams; inpatient treatment uses higher doses.

ance to this effect often develops. Increased ability to concentrate and improvement in sleep is seen with the TCAs. The antidepressant action can take up to 1 month to fully develop.

Adverse reactions

The widely diverse effects associated with the tricyclic antidepressants resemble those of the antipsychotic agents.

1. CNS effects. Almost all of the TCAs induce some degree of sedation and some of them can produce tremors. The latter effect is not caused by extrapyramidal stimulation and therefore does not respond to antiparkinson medication. It consists of a fine tremor in the upper extremities (arms or hands) and occurs in at least 10% of the patients treated with these drugs.

2. Autonomic nervous system effects. The peripheral effects of the TCAs are primarily on the autonomic nervous system. These agents possess

distinct anticholinergic effects resulting in xerostomia, blurred vision, tachycardia, constipation, and urinary retention. Tolerance to these effects develops with continued use. Although the TCAs initially produce orthostatic hypotension like the phenothiazines, tolerance to this effect occurs.

3. Cardiac effects. The most serious peripheral side effect associated with the TCAs is cardiac toxicity. Myocardial infarction and congestive heart failure have occurred during the course of treatment. Arrhythmias and episodes of tachycardia can be caused by the antimuscarinic (anticholinergic, atropine-like) effects of the TCAs.

4. Dependence or withdrawal. Rarely, TCAs have been found to produce psychic or physical dependence. Slight withdrawal effects after abrupt discontinuation have been reported. Tolerance develops to many of the side effects, although not to the antidepressant effect.

Drug interactions

Unlike the phenothiazines, the TCAs potentiate the behavioral actions of the amphetamines and other CNS stimulants. TCAs potentiate the pressor effect of injected sympathomimetics. These agents also interact with the monoamine oxidase (MAO) inhibitors, resulting in severe toxic reactions. TCAs may be displaced from plasma protein binding sites by phenytoin. TCAs may be metabolized more quickly because of induction of hepatic microsomal enzymes by the barbiturates, carbamazepines, and cigarette smoking. They may interfere with the antihypertensive effects of guanethidine and clonidine. Additive anticholinergic effects are seen if they are administered with another agent with anticholinergic action.

Poisoning

Accidental poisoning with the TCAs has become more common, and such an overdose can be lethal. The effects of acute poisoning consist of severe hypertension, cardiac arrhythmias, hyperpyrexia, convulsions, coma, and respiratory failure. Survivors may have permanent myocardial damage. The treatment is symptomatic and should be conservative in view of the interactions with other CNS vasopressor agents. Activated charcoal or gastric lavage may be helpful. Physostigmine has been reported to be effective in treating mild poisoning by tricyclic antidepressants.

Uses

Tricyclic antidepressants can be used alone or in combination with the phenothiazines or ECT in the treatment of depression. In patients who are suicide risks, the long onset of action of the tricyclic antidepressants (several weeks) requires the use of ECT during the initial phase of drug treatment. These agents, after several weeks are allowed for the development of their effects, can prevent relapse and thus provide long-term control of depression.

The tricyclic antidepressants are often combined with one of the phenothiazines in the treatment of combination psychoses, neuroses, and anxieties. One example is a combination of perphenazine and amitriptyline (Triavil, Etrafon). Comments relating to the dental implications of both the TCAs and the phenothiazines apply to patients taking this type of product. TCAs have been used with some success to control nocturnal enuresis (incontinence) in children.

Dental implications

1. Sympathomimetic amines. Vasoconstrictors (sympathomimetic amines) must be used with caution in the local anesthetic solution administered to patients taking TCAs. They may potentiate vasopressor (increased blood pressure) response to epinephrine. In the usual therapeutic doses the sympathetic amines present in a local anesthetic solution can be safely administered to patients without preexisting arrhythmias.

2. Xerostomia. The anticholinergic effect of these agents is additive with that of other agents producing dry mouth. The hygienist should question patients about the products they use to alleviate this troublesome side effect and suggest alternatives such as artificial saliva or sugarless gum.

3. Tremors. The fine tremors associated with use of the TCAs may make it difficult for patients to maintain good oral hygiene.

Monoamine oxidase inhibitors

Monoamine oxidase inhibitors (MAOIs) include a large variety of drugs that have the ability to inhibit monoamine oxidase and thus block the metabolism (oxidative deamination) of the naturally occurring amines norepinephrine and epinephrine. The MAOIs in current use for the treatment of depression are listed in Table 17-2. Another MAOI, pargyline (Eutonyl) is used to treat hypertension. They possess many adverse effects, and an overdose can lead to a severe toxic reaction. Because the enzymes inhibited by the MAOIs inactivate many endogenous amines, the action of any exogenous sympathomimetic amine is potentiated (i.e., it is not metabolized as quickly). The MAOIs interact with many drugs, such as amphetamine, and with foods such as cheeses, wines, and fish, precipitating a hypertensive crisis and even death. Because of the potential for life-threatening situations, patients taking MAOIs should not be given any drug unless the prescriber has first consulted a reference source on drug interactions.

Atypical antidepressants

Trazodone. Trazodone (Desyrel) is an antidepressant unrelated chemically to the TCAs. It appears to have antidepressant effects equivalent to those of the TCAs. Its advantages include that it is less cardiotoxic and produces fewer anticholinergic effects (e.g., xerostomia). Its disadvantages include that being a newer drug its side effects profile may be somewhat unknown, it is highly sedative, and it has been associated with painful priapism requiring surgical intervention and leaving some patients permanently impotent.

Fluoxetine. Fluoxetine (Prozac) is unrelated chemically to any other antidepressant. Its antidepressant action is also equivalent to that of the TCAs. Its advantage is that it more commonly produces CNS stimulation rather than sedation, and weight loss rather than weight gain as with the TCAs may occur. Being a new drug, the side effect profile of fluoxetine needs to be clarified. Commonly reported side effects include headache, nervousness, insomnia, nausea, anorexia, excessive sweating, asthenia, and upper respiratory tract infections. Oral side effects include dry mouth (10%), tongue edema, aphthous stomatitis, and change or loss of taste.

Lithium

Lithium (Eskalith, Lithobid) is used in the treatment of manic depressive illness, which is characterized by cyclic recurrence of mania alternating with depression. The side effects, which can be minimized by monitoring serum lithium levels, include polyuria, fine hand tremor, thirst, and, in more severe cases, slurred speech, ataxia, nausea, vomiting, and diarrhea. Patients undergoing lithium therapy should be observed for signs of overdose toxicity, which may be exhibited by CNS symptoms including muscle rigidity, hyperactive deep reflexes, excessive tremor, and muscle fasciculations. Some nonsteroidal antiinflammatory agents can alter lithium levels substantially. of lithium (avoid NSAIDs)

Be cautious when rec. pain relievers

REVIEW QUESTIONS

1. Explain the difference between the neuroses and the schizophrenias.
2. Name three commonly used phenothiazines.
3. State the major pharmacologic effect of the phenothiazines.
4. State the adverse reactions attributable to the phenothiazines.
5. Describe the following adverse reactions, including methods of recognition in the dental office:
   a. Orthostatic hypotension
   b. Extrapyramidal symptoms
   c. Tardive dyskinesia
   d. Anticholinergic effects
6. Name three uses for the phenothiazines.
7. List four ways in which you would handle a patient taking antipsychotic agents differently from unmedicated patients.
8. Explain the drug interactions between epinephrine and the phenothiazines and the tricyclic antidepressants.
9. List three adverse reactions associated with the tricyclic antidepressants.
10. Describe two ways in which you would treat a patient taking antidepressants differently from an unmedicated patient.
11. State the agent used in the treatment of poisoning by tricyclic antidepressants.
12. Name two new antidepressants and describe one advantage of each.
13. Name the agent used to treat bipolar affective disorders and describe its effect on saliva.

Chapter 18

11/3/93

Autacoids and antihistamines

The term "autacoids" is derived from the Greek *autos* ("self") and *akos* ("remedy"). Although the agents in this class possess widely differing pharmacologic actions, they all occur naturally in the body, and their exact functions are not yet understood. These substances and their potential antagonists hold great promise for the future. Together with histamine the following groups of compounds fall into the class of autocoids: prostaglandins, thromboxanes, leukotrienes, and kinins.

HISTAMINE

Histamine is a rather ubiquitous biogenic amine. Although many of its peripheral actions are well-known, its precise physiologic function, particularly in the central nervous system (CNS), is not clear. The structure of histamine is as follows:

$$\text{HN} \diagdown \text{N} - \text{CH}_2 - \text{CH}_2 - \text{NH}_2$$

Almost all mammalian tissues contain or can synthesize histamine. In humans histamine is stored in the mast cells in the intestinal mucosa and in the CNS. When an allergic reaction occurs, the mast cells degranulate and histamine is released. Histamine is released from the tissues in the body by normal reactions, abnormal reactions, or the administration of certain drugs. The amount of histamine released in these reactions determines the effects seen in the patient.

Pharmacologic effects

In humans histamine causes the following effects:
1. Vasodilation

2. Increased capillary permeability
3. Bronchoconstriction
4. Increased gastric acid secretion
5. Pain or itching in cutaneous nerve endings

With the synthesis of agents that can block some of histamine's effects, the concept of histamine receptors has been advanced. The histamine receptors are termed H_1 and H_2. The H_1 receptors are primarily related to vasodilation, increased capillary permeability, and bronchoconstriction. The H_2 receptors are responsible for stimulating gastric acid secretion.

Histamine's actions may be mediated by activation of H_1 receptors, H_2 receptors, or both. Agents that block or antagonize the effects of one or the other of these receptors are referred to as H_1 blockers or H_1 antagonists and H_2 blockers or H_2 antagonists.

Adverse reactions

When an allergic reaction or anaphylaxis occurs, an antigen-antibody reaction causes the release of histamine and other autacoids. Anaphylaxis is a serious and sometimes fatal reaction to a foreign protein or drug introduced into the body. Difficulty in breathing, convulsions, lapse into unconsciousness, and death can ensue. The predominant feature in this syndrome is bronchoconstriction.

In addition to bronchoconstriction, the action of histamine during an anaphylactic reaction includes vasodilation and increased capillary permeability, both of which lead to decreased blood pressure followed by shock and cardiovascular collapse. Other symptoms of anaphylaxis include apprehension, paresthesia, urticaria, edema, choking, cyanosis, cough, and wheezing. Fever,

[handwritten at top: use of histamine: 1) Achlorhydria - production of acid 2) Pheochromocytoma - col. ...skin]

shock, loss of consciousness, coma, convulsions, and death may result.

Although the treatment of anaphylaxis is described in Chapter 23, it is discussed here in relation to its cause. The drug of choice for anaphylaxis is epinephrine, a physiologic antagonist, rather than an antihistamine, a pharmacologic antagonist. The reason for this is that antihistamines antagonize only some of the effects of histamine and they work only competitively.

Uses

Histamine's only clinical uses are in the diagnosis of achlorhydria and pheochromocytoma.

ANTIHISTAMINES (H_1 RECEPTOR ANTAGONISTS)

Antihistamines are widely used drugs and the dental hygienist should be familiar with them for the following reasons:

1. Many patients have seasonal allergic reactions (e.g., hay fever) that make dental treatment difficult. The dentist may prescribe antihistamines to make breathing easier during dental procedures.
2. A mild allergic reaction to a drug may have to be treated with antihistamines in the dental office.
3. Patients receiving long-term antihistamine therapy may have side effects like xerostomia.
4. Antihistamines interact with many other drug groups.

The older H_1 receptor antagonists, also called H_1 blockers, have antihistaminic, anticholinergic, antiserotonergic, sedative, and other effects, whereas the newer **nonsedating H_1 blockers** with more specific peripheral H_1 antagonistic effect produce less sedation (termed nonsedating). These are discussed separately.

The older antihistamines (H_1 blockers) have a chemical structure similar to that of histamine. Table 18-1 gives the chemical group of various antihistamines, some examples of each group, and some properties of each group.

Pharmacologic effects

The older H_1 antagonists have a broad spectrum of pharmacologic actions that can be divided into those caused by blocking histamine at the H_1 receptor and those independent of this effect.

1. H_1 blocking effects. As H_1 antagonists, these drugs competitively block or antagonize histamine's effect on the following:
   a. Capillary permeability
   b. Vascular smooth muscle (vessels)
   c. Nonvascular (bronchiolar) smooth muscle. Since other autacoids are also released in an anaphylactic reaction, antihistamines are not effective in counteracting the bronchoconstriction present during that reaction.
   d. Nerve endings. The antihistamines can suppress the itching and pain associated with this histamine-mediated reaction at the cutaneous nerve endings.

2. CNS depression. These antihistamines produce varying degrees of CNS depression. Because of this effect, they are the principal agent in certain over-the-counter (OTC) sleep aids.

3. CNS stimulation. CNS excitation or stimulation can occur in some cases. It is more common in children, elderly patients, and those who abuse antihistamines or use a larger dose than prescribed. Symptoms include restlessness, excitation, and, in severe cases, convulsions.

4. Anticholinergic effects. Cholinergic blockade, similar to that with atropine, can produce xerostomia. This can cause an increased caries rate in patients taking antihistamines on a long-term basis.

5. Antiemetic effects. Some groups of antihistamines (the ethanolamines and the piperazines, Table 18-1) have pronounced anti–motion sickness activity. These agents are also effective in controlling labyrinthine-induced nausea and vomiting. This antiemetic effect makes these agents useful in dentistry to reduce postoperative nausea and vomiting.

6. Local anesthesia. Although antihistamines are not as effective as the other local anesthetics, they can be administered topically or by injection to provide some local anesthesia.

Table 18-1. Properties of antihistamines (H_1 blockers)

Group (Example)	Usual adult dose (mg)	Dosing interval (hr)	Special properties	Other group members
Alkylamines				
Chlorpheniramine (Chlor-Trimeton)	4	4–6	Low incidence of moderate sedation; available OTC	Brompheniramine (Dimetane) Triprolidine (Actidil)
Ethanolamines				
Diphenhydramine (Benadryl)	25–50	4–6	High incidence of prounced sedation; antipruritic property; high anti–motion sickness action	Dimenhydrinate (Dramamine) Carbinoxamine (Clistin) Clemastine (Tavist)
Ethylenediamine				
Tripelennamine (Pyribenzamine)	25–50	4–6	Moderate incidence of pronounced sedation; gastrointestinal irritation	Pyrilamine
Phenothiazines				
Promethazine (Phenergan)	12.5–25.0	6–24	Pronounced sedation; excellent antiemetic; phenothiazine side effects	Trimeprazine (Temaril) Methdilazine (Tacaryl)
Piperidines				
Cyproheptadine (Periactin)	4	8	Little sedation	Azatadine (Optimine) Diphenylpyraline (Hispril) Phenindamine (Nolahist)
Piperazines				
Hydroxyzine (Vistaril, Atarax)	10–25	4–6	Low incidence of moderate sedation; antipruritic; other members used for anti–motion sickness	Meclizine (Bonine, Antivert) Cyclizine (Merezine)
Miscellaneous				
Terfenadine (Seldane)	60	12	Claims to be nonsedating; new members to be released; expensive	

OTC, Over the counter.

Adverse reactions

1. CNS depression. The most common side effect associated with the older antihistamines is sedation, which may be accompanied by dizziness, tinnitus, uncoordination, blurred vision, and fatigue. Patients who are given antihistamines should be warned against operating a motor vehicle. Sedation with antihistamines is additive with that caused by other CNS depressant drugs.

2. Gastrointestinal effects. Gastrointestinal tract complaints commonly associated with the antihistamines include anorexia, nausea, vomiting, constipation, and xerostomia.

Toxicity

Antihistamine poisoning has become more common in recent years because of these agents' easy accessibility in OTC preparations promoted as sleep aids. Excitation predominates in small children, and sedation can occur in adults. Death is usually due to coma with cardiovascular and respiratory collapse. The treatment is conservative and directed at specific symptoms.

Uses

1. Control of allergic reactions. Certain allergic reactions such as allergic rhinitis and seasonal hay fever can be controlled by H_1 antihistamines. With continued use, tolerance can develop to the effects of a particular antihistamine. Changing to an agent in another group can often restore the effects desired. These agents are not useful in the treatment of the common cold. Acute urticarial attacks can be treated with antihistamines to relieve itching, edema, and erythema. In the treatment of anaphylaxis the physiologic antagonist epinephrine rather than the antihistamines is indicated first. The xanthines (aminophylline) are also more effective than the antihistamines in producing bronchodilation in acute anaphylaxis. Certain allergic oral ulcers can be treated by the topical use of antihistamines. The potential hazard of a sensitivity reaction induced by topical administration must be weighed against the benefit of such treatment. These agents also produce some local anesthetic effect when applied topically.

2. Treatment of nausea and vomiting. Because of the antiemetic action of the antihistamines, they are used to prevent and treat motion sickness and to control postoperative vomiting and vomiting induced by radiation therapy. The nausea and vomiting associated with pregnancy should not be treated with antihistamines because of these agents' potential for fetal harm.

3. Preoperative sedation. The use of the older H_1 antihistamines in dentistry is primarily based on their CNS effects. They are employed for preoperative sedation because of their sedative and antiemetic effects. Hydroxyzine and promethazine are particularly useful for this purpose (see Table 18-1).

4. OTC sleep aids. Agents used as OTC sleep aids include diphenhydramine (Nytol, Compoz) or pyrilamine (Dormarex, in Quiet World).

5. Local anesthesia. Although not as effective as the local anesthetics usually employed, antihistamines such as diphenhydramine (Benadryl) can be used by injection to provide some degree of local anesthesia. This may be necessary when patients have exhibited allergies to the normally used local anesthetic agents.

Peripheral (nonsedating) H_1 receptor antagonists

Chemically, members of the nonsedating H_1 receptor antagonists do not have any common denominator. They are quite different in origin, chemical structure, solubility, and metabolic effects. They all share the specific blocking action of peripheral H_1 receptors, and they do not cross the blood-brain barrier in usual therapeutic doses. Terfenadine is discussed as a prototype, since it is the only member available in the United States.

Terfenadine (Seldane)

Terfenadine may be regarded as the most specific H_1 antagonist currently available. It does not appear to have significant antiserotonergic, anticholinergic, or antiadrenergic activity. It is readily absorbed from the gastrointestinal tract, and peak plasma concentrations are reached by 1 to 2 hours after a single oral dose. It is metabolized in the liver and excreted in urine and feces. Terfenadine has been found most effective in the treatment of allergic rhinitis. It may also be effective in treating chronic idiopathic urticaria, enabling discontinuance of corticosteroid therapy in some cases. Terfenadine neither impairs psychomotor performance, nor enhances the depressant effect of concomitantly administered alcohol or benzodiazepines. Terfenadine can be considered a major breakthrough for control of allergic rhinitis in patients for whom the sedative effect of the older antihistamines constitutes a disturbing side effect. It is very expensive relative to the older antihistamines.

Comparison of H_1 antagonists

Terfenadine will take its place as a valuable adjunct in the therapy of seasonal and perennial rhinitis, as well as certain forms of urticaria. It is likely that the nonsedating H_1 antagonists will eventually replace the older H_1 antagonists for these conditions. In dentistry, however, the place of the older H_1 receptor blockers rests assured, since for the treatment of the dental patient these compounds are used as much for their side effects as for their antihistaminic action.

H_2 receptor antagonists

H_2 blocking agents, such as cimetidine (Tagamet), inhibit the action of histamine at the H_2 receptors. Because they are used to treat gastrointestinal problems, they are discussed in Chapter 22.

OTHER AUTACOIDS
Prostaglandins and thromboxanes

The family of prostaglandins, the thromboxanes together with the leukotrienes, are often referred to as *eicosanoids*, because they all derive from arachidonic acid. They are among the most common autacoids and have been found in most body tissues and fluids. They are produced in the body in response to many different stimuli, and in small quantities they produce a large spectrum of effects on many different body systems.

The family of prostaglandins (PG) is divided into six main series of agents, A, B, C, D, E, and F, of which the last two are predominant. These main groups are further subdivided and give rise to an extensive and complicated series of compounds.

Until recently PGEs and PGFs were the most abundant and most intensively studied prostaglandins. Now many new prostaglandins (PGG_2 and PGH), thromboxanes (TXA_2 and TXB_2), and prostacyclin (PGI_2) have become of central interest.

The pharmacologic effects of the prostaglandins encompass many diverse actions. Not only is there a wide spectrum of action, but different prostaglandins have different activities in both amount and kind, including vasodilation, increased heart rate and cardiac output, uterine contraction, increased capillary permeability, alteration of smooth muscle contraction, inhibition of gastric secretion and increased mucus secretion in the intestines, increased renal blood flow, sedation, stimulation of pain fibers, and effects on a number of endocrine gland secretions.

An example of opposing actions of the prostaglandins is as follows: thromboxane, produced by platelets, stimulates platelet aggregation and is a vasoconstrictor; while prostacyclin, produced by the vessel walls, inhibits platelet aggregation and is a vasodilator. A normal balance between these two agents exists.

Prostaglandins are important in dentistry because they have been implicated in periodontal disease. At least two stages of periodontal disease may involve prostaglandins. The first is the inflammation of the gingiva with its resultant erythema, edema, and increase in gingival exudate. Prostaglandins, thought to be mediators of the inflammatory response in oral soft tissues, may be involved in this initial stage of periodontal disease. The second is the resorption of alveolar bone with tooth loss. They also prevent the synthesis of new bone by inhibiting osteoblastic activity.

Since the prostaglandins have many activities, it is likely that they have no single receptor. They are released by mechanical, thermal, chemical, bacterial, or traumatic injuries. Their role seems more important in chronic inflammation, and this may be their involvement in periodontal disease.

The only therapeutic use of the prostaglandins is inducing mid-trimester abortions. They are used by intraamniotic injection ($PGF_{2\alpha}$) or by vaginal suppository (PGE_2). Currently, prostaglandins are being studied in the prevention of ulcers and the treatment of bronchial asthma and hypertension. The administration of prostaglandin antagonists may prove useful in the treatment of certain pathologic conditions. This seems reasonable in view of the many effects of the prostaglandins in the body.

It has been shown that aspirin and certain other nonsteroidal anti-inflammatory drugs interfere with the synthesis and release of the prostaglandins. There is also some evidence that certain phenolic compounds such as eugenol (clove oil) inhibit prostaglandin. Since prostaglandins are involved in inflammation, agents that inhibit the prostaglandins may be useful in the treatment of inflammation.

Leukotrienes

Another complex group of autacoids is also derived from arachidonic acid and these substances are collectively known as the leukotrienes. Although they show considerable species variation, their dominant action in humans is powerful bronchoconstriction. In that effect, leukotrienes are far more potent than histamine. They also contract other smooth muscle like the uterus or gastrointestinal tract. Extensive research is devoted to these substances and great progress can be expected, potentially in the treatment of asthma and other forms of bronchoconstriction.

Kinins

Kinins are polypeptides that are distributed in a great variety of body tissues. Two members of this group, kallidin and bradykinin, are found in plasma and may play a role in dental diseases. These agents are formed by the action of certain proteolytic enzymes (kininogenases) such as kalli-

krein on their common precursor, kinogen. Other kininogenases include trypsin, plasmin, and certain snake venoms.

The plasma kinins may be involved in shock and acute or chronic allergic or inflammatory conditions such as anaphylaxis and arthritis. Their effects on the body include vasodilation, increased capillary permeability, edema, pain resulting from action on nerve endings, and contraction or relaxation of nonvascular smooth muscles. The kinins apparently mediate pulpal pain and are implicated in the control of the synthesis of endogenous analgesics, particularly the endorphins, during caries formation. It is possible that inhibitors of kinins may be useful dental therapeutic aids in the future.

Although no specific antagonists of the kinins are yet available, some drugs are known to inhibit kinin-evoked responses. For example, salicylates (aspirin) and glucocorticoids (steroids) may inhibit kallikrein activation and may play a role in future therapy. The synthesis of antagonists to the autacoid kinins and their possible clinical use are currently being investigated.

REVIEW QUESTIONS

1. Define the term "autacoid."
2. Name the major pharmacologic effects of histamine.
3. Describe the effects of stimulation of H_1 and H_2 receptors.
4. Explain why the older antihistamines are called H_1 antagonists or blockers.
5. Explain the pharmacologic effects of the older antihistamines.
6. Describe the effects of the antihistamines that are related to their action on the CNS.
7. Explain the major adverse reactions associated with antihistamines.
8. Discuss the therapeutic uses of all antihistamines. Name a specific use for the antihistamines in dentistry.
9. Name a "newer" antihistamine and explain one advantage and disadvantage it possesses.
10. Describe why the prostaglandins have taken on increased importance to the dental profession.
11. Name two types of drugs that inhibit the synthesis of prostaglandin and give one example of each type. Explain how this action is used therapeutically.

Adrenocorticosteroids

The term "adrenocorticosteroids" (adrenal corticosteroids, corticosteroids) refers to a group of agents that are secreted by the adrenal cortex. The dental hygienist should be aware of the effects, adverse reactions, and dental implications of these agents for at least the following reasons:

1. Use in dentistry. Some of these compounds are used topically or systemically for the treatment of oral lesions.

2. Long-term therapy. The adrenocorticosteroids, or "steroids" as they are commonly called, are prescribed for many patients with chronic systemic diseases such as asthma or arthritis. These agents can cause a variety of adverse reactions that may influence the patient's dental treatment.

MECHANISM OF RELEASE

The adrenocorticosteroids are naturally occurring compounds secreted by the adrenal cortex. Their release is triggered by a series of events (Fig. 19-1). First a stimulus such as stress causes the hypothalamus (1) to release corticotropin-releasing factor (CRF), which acts (2) on the pituitary gland. Under the influence of CRF the pituitary gland secretes adrenocorticotropic hormone (ACTH) (3), which stimulates the adrenal cortex to release hydrocortisone (4). Hydrocortisone then acts on both ACTH (5) and CRF (6) to inhibit the release of these agents. This mechanism is called negative feedback.

Exogenous steroids act in the same way as hydrocortisone; that is, they inhibit the release of CRF and ACTH. With long-term administration of steroids, ACTH release is suppressed and there is atrophy of the adrenal gland. If the administration of exogenous steroid is then abruptly stopped, a relative steroid deficiency results. This can cause severe problems including adrenal crisis.

CLASSIFICATION

The adrenocorticosteroids can be divided into two major groups, the glucocorticoids, which affect intermediate carbohydrate metabolism, and the mineralocorticoids, which affect the water and electrolyte composition of the body. The major glucocorticoid present in the body is cortisol (hydrocortisone). Without stress, the normal adult secretes about 20 mg of hydrocortisone daily. A 10-fold increase can occur with stress. Maximal secretion occurs between 4 AM and 8 AM in people with a normal schedule. The chemical structures of the synthetic agents and the naturally occurring adrenocorticosteroids such as hydrocortisone are similar. Many chemical modifications have been made in an attempt to produce synthetic glucocorticoids with fewer adverse reactions and more specific activity.

Although the term "adrenocorticosteroids" refers to those steroids secreted by the adrenal cortex and includes both the glucocorticoids and the mineralocorticoids, this chapter deals primarily with the glucocorticoids because of their more frequent use.

DEFINITIONS

The following terms are used in this chapter:

steroids Chemical substances comprising many body constituents and drugs, each containing a certain chemical structure.

adrenocorticosteroids or **corticosteroids** Steroidal components released from the adrenal cortex, including glucocorticoids and mineralocorticoids.

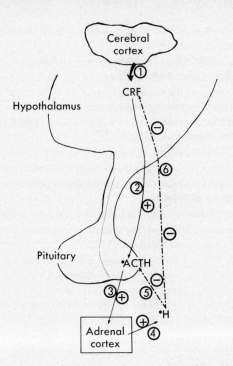

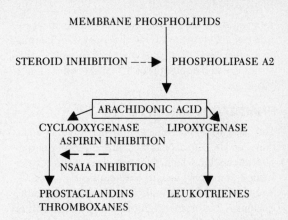

Fig. 19-2. Effect of glucocorticoid on prostaglandins and leukotrienes. (From Holroyd, S.V., Wynn, R.L., and Requa-Clark, B.: Clinical pharmacology in dental practice, ed. 4, St. Louis, 1988, The C.V. Mosby Co.)

Fig. 19-1. Control of the release of adrenocorticosteroids. *1*, Stimuli (such as stress) from the cerebral cortex releases corticotropin releasing factor (CRF); *2*, CRF stimulates the pituitary to release adrenocorticotropic hormone (ACTH); *3*, ACTH stimulates the adrenal cortex to secrete hydrocortisone (H); and *4*, H inhibits the secretion of *5*, ACTH, and *6*, CRF.

glucocorticoids Adrenocorticosteroids that primarily affect carbohydrate metabolism.

mineralocorticoids Adrenocorticosteroids that affect the body's sodium and water balance (fluid levels).

adrenocorticotropic hormone (ACTH) Agent secreted by the pituitary that causes the release of hormones from the adrenal cortex.

Addison's disease Deficiency of the adrenocorticosteroids.

Cushing's syndrome Excess of the adrenocorticosteroids.

ROUTES OF ADMINISTRATION

The glucocorticoids are available in a wide variety of dosage forms. They are routinely used topi-cally, orally, intramuscularly, and intravenously. Systemic effects are commonly obtained when the drug is administered orally or parenterally, but topical administration can also cause systemic effects. If a large quantity of a steroid is applied topically, especially if the skin is denuded or an occlusive dressing such as Saran Wrap is applied, systemic effects can occur.

MECHANISM OF ACTION

The mechanism of action of the steroids involves binding to a specific receptor, forming a steroid-receptor complex. The complex then enters the nucleus and alters gene expression, resulting in the regulation of many cellular processes. Because of this mechanism, a lag time exists in the action of the steroids, and the relationship between their effects and blood level is poor. The antiinflammatory action of the glucocorticoids results from their inhibition of arachidonic acid metabolism. They induce the synthesis of a protein that inhibits phospholipase A2, decreasing the production of both prostaglandins and leukotrienes (Fig. 19-2). These agents, responsible for the delayed phase of acute inflammation, act synergistically. Other antiinflammatory effects of the corticosteroids include their effects on the im-

[handwritten: Hypokalemia = low potassium]

mune system that result in a **decrease** in accumulation of neutrophils at the site of inflammation, and also of monocytes and lymphocytes, with a greater depletion of T lymphocytes than B lymphocytes.

PHARMACOLOGIC EFFECTS

The pharmacologic effects and the adverse reactions of the corticosteroids are closely related. The effects for which they are used include their antiinflammatory action and suppression of allergic reactions. They also suppress the immune response. The corticosteroids are palliative rather than curative. The glucocorticoid effects and the mineralocorticoid effects are listed below. Many of these effects produce adverse reactions and are discussed in the section below.

   Glucocorticoid effects
   Broad
      Carbohydrate metabolism
      Antiinflammatory
      Antiallergenic
      Enzyme action
      Membrane function
      RNA synthesis
   Catabolic
      Increase gluconeogenesis
      Decrease glucose use
      Inhibit protein synthesis
      Increase protein catabolism
      Decrease growth
      Decrease resistance to infection
   Mineralocorticoid effects
   Increase sodium retention
   Increase potassium loss
   Edema and hypertension

[handwritten: Never give for viral infections!]

[handwritten: due to reduced inflammation delayed healing]

ADVERSE REACTIONS

The adverse reactions of the corticosteroids are proportional to the dosage, frequency and time of administration, and the duration of treatment. With prolonged therapy with high enough doses the following side effects occur:

1. Metabolic changes. Moon face (round), buffalo hump (fat deposited on back of the neck), truncal obesity, weight gain, and muscle wasting give patients the Cushing's syndrome appearance. Bruising, hyperglycemia (toward diabetes), osteo-

porosis, impaired wound healing, and abdominal striae also occur.

2. Infections. Corticosteroids decrease resistance to infection. Because of their antiinflammatory action, they may also mask its symptoms. Patients taking long-term glucocorticoid therapy are given isoniazid (INH), an antituberculosis agent, to prevent tuberculosis.

3. CNS effects. Changes in behavior and personality including euphoria (with increasing dose), agitation, psychoses, and depression (with decreasing dose) can occur.

4. Osteoporosis. Thinning bones can result in fractures in patients on chronic steroids who have not undergone trauma.

5. Other effects. Because corticosteroids can increase intraocular pressure, glaucoma may be exacerbated. Hyperglycemia may be aggravated or initiated. More antidiabetic medication may be required. Because the steroids stimulate stomach acid secretion, they may exacerbate ulcers.

6. Electrolyte and fluid balance. The glucocorticoids that possess some mineralocorticoid action can produce sodium and water retention. Hypertension or congestive heart failure may be exacerbated. Hypokalemia may also result.

7. Adrenal crisis. If adrenal suppression is present and a patient undergoes a stressful situation, adrenal crisis could result. The adrenal gland is unable to respond with additional steroid in this situation. Weakness, syncope, cardiovascular collapse, and death could ensue.

8. Dental effects. Oral tissue changes may occur in patients taking corticosteroids. Osteoporosis, affecting the alveolar bone, could result in tooth loss.

USES
Medical uses

[handwritten: Treats effects But doesn't cure.]

The adrenocorticosteroids are generally used in medicine for one of the following reasons:

1. Replacement therapy. Patients with hypofunction of the adrenal cortex (Addison's disease) need replacement of glucocorticoid and mineralocorticoid activity. Usually, hydrocortisone is used to restore glucocorticoid activity and desoxy-

corticosterone is used to restore mineralocorticoid activity. Patients with hyperfunction of the adrenal cortex (Cushing's syndrome) may have a majority of the gland removed surgically. In this case replacement therapy is needed.

2. Emergencies. The corticosteroids are used in emergency situations for the treatment of shock or adrenal crisis, as discussed in Chapter 23.

3. Anti-inflammatory effects. The most extensive use of the corticosteroids in both medicine and dentistry is in the treatment of a wide variety of inflammatory and severe allergic conditions. These agents are not curative but merely ameliorate symptoms because of their antiinflammatory activity. Some conditions that have been treated with corticosteroids are rheumatoid arthritis, rheumatic fever, systemic lupus erythematosus, scleroderma, inflammation of the joints and soft tissues, acute bronchial asthma, severe and acute allergic reactions, and severe allergic dermatoses.

Dental uses

Because of the adrenocorticosteroids' antiinflammatory action, they are administered topically, intraarticularly, or orally in the following dental situations:

1. Oral lesions. Systemically administered steroids are often effective in the treatment of oral lesions associated with noninfectious inflammatory diseases, including erythema multiforme, lichen planus, pemphigus, desquamative gingivitis, and benign mucous membrane pemphigoid (BMMP).

2. Temporomandibular joint (TMJ) arthritis. The TMJ affected with arthritis also responds to the systemic administration of steroids. If this is the only joint affected, an intraarticular injection can often decrease the pain and improve the joint movement.

3. Oral surgery. Adrenocorticosteroids have been used in oral surgery to reduce edema, trismus, and pain. Although the decrease in postoperative edema can be easily documented, the magnitude of the benefit must be weighed against the potential risk. The safety and effectiveness of these agents have been evidenced primarily by clinical observation rather than by controlled double-blind studies.

4. Pulp procedures. Adrenocorticosteroids have been used in pulp capping, pulpotomy procedures, and the control of hypersensitive cervical dentin. Their use in these situations is currently empirical or experimental.

5. Aphthous stomatitis. The evidence for the benefit of adrenocorticosteroids in the treatment of aphthous stomatitis seems clear. Triamcinolone acetonide (Kenalog in Orabase) has been advocated. Other topical steroids can be used.

Although there has been mixed success in the use of steroids in dentistry, double-blind controlled studies are needed to determine unequivocally their proper place in the therapeutic armamentarium.

CORTICOSTEROID PRODUCTS

In Table 19-1 selected synthetic corticosteroids are arranged according to their duration of action—short, intermediate, and long. The relative antiinflammatory and salt-retaining activity and equivalent oral dose are given, with hydrocortisone arbitrarily assigned the value of 1. The other agents are then given values in relation to those of hydrocortisone. For example, prednisone, with an antiinflammatory activity of 4, has 4 times as much antiinflammatory action as hydrocortisone or requires ¼ as much agent to have the same effect. The mineralocorticoid, or salt-retaining properties of the glucocorticoids are also compared with that of hydrocortisone. For example, triamcinolone does not increase salt retention, whereas hydrocortisone does.

Table 19-1 lists the equivalent oral dose in milligrams based on 20 mg of hydrocortisone, the amount normally secreted daily by an adult without stress. By looking at Table 19-1, one can see that 0.75 mg of dexamethasone or 5 mg of prednisone is approximately equivalent to 20 mg of hydrocortisone.

DENTAL IMPLICATIONS

1. Gastrointestinal effects. Because the adrenocorticosteroids stimulate acid secretion, patients

Table 19-1.   Relative activity of glucocorticosteroids

Drug	Activity		Equivalent oral dose (mg)
	Anti-inflammatory	Salt-retaining	
Glucocorticoids			
Short acting			
Hydrocortisone	1	1	20
Prednisone (Deltasone)	4	0.8	5
Intermediate acting			
Triamcinolone (Aristocort, Kenacort, Kenalog, Mycolog)	5	0	4
Long acting			
Betamethasone (Celestone, Valisone)	25	0	0.6
Dexamethasone (Decadron, Hexadrol)	30	0	0.75

taking these agents should avoid other ulcerogenic medication such as the salicylates.

2. Elevated blood pressure. The blood pressure of patients taking corticosteroids should be measured, since these agents can exacerbate hypertension.

3. Infection. Owing to the antiinflammatory activity of the adrenocorticosteroids, they may mask the symptoms of an infection or decrease a patient's resistance to infection.

4. Behavioral changes. A patient's bizarre behavior may be explained by the presence of, or withdrawal from, adrenocorticosteroids.

5. Osteoporosis. Dental radiographs may demonstrate osteoporosis in patients taking adrenocorticosteroids.

6. Glaucoma. Other agents that can induce or exacerbate glaucoma, such as the anticholinergics, should be used with great caution in patients taking adrenocorticosteroids.

7. Delayed wound healing. Since the adrenocorticosteroids cause delayed wound healing, special precautions should be taken when surgical procedures are performed.

8. Adrenal crisis. Patients undergoing long-term therapy with the adrenocorticosteroids may not be able to respond with the release of hydrocortisone in a stressful situation such as a dental appointment. It may be necessary for the physi-

cian to increase the dosage of the adrenal steroids.

The Rule of Two's states that adrenal suppression may occur if a patient is taking more than 20 mg of cortisone (or equivalent) daily, for 2 weeks within 2 years of dental treatment. Another suggestion includes doubling the dose of steroids for patients taking between 20 and 40 mg of hydrocortisone (or equivalent) and giving the usual daily dose for patients taking over 40 mg daily. It is better to give additional steroids because a one-time increase in steroids produces no additional adverse effects over the usual doses.

See earlier section on dental uses of corticosteroids.

REVIEW QUESTIONS

1. Compare and contrast the activity of the glucocorticoids and mineralocorticoids.
2. Explain the relative salt-retaining, antiinflammatory, and topical activity of the steroids. Describe the calculations used to determine relative potency.
3. List and explain the routes of administration for the steroids used in dentistry.
4. Enumerate the major pharmacologic effects and adverse reactions associated with the glucocorticoids.
5. Describe the three major uses of the steroids in medicine.
6. List the contraindications and cautions associated with the adrenocorticosteroids and explain how these adverse effects are related.

7. Describe how the adverse effects of the adrenocorticosteroids can be minimized or treated. Include the rationale for the administration of isoniazid (INH) and antacid.

8. Explain how to evaluate a patient undergoing steroid therapy and how to determine whether the patient's physician should be consulted. State what problems could arise from dental treatment and how these adverse effects could be monitored.

9. Compare and contrast the glucocorticoids available, and state the agent used for various dental conditions.

10. Define the terms "Cushing's syndrome" and "Addison's disease."

11. Explain the term "equivalent oral dose" and calculate the minimum dose of agents that can cause Cushing's syndrome. Remember that 100 mg of hydrocortisone or its equivalent can produce this effect.

12. Describe the "Rule of Two's."

Chapter 20

Other hormones

Hormones are secreted by endocrine glands and transported by the blood to target organs where they are biologically active. Endocrine glands include the pituitary, thyroid, parathyroids, pancreas, adrenals, gonads, and placenta. They help maintain homeostasis by regulating body functions and are controlled themselves by feedback systems. Drugs that effect the endocrine system include the active principles of the endocrine glands, synthetic hormone agonists and antagonists, and substances that influence the synthesis and secretion of hormones. The most important clinical application of these drugs is their use in replacement therapy, such as in the treatment of diabetes mellitus or myxedema. Additional applications include diagnostic procedures, contraception, and the treatment of glandular hyperfunction, cancer, and other systemic disorders.

PITUITARY HORMONES

The pituitary gland (hypophysis) is a small endocrine organ located at the base of the brain. It has been called the master gland because of its regulatory effect on other endocrine glands and organs of the body. It secretes peptide hormones that regulate the thyroid, adrenal, and sex glands; the kidney and uterus; and growth. In addition to their regulatory effect, the pituitary hormones have a trophic effect that is necessary for the maintenance of many systems. For example, without the gonadotropins, the entire reproductive system fails; without growth hormone and thyrotropin, normal growth and development are impossible. The secretion of pituitary hormones is influenced by peripheral endocrine glands via hormonal feedback mechanisms and by neurohumoral substances from the hypothalamus.

There are two parts to the pituitary gland, the anterior lobe (adenohypophysis) and the posterior lobe (neurohypophysis).

The anterior lobe secretes growth hormone (GH), or somatotropin; luteinizing hormone (LH); follicle-stimulating hormone (FSH); thyroid-stimulating hormone (TSH), or thyrotropin; adrenocorticotropic hormone (ACTH), or corticotropin; and prolactin (Fig. 20-1).

The posterior pituitary gland secretes antidiuretic hormone (ADH, vasopressin) and oxytocin.

Pituitary deficiency (hypopituitarism) can produce a loss of secondary sex characteristics, decreased metabolism, dwarfism, diabetes insipidus, hypothyroidism, Addison's disease, loss of pigmentation, thinning and softening of the skin, decreased libido, and retarded dental development.[1] Hypersecretion of pituitary hormones can produce sexual precocity, goiter, Cushing's disease, acromegaly, and giantism.

Genetic engineering can now produce human growth hormone. It is used medically to treat children who lack it and illicitly by body builders and weight lifters to develop muscles. FSH, which stimulates follicle growth, and LH, which induces ovulation, are used in the treatment of infertility. Vasopressin is used intranasally to treat diabetes insipidus. Oxytocin, either by injection or intranasally, is used to induce labor and control postpartum hemorrhage. TSH is used to test thyroid function and ACTH to test the adrenal cortex.

THYROID HORMONES

Thyroxine (T_4) and triiodothyronine (T_3) are iodine-containing hormones synthesized and secreted by the thyroid gland. Both act on virtually

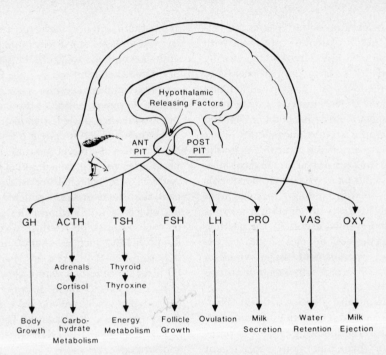

Fig. 20-1. Pituitary hormones. Hormones and actions are not all-inclusive. ANT PIT, Anterior pituitary; POST PIT, posterior pituitary; GH, growth hormone; ACTH, adrenocorticotropic hormone; TSH, thyroid-stimulating hormone; FSH, follicle-stimulating hormone; LH, luteinizing hormone; PRO, prolactin; VAS, vasopressin; OXY, oxytocin.

every tissue and organ system of the body and are important for energy metabolism, growth, and development. Vulnerability to stress, altered drug response, and altered orofacial development are all possible manifestations of thyroid dysfunction.

Thyroid hormone is synthesized from iodine and tyrosine and stored as a complex protein until stimulated to be released by TSH. The actions of the thyroid hormones include those on growth and development, calorigenic effects, and metabolic effects. In frogs, thyroid can transform a tadpole into a frog.

Iodine

Normal thyroid function requires an adequate intake of iodine (approximately 125 µg per day). Without it, normal amounts of hormone cannot be made, TSH is secreted in excess, and the thy-

roid hypertrophies. This thyroid hypertrophy is called simple or nontoxic goiter. Because iodine is not abundant in most foods, simple goiter is quite prevalent in some areas of the world. Marine life is the only common food that is naturally rich in iodine. Iodized salt has decreased the incidence of simple goiter in many countries. Simple goiter resulting from iodine deficiency is treated with the appropriate dose of either a saturated solution of potassium iodide or Lugol's solution, containing 5% iodine and 10% potassium iodide.

Hypothyroidism

In the small child, thyroid hypofunction is referred to as cretinism. In the adult it is called myxedema, or simple hypothyroidism. The main characteristic is mental and physical retardation.

Such patients are usually drowsy, weak, and listless and exhibit an expressionless, puffy face with edematous tongue and lips. Oral findings usually include delayed tooth eruption, malocclusion, and increased tendency to develop periodontal disease.[3] The teeth are usually poorly shaped and carious. The gingiva is either inflamed or pale and enlarged. The cretin is often uncooperative and difficult to motivate for plaque control. Diagnostic radiographs and routine dental prophylaxis may require special assistance. Hypothyroid patients have a difficulty in withstanding stress and tend to be abnormally sensitive to all central nervous system (CNS) depressants, especially the narcotic analgesics. If used, their dosages should be adjusted. Pregnant women with hypothyroidism tend to produce offspring with larger maxillary and mandibular teeth.[4]

Thyroid hypofunction is rationally and effectively treated by oral administration of exogenous thyroid hormones. The following is a list of preparations used for thyroid hormone replacement therapy:

Levothyroxine sodium (Synthroid)
Liothyronine sodium (Cytomel)
Liotrix (Euthroid)
Thyroglobulin (Proloid)
Thyroid tablets (Thyrar)
Thyroid

Hyperthyroidism

Diffuse toxic goiter (Graves' disease) and toxic nodular goiter (Plummer's disease) are the two forms of thyroid hyperfunction. Diffuse toxic goiter is characterized by a diffusely enlarged, highly vascular thyroid gland; it is common in young adults, and is considered to be a disorder of the immune response. Toxic nodular goiter is characterized by nodules within the gland that spontaneously secrete excessive amounts of hormone while the rest of the glandular tissue is atrophied. It occurs primarily in older patients and usually arises from long-standing nontoxic goiter.

The adverse effects from excessive levels of circulating thyroid hormone, or thyrotoxicosis, include excessive production of heat, increased sympathetic activity, increased neuromuscular activity, increased sensitivity to pain, ophthalmopathy, exophthalmos (protruding eyes), and anxiety. Oral manifestations include accelerated tooth eruption, and marked loss of the alveolar process, diffuse demineralization of the jawbone, and rapidly progressing periodontal destruction.

The cardiovascular system is especially hyperactive because of a direct inotropic effect, increased peripheral oxygen consumption, and increased sensitivity to catecholamines.[5,6] Epinephrine is contraindicated in these patients. The potentiating effects of thyroid hormones and epinephrine on each other could result in severe cardiovascular problems, such as angina, arrhythmias, and hypertension. β-Blockers are therapeutically useful if such a condition does arise.

In addition to their increased sensitivity to pain, hyperthyroid persons have an increased tolerance to CNS depressants. They may require higher than usual doses of sedatives, analgesics, and local anesthetics.

No treatment should be begun for any patient with a visible goiter, exophthalmos, or a history of taking antithyroid drugs until approval is obtained from the patient's physician. Medical management of the condition is important before any elective surgery is performed. Even in controlled patients who are considered to be euthyroid, stress should be kept at a minimum, preoperative sedation should be considered, and the dental hygienist should be alert for signs of hypothyroidism or hyperthyroidism.

Treatment of hyperthyroidism usually includes one of the following four catagories:

1. Antithyroid drugs
2. Iodide
3. Radioactive iodine
4. Thyroidectomy

Antithyroid drugs interfere directly with the synthesis of thyroid hormones by inhibiting the iodination of tyrosine moieties and the coupling of the iodotyrosines. Untoward reactions are relatively few, but the most serious is agranulocytosis, which can lead to poor wound healing, oral ulceronecrotic lesions, and oral infections. Paresthesia of facial areas and loss of taste are also seen. Not only are antithyroid drugs used over prolonged periods to bring a hyperactive thyroid to the euthyroid state, but they are also given before thyroidectomy to reduce the possibility of thyroid storm, a life-threatening acute form of thyrotoxicosis. Antithyroid drugs include propylthiouracil (Propacil) and methimazole (Tapazole).

Iodide in high concentrations suppresses the thyroid in a still poorly understood manner. It may produce gingival pain, excessive salivation, and sialadenitis as side effects. Radioactive iodine is sequestered by the gland and results in localized destruction of thyroid tissue.

Thyroidectomy is the surgical approach to hyperthyroidism. Both radioactive iodine and thyroidectomy usually result in hypothyroidism and thyroid supplements are often required.

PANCREATIC HORMONES

The two primary hormones secreted by the islets of Langerhans of the pancreas are insulin and glucagon. Insulin promotes fuel storage, whereas glucagon promotes fuel mobilization in the body.

Diabetes mellitus

Diabetes mellitus results in almost all instances from inadequate or poorly timed secretion of insulin from the pancreas. It is primarily characterized by hyperglycemia and glycosuria. Other characteristics include hyperlipemia, azoturia, ketonemia, and, when the deficiency is severe, ketoacidosis. Patients usually experience general weakness, weight loss, polyphagia, polydipsia, and polyuria.

Diabetes mellitus is currently classified as insulin dependent (type I, IDDM), noninsulin dependent (type II, NIDDM), or other (e.g., drug induced). Insulin-dependent (previously called juvenile-onset) diabetes usually develops in persons younger than 20 years and is associated with a complete lack of insulin secretion, rapid development, and severity of symptoms. Noninsulin-dependent (previously called maturity-onset) diabetes, which usually develops in persons older than 40 years, is associated with the ability of the

pancreas to secrete some insulin, and involves a slower onset and less severe symptoms.

Uncontrolled diabetes produces a pronounced susceptibility to dental caries. This is caused mainly by decreased salivary flow and increased levels of carbohydrates in the parotid saliva.[7] Since the start of the widespread use of insulin, however, most studies have failed to demonstrate an increased incidence of caries in treated patients.[8] Some investigators have even found fewer cavities in treated diabetic children than in healthy controls.[9] Dietary restrictions may be the reason for the lower incidence of caries.

Diabetes mellitus also affects the dental development of children.[10] Diabetic children have been shown to differ from normal children in the median ages at which they lose their deciduous teeth and gain their permanent teeth.

Uncontrolled or undiagnosed diabetics are more prone to periodontal disease.[11-13] However, the periodontal status of the well-controlled diabetic has been somewhat more controversial. Despite the fact that some investigators reported a lack of correlation between diabetes and increased periodontal disease, many other studies have resulted in the opposite conclusion. After an extensive review of the literature, especially those studies of sound design, Murrah[14] concluded that increased periodontal disease does occur in the diabetic person, whether or not he or she is well controlled.

Periodontal findings include inflammatory and degenerative changes ranging from mild gingivitis to painful periodontitis with a widened periodontal ligament, multiple abscesses, putrescent exudates from periodontal pockets, and increased tooth mobility caused by destruction of supporting alveolar bone. Even though it may be more severe, diabetic periodontal disease appears to be similar to that found in nondiabetics. The diabetic state probably serves as a predisposing factor that can accelerate the periodontal destruction originated by microbial agents.[11] The proposed etiology for the periodontal changes seen in the diabetic includes microangiopathy of the tissues, thickening of capillary basement membranes, changes in glucose tolerance factor (GTF) (more glucose), altered polymorphonuclear leukocyte function and enhanced collagenase activity.

Dental appointments should not interfere with meals and should involve minimal stress. In controlled diabetics, oral surgical procedures should be performed 1½ to 2 hours after the patient has eaten a normal breakfast and taken regular antidiabetic medication. Following surgery, the patient should receive an adequate caloric intake to prevent hypoglycemia.[15,16]

Diabetics have fragile blood vessels and other vascular problems that result in delayed wound healing and a tendency to develop infections; therefore surgical therapy should be approached with caution. Sealing and soft tissue curettage are usually well-tolerated.[17] Antibiotic therapy may be considered in selected patients. If infection ensues it should be aggressively treated. Measures to reduce the possibility of infection should be used whenever possible.[18]

Drugs that may decrease insulin release or increase insulin requirements, such as epinephrine, glucocorticoids, or opioid analgesics, should be used with caution in the diabetic patient. Caution should also be exercised with general anesthetics because of the possibility of acidosis.

Antidiabetic agents

Dietary control is still an important component of all antidiabetic therapy. In addition, the patient may be taking either insulin or an oral antidiabetic agent.

Insulin

Insulin is usually administered by subcutaneous injection. The older preparations were prepared from beef or pork pancreases and differed their onset and duration of action. Table 20-1 lists insulin preparations, their peak effect, and duration of action. Human insulin is now available and produced by two different processes. With recombinant deoxyribonucleic acid (DNA) synthesis human insulin can be made by *Escherichia coli*. The other process uses transpeptidation of pork insulin. The most common combination of insulins used in clinical practice is NPH (isophane insulin suspension) or Lente (insulin zinc suspension) plus regular insulin. Human insulin is available in both NPH and regular.

The most common complication in the diabetic dental patient on insulin is a hypoglycemic reaction. This can be caused by an unintentional insulin overdosage (**insulin shock**), failure to eat, or

Table 20-1. Insulin preparations

Action	Preparation	Peak (hr)	Duration (hr)
Rapid	Insulin Injection (Regular, Humulin R*)	2–5	6–8
	Prompt Insulin Zinc Suspension (Semilente, Semitard)	5–10	12–16
Intermediate	Isophane Insulin Suspension (NPH, Humulin N*)	8–12	24
	Insulin Zinc Suspension (Lente, Lentard, Monotard, Humulin L*)	7–15	24
Long	Protamine Zinc Insulin Suspension (PZI)	14–20	36
	Extended Insulin Zinc Suspension (Ultralente, Ultratard)	10–30	>36

*Human insulin.

increased exercise or stress. Symptoms that can be explained by an increased release of epinephrine from the adrenals include sweating, weakness, nausea, and tachycardia. Symptoms caused by glucose deprivation of the brain include headache, blurred vision, mental confusion, incoherent speech, and eventually coma, convulsions, and death. Treatment of hypoglycemic reactions in their early stages, when the patient is awake, includes fruit juice or soluble carbohydrates. When the patient is unconscious, treatment consists of intravenous (IV) glucose, dextrose, or glucagon (these items should be readily available in the dental office for emergencies).[19]

It is often difficult clinically to distinguish insulin hypoglycemia from severe diabetic ketoacidosis. A few grams of sugar, however, added to diabetic acidosis will produce no harm. Insulin should never be administered in a dental office emergency.

Oral antidiabetic agents

The sulfonylureas are the primary oral antidiabetic agents. Their effectiveness is based on their ability to stimulate the secretion of insulin from the beta cells. They are indicated for non-insulin-dependent diabetics who cannot be treated with diet alone and are unable or unwilling to take insulin. Side effects include blood dyscrasias, gastrointestinal disturbances, cutaneous reactions, and liver damage. Hypoglycemic reactions may occur and are most often seen in patients over 50 years of age with impaired hepatic or renal function. The same dental precautions are in order as for patients taking insulin. Drugs of interest to the dentist that may interact with the sulfonylureas to increase the risk of hypoglycemia include salicylates, sulfonamides, phenylbutazone, barbiturates, and alcohol. Table 20-2 lists the first- and second-generation sulfonylureas, their average daily dose, and duration of action.

Glucagon

Glucagon is produced by the pancreatic alpha cells and promotes fuel mobilization. Its role is antagonistic to that of insulin. The only clinical use for glucagon is the treatment of hypoglycemia.

FEMALE SEX HORMONES

The female sex hormones, estrogen and progesterone, are secreted primarily by the ovaries but also by the testes and placenta. They are largely responsible for producing the female sex characteristics, developing the reproductive system, and preparing it for conception. They also influence other tissues including the gingiva. For example, changes in sex hormone levels during the life of the female are related to the development of gingivitis at puberty (puberty gingivitis), during pregnancy (pregnancy gingivitis), and after menopause (chronic desquamative gingivitis).[20,21] Conscientious plaque control helps to minimize these conditions. The increase in gingival inflammation may occur even with a decrease in the amount of plaque.[22] This may be a result of increased levels of prostaglandin E (PGE), estradiol,[24] and progesterone[23] in the saliva.

Table 20-2. Oral hypoglycemic agents (sulfonylureas)

Agent	Average daily dose (mg)	Duration (hr)
First generation		
Tolbutamide (Orinase)	1000	6–12
Acetohexamide (Dymelor)	500	12–24
Tolazamide (Tolinase)	250	10–16
Chlorpropamide (Diabinese)	250	60
Second generation		
Glyburide (DiaBeta, Micronase)	5	24
Glipizide (Glucotrol)	5	10–24

Estrogen and progesterone levels vary daily. These changes are dependent on the gonadotropic hormones FSH and LH. The interrelationship among these four hormones during the female sexual cycle is as follows: On day 1 of an average 28-day cycle, when the menstrual flow begins, the secretions of FSH and LH are beginning to increase. This release is caused by a reduction in the blood levels of estrogen and progesterone, which normally inhibit their release. In response to increased FSH, an ovarian egg matures, and the follicle in which it is contained grows in size and begins to produce and secrete estrogen. For reasons not entirely understood, on approximately day 12, the rate of secretion of FSH and LH increases markedly to cause a rapid swelling of the follicle that culminates in ovulation on day 14. Following ovulation, LH causes the secretory cells of the follicle to develop into a corpus luteum that secretes large quantities of estrogen and progesterone. This causes a feedback decrease in the secretion of both FSH and LH. On approximately day 26, the corpus luteum completely degenerates. The resultant decrease in estrogen and progesterone leads to menstruation and increased release of FSH and LH. The FSH initiates growth of new follicles to begin a new cycle.

Estrogens

In addition to their role in the female sexual cycle, estrogens are largely responsible for the changes that take place at puberty in girls. They promote the growth and development of the vagina, uterus, fallopian tubes, breasts, and axillary and pubic hair. They increase the deposition of fat in subcutaneous tissues and increase the retention of salt and water. They also cause increased osteoblastic activity and early fusion of the epiphyses.

The most potent endogenous estrogen is 17β-estradiol. The liver readily oxidizes it to estrone, which in turn can be hydrated to estriol. Because synthetic estrogens can be administered orally, they are used for therapy and contraception.

Some representative examples are:

Diethylstilbestrol (Stilphostrol)
Estradiol (Estrace, Estraderm)
Conjugated estrogens (Premarin)
Esterified estrogens (Menest)
Ethinyl estradiol (Estinyl)

In addition to their presence in oral contraceptives, estrogens are used to treat menstrual disturbances (dysmenorrhea, dysfunctional uterine bleeding), osteoporosis, atrophic vaginitis, nondevelopment of the ovaries, hirsutism, cancer, and symptoms of menopause, particularly vasomotor instability (hot flashes, night sweats). Estradiol transdermal system (Estraderm) is applied to the skin twice a week to treat the vasomotor symptoms of menopause. The postcoital or "morning-after" pill contains diethylstilbestrol (DES) alone. This preparation has serious side effects but is useful in emergencies such as rape or incest.

The most common side effect of estrogen therapy is nausea and vomiting. With continued treatment, tolerance develops and these symptoms usually disappear. Other side effects include uterine bleeding, vaginal discharge, edema, thrombophlebitis, weight gain, and hypertension. Estrogen therapy may also promote endometrial carcinoma in postmenopausal women.[25] This risk may be minimized by administration of a progestin (medroxyprogesterone [Provera]) for the last 10 days of the cycle. No increased risk of breast cancer has been demonstrated. The incidence of vaginal and cervical carcinoma has been shown to increase in the female offspring of women given DES. Other side effects are discussed in the section on oral contraceptives.

Progestins

The corpus luteum is the primary source of progesterone during the normal female sexual cycle. Progesterone promotes secretory changes in the endometrium and prepares the uterus for implantation of the fertilized ovum. If implantation does not occur by the end of the menstrual cycle, progesterone secretion declines, and the onset of menstruation occurs. If implantation takes place, the developing trophoblast secretes chorionic gonadotropin, which sustains the corpus luteum, thus maintaining progesterone and estrogen levels and preventing menstruation. Other effects of progesterone include suppression of uterine contractility, proliferation of the acini of the mammary gland, and enhancement of transplantation immunity to prevent immunologic rejection of the fetus.[26]

In addition to progesterone, which is given parenterally, there are many orally active progestins, or progestational agents that have the same action. Medroxyprogesterone (Provera) is one example. Progestin-only minipills containing either norethindrone (Micronor) or norgestrel (Ovrette) are used for contraception in patients in whom estrogens are containdicated. They must be taken each day of the month and are slightly less effective than the combination products. An intrauterine device (IUD) impregnated with a progestational agent (Progestasert) is also available for contraception.

Uses of progestational agents include the treatment of endometriosis, dysmenorrhea, dysfunctional uterine bleeding, and premenstrual tension. The primary use is for oral contraception or with estrogen for postmenopausal symptoms.

Oral contraceptives

Oral contraceptives contain estrogens and progestins, either alone or in combination. The combination preparation is the most common and about 99% effective. Preparations that contain a progestin alone (the minipill) are slightly less effective, produce less regular menstrual cycles, but do not have most of the side effects of the combination preparation. The compounds most commonly found in oral contraceptives are the estrogens, ethinyl estradiol and mestranol; and the progestins, norgestrel, norethindrone, and norethynodrel. Examples of commonly used oral contraceptives include Ortho-Novum, Lo-Ovral, Norinyl, Ovral, Nordette, and Ovcon.

The combination type of oral contraceptive is taken between days 5 and 25 of the menstrual cycle. Three different formulations exist: the fixed combination, the biphasic, and the triphasic (three different types of tablets with varying amounts of the estrogenic and progestogenic component).

Oral contraceptives interfere with fertility by inhibiting the release of FSH and LH and therefore preventing ovulation. Early follicular FSH and midcycle FSH and LH increases are not seen. In addition, these contraceptive agents interfere with impregnation by altering the endometrium and the secretions of the cervix.

Two major side effects that have been attributed to oral contraceptives are their carcinogenicity and their tendency to produce thrombophlebitis and thromboembolism. The substantiation of these claims, however, is still controversial. The minor side effects of nausea, dizziness, headache, weight gain, and breast discomfort resemble those during early pregnancy and are mainly attributable to the estrogen in the preparation. These effects usually last only several weeks. Others include blood pressure elevation and liver damage. Previous studies have shown that oral contraceptives produce increased gingival fluid,[23] hyperplastic gingivitis,[27] and gingival inflammation similar to that seen in pregnancy.[28] However, Knight and Wade[29] failed to show any significant differences among plaque scores, gingival scores, or loss of attachment when comparing users and nonusers of oral contraceptives. This discrepancy may be based partly on differences in dose between the two studies. Also, this effect may not be evident in all users but may be of clinical significance only in those persons who are highly susceptible to oral soft tissue disorders. In any case the dental hygienist should be aware that oral contraceptives do have the potential to cause or aggravate gingival inflammation.

Oral contraceptives are also associated with a significant increase in the frequency of dry socket after extractions.[30,31] This risk can be minimized by performing extractions during days 23 through 28 of the tablet cycle. Contraindications for the use of oral contraceptives include thromboembolic disorders, significant dysfunction of the liver, known or suspected carcinoma of the breast or other estrogen-dependent neoplasm, and undiagnosed genital bleeding.

In light of the increased use of antibiotics in periodontal therapy, an important antibiotic–oral contraceptive interaction must be mentioned. Certain antibiotics, including tetracycline and ampicillin, have been shown to interact with oral contraceptives to produce a decrease in oral contraceptive efficacy.[32] They do so indirectly by suppressing the intestinal flora and thus diminishing the availability of hydrolytic enzymes to regenerate the parent steroid molecule. Consequently, plasma concentrations of the steroids are abnormally low, and the steroid is cleared more rapidly from the body than under normal circumstances. The most frequent recommendation is to advise the patient to use an additional method of contraception during the time of concurrent drug use. Other suggestions include the substitution of topical for systemic antibiotics, if possible, and the use of oral contraceptives with higher levels of the estrogen component. The latter suggestion should only be undertaken by the patient's physician.[32] Documentation in the dental chart that the patient was informed about the rare chance of a drug interaction between oral contraceptives and antibiotics should be done in our litigation-conscious society.

MALE SEX HORMONES

The main androgen, testosterone, has both androgenic and anabolic effects. It produces the development of secondary male sex characteristics. Its anabolic action results in an increase in tissue protein and nitrogen retention in the body. Other actions include increased osteoblastic activity, epiphyseal closure, and an increase in sebaceous gland activity. "Puberty gingivitis" can occur related to hormonal changes. Treatment includes subgingival debridement and oral hygiene instructions.

Androgenic steroids are used medically in the treatment of breast cancer and as replacement therapy and illicitly for muscle mass gain. The possibility of their use as a male oral contraceptive is being investigated. Examples of androgenic steroids include methyltestosterone (Metandren) and fluoxymesterone (Halotestin), and anabolic steroids include methandrostenolone (Dianabol) and nandrolone decanoate (Deca-Durabolin). Danazol (Danocrine), another androgenic agent, is used to treat endometriosis and fibrocystic breast disease in women.

The androgens, used extensively by body builders and weight lifters, have been associated with hepatotoxicity, cholestatic jaundice, and malignant liver tumors. In the female, their side effects include virilism, resulting in hirsutism, acne, and a deepening voice. Male-pattern baldness and impotence have also been reported. Considering the potential for side effects, the illicit use of these agents is difficult to understand.

CLOMIPHENE (CLOMID, SEROPHENE)

Clomiphene has the ability to induce ovulation in some anovulatory women. Clomiphene reduces the number of estrogenic receptors (antiestrogen) by binding to them. The hypothalamus and pituitary then falsely interpret the situation as estrogen levels that are low and increase their secretion of LH, FSH, and gonadotropins. Ovarian stimulation then results. It is used to treat infertility in females and has been used experimentally for males also. The chance of multiple pregnancies increases about six times with clomiphene treatment. Dental patients being treated with clomiphene should be considered to be pregnant, unless otherwise known.

REVIEW QUESTIONS

1. List one drug group to which patients with hypothyroidism (uncontrolled) and hyperthyroidism (poorly controlled) may have an altered response.
2. Name these diseases:
   a. Hypothyroidism in children
   b. Hypothyroidism in adults
   c. Excessive circulation of thyroid hormone
3. Describe the two situations that can occur when insulin and glucose are not in balance in the diabetic patient.
4. Explain the oral manifestations of diabetes and explain their causes.

5. Describe the types of insulin and state their most common usage pattern.
6. Name three oral hypoglycemic agents and state two side effects of this group of drugs.
7. State what two drug groups are combined to produce the common birth control pill. State what dental drugs may reduce their efficacy.
8. State the relationship between birth control pills and oral manifestations and the incidence of dry socket.
9. Discuss the potential problems with the use of androgenic steroids for body building.

REFERENCES

1. Saadoun, A.: Diabetes and periodontal disease: a review and update, J. West. Soc. Periodont. Abstr. **28**:116, 1980.
2. Faulconbridge, A., et al.: The dental status of a group of diabetic children, Br. Dent. J. **151**:253, 1981.
3. Mattson, L., and Koch, G.: Caries frequency in children with controlled diabetes, Scand. J. Dent. Res. **83**:327, 1975.
4. Murrah, V.A.: Diabetes mellitus and associated oral manifestations: a review, J. Oral Pathol. **14**:271, 1985.
5. Kalkwarf, K.L.: Effect of oral contraceptive therapy on gingival inflammation in humans, J. Periodontal. **49**:560, 1978.
6. Knight, G.M., and Wade, A.B.: The effects of hormonal contraceptives on the human periodontium, J. Periodont. Res. **9**:18, 1974.
7. Catellani, J.E., et al.: Effect of oral contraceptive cycle on dry socket (localized alveolar osteitis), J. Am. Dent. Assoc. **101**:777, 1980.
8. Barnett, M.L.: Inhibition of oral contraceptive effectiveness by concurrent antibiotic administration: a review, J. Periodontol. **56**(1):18, 1985.
9. Mattson, L., and Koch, G.: Caries frequency in children with controlled diabetes, Scand. J. Dent. Res. **83**:327, 1975.
10. Adler, P., Wegener, H., and Bohatka, L.: Influence of age and duration of diabetes on dental development in diabetic children, J. Dent. Res. **52**:535, 1973.
11. Sznojder, N., et al.: Periodontal findings in diabetic and nondiabetic patients, J. Periodontol. **49**:445, 1978.
12. Cohen, D.W., et al.: Studies on periodontal patterns in diabetes mellitus, J. Periodont. Res. **4**(suppl.):35, 1969.
13. Belting, C.M., Hinicher, J.J., and Dummett, C.O.: Influence of diabetes mellitus on the severity of periodontal disease, J. Periodontal. **35**:476, 1964.
14. Murrah, V.A.: Diabetes mellitus and associated oral manifestations: a review, J. Oral Pathol. **14**:271, 1985.
15. Martin, L.R., and Portera, J.J.: Dental awareness and

management of the diabetic patient, J. Miss. Dent. Assoc. **36**:20, 1979.
16. Lane, D.S.: Dental considerations of diabetes mellitus, Dent. Hyg. **53**:306, 1979.
17. Bay, I., Ainamo, J., and Gad, T.: The response of young diabetics to periodontal treatment, J. Periodontol. **45**:806, 1974.
18. Rothwell, B.R., and Richard, E.L.: Diabetes mellitus: medical and dental considerations, Spec. Care Dent. **4**(2):58, 1984.
19. Seltzer, H.S.: Drug-induced hypoglycemia: a review based on 473 cases, Diabetes **21**:955, 1972.
20. Lindhe, J., and Hugoson, A.: The influence of estrogen and progesterone on gingival exudation of regenerating dentogingival tissues, Paradontology **23**:16, 1969.
21. Lindhe, J., Attstroem, R., and Bjoern, A.: The influence of progestogen on gingival exudation during menstrual cycles: longitudinal study, J. Periodont. Res. **4**:97, 1969.
22. O'Neil, T.C.: Plasma female sex hormone levels and gingivitis in pregnancy, J. Periodontol. **50**:279, 1979.
23. Grower, M.F., et al.: Cyclic AMP content of gingival fluid in women taking oral contraceptives, J. Oral Pathol. **4**:291, 1975.
24. Zaki, K., et al.: Salivary female sex hormone levels and gingivitis in pregnancy, Biomed. Biochim. Acta **43**(6):749, 1984.
25. Greenwald, P., et al.: Vaginal cancer after maternal treatment with synthetic estrogens, N. Engl. J. Med. **285**:390, 1971.
26. Siiteri, P.K., et al.: Progesterone and maintenance of pregnancy: is progesterone nature's immunosuppressant? Ann. N.Y. Acad. Sci. **286**:384, 1977.
27. Kaufman, A.Y.: An oral contraceptive as an etiologic factor in producing hyperplastic gingivitis and a neoplasm of a pregnancy tumor type, Oral Surg. **28**:666, 1969.
28. Kalkwarf, K.L.: Effect of oral contraceptive therapy on gingival inflammation in humans, J. Periodontol. **49**:560, 1978.
29. Knight, G.M., and Wade, A.B.: The effects of hormonal contraceptives on the human periodontium, J. Periodont. Res. **9**:18, 1974.
30. Catellani, J.E.: Review of factors contributing to dry socket through enhanced fibrinolysis, J. Oral Surg. **37**:42, 1979.
31. Catellani, J.E., et al.: Effect of oral contraceptive cycle on dry socket (localized alveolar osteitis), J. Am. Dent. Assoc. **101**:777, 1980.
32. Barnett, M.L.: Inhibition of oral contraceptive effectiveness by concurrent antibiotic administration: a review, J. Periodontol. **56**(1):18, 1985.

Chapter **21**

Antineoplastic drugs

Antineoplastic agents, agents used to treat malignancies, are prescribed primarily by physicians. Dental hygienists may treat these patients either before these agents are used or during their use. For this reason, the dental hygienist needs to be familiar with the side effect of these agents, especially oral manifestations, and their management.

USE OF ANTINEOPLASTIC AGENTS

Antineoplastic agents, sometimes called cancer chemotherapeutic agents, are used clinically to destroy and suppress the growth and spread of malignant cells. These agents are used either alone or in combination with radiation and surgery, depending on the type of malignancy being treated. For certain malignancies, for example, the leukemias, choriocarcinoma, multiple myeloma, and Burkitt's lymphoma, drugs are considered the primary agents. Often antineoplastic agents, added to either surgery and/or irradiation, may effect a cure that each procedure alone could not.

The current philosophy for the use of the antineoplastic agents involves treating the initial stages very aggressively. This approach promises more chance of controlling and curing the disease, but also more side effects including those involving the oral cavity.

MECHANISMS OF ACTION

The efficacy of antineoplastic agents is based primarily on their ability to interfere with the metabolism or the reproductive cycle of the tumor cells, thereby destroying them. The reproductive cycle of a cell is considered to consist of four stages (Fig. 21-1):

1. G_1 ("gap" 1), which is the postmitotic or pre-DNA synthesis phase
2. S, which is the period of deoxyribonucleic acid (DNA) synthesis
3. G_2 ("gap" 2), which is the premitotic or post-DNA synthesis phase
4. M, which is the period of mitosis

Cells in a resting stage, or not in a process of cell division, are described as being in the G_0 stage. Cells enter the cycle from the G_0 stage. In some tumors a large proportion of the cells may be at the G_0 level.

Most antineoplastic agents are labeled either "cycle dependent," indicating that they are effective only at specific stages in the mitotic cycle, or "cycle independent," indicating that they are effective at all levels of the cycle. For example, the alkylating agents interfere with the malignant cells during all phases of the reproductive cycle, as well as the resting stage (G_0), and therefore are classified as cycle independent.

Agents of widely different mechanisms of action are often employed together to inhibit the reproduction of neoplastic cells in all phases and to gain therapeutic advantage for the host. Mixtures of these agents may act synergistically, leading to enhanced cytotoxicity with fewer side effects. This is the rationale for combination drug therapy.

CLASSIFICATION

The antineoplastic agents are divided into groups depending on their mechanism and site of action. The alkylating agents (Table 21-1) contain alkyl radicals that react with DNA in all cycles of the cell, preventing reproduction. The antimetabolites (Table 21-2) attack the cells in the S period

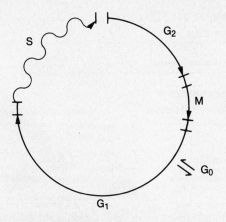

Fig. 21-1. Diagrammatic representation of the cell cycle. (Modified from Holroyd, S.V., Wynn, R.L., and Requa-Clark, B.: Clinical pharmacology in dental practice, ed. 4, St. Louis, 1988, The C.V. Mosby Co.)

Table 21-1. Major alkylating agents and their general uses as antineoplastics

Drug	Use
Nitrogen mustards	
Mechlorethamine (Mustargen)	Hodgkin's disease and other lymphomas
Cyclophosphamide (Cytoxan)	Lymphomas
Chlorambucil (Leukeran)	Chronic lymphocytic leukemia; primary macroglobulinemia
Melphalan (Alkeran)	Hodgkin's disease and other lymphomas
Nitrosoureas	
Carmustine (BiCNU)	
Lomustine (CeeNU)	
Semustine (Methyl-CeeNu)	Hodgkin's disease, other lymphomas, and myeloma
Busulfan (Myleran)	Chronic granulocytic leukemia

From Holroyd, S.V., Wynn R.L., and Requa-Clark, B.: Clinical pharmacology in dental practice, ed. 4, St. Louis, 1988, The C.V. Mosby Co.

of reproducing by interfering with purine or pyrimidine synthesis. Plant alkaloids (Table 21-3) act by arresting cells in metaphase. Because of their low bone marrow toxicity, they are often used in combination. Antibiotics (Table 21-3) are cell-cycle nonspecific and are effective for solid tumors. Other agents (Table 21-3) include hormones, such as prednisone, which interrupt the cell cycle at the G_1 stage. Both androgens and estrogens are used for palliation in inoperable breast cancer. Cisplatin, a heavy metal complex of platinum, is cell-cycle nonspecific. Tamoxifen, an antiestrogenic substance, is used to manage breast cancer.

ADVERSE DRUG EFFECTS

Rapidly growing cells, such as neoplastic cells, are more susceptible to inhibition or destruction by antineoplastic agents. The most serious difficulty in antineoplastic therapy stems from the lack of selectivity between tumor tissue and normal tissue. Some normal cells exhibit a faster reproduction cycle than do slowly growing tumor cells. In an effort to eradicate a malignancy, certain normal cells are also destroyed, resulting in adverse effects. Because the cells of the gastrointestinal

tract, bone marrow, and hair follicles are among the faster growing normal cells, the early side effects are associated with these tissues.

The principal adverse effects are as follows:

1. **Bone marrow suppression.** This results in leukopenia, thrombocytopenia, and anemia. The degree of cytopenia that results depends on the drugs being employed, the condition of the bone marrow at the time of administration, and other contributing factors.

2. **Gastrointestinal effects.** Disturbances may occur from sloughing of the gastrointestinal mucosa. Clinically, these disturbances are expressed as nausea, stomatitis, vomiting, and hemorrhagic diarrhea.

3. **Dermatologic effects.** Cutaneous reactions vary from mild erythema and maculopapular eruptions to exfoliative dermatitis and Stevens-Johnson syndrome. Alopecia is frequent, but the

Table 21-2. Antimetabolites and their general uses as antineoplastics

Drug	Use
Folic acid analog	
Methotrexate (Amethopterin)	Acute lymphoblastic leukemia in children
Pyrimidine analogs	
Fluorouracil (5-FU)	
Floxuridine (FUDR)	Carcinoma of the breast, GIT, ovary, cervix, and prostate
Cytosine arabinoside (Cytosar-U)	Induction of remission in acute leukemia in children and adults
Purine analogs	
Mercaptopurine (Purinethol)	Leukemia in children and adults
Thioguanine (TG)	Acute leukemia and induction of remissions in acute granulocytic leukemia

From Holroyd, S.V., Wynn, R.L., and Requa-Clark, B.: Clinical pharmacology in dental practice, ed. 4, St. Louis, 1988, The C.V. Mosby Co.
GIT, Gastrointestinal tract.

Table 21-3. Miscellaneous antineoplastics and their uses

Antineoplastic	Use
Plant alkaloids	
Vinblastine (Velban)	Metastatic testicular tumor
Vincristine (Oncovin)	Hodgkin's disease and other lymphoma
Antibiotics	
Dactinomycin (Actinomycin D)	Wilms' tumor in children
Doxorubicin (Adriamycin)	Acute leukemias and malignant lymphoma
Bleomycin sulfate (Blenoxane)	Testicular carcinoma
Mitomycin (Mutamycin)	Gastric adenocarcinoma
Hormones	
Adrenocorticosteroids	Acute leukemias
Androgens and estrogens	Breast carcinoma
Progestin	Endometrial carcinoma
Other	
L-Asparaginase	Acute lymphoblastic leukemia
Cisplatin (Platinol)	Testicular tumor
Tamoxifen	Breast carcinoma

Modified from Holroyd, S.V., Wynn, R.L., and Requa-Clark, B.: Clinical pharmacology in dental practice, ed. 4, St. Louis, 1988, The C.V. Mosby Co.

hair usually regrows when therapy is discontinued.

4. Hepatoxicity. Liver problems occur principally with the antimetabolites, for example, methotrexate, but may occur with other agents as well.

5. Neurologic effects. Neurotoxic effects such as peripheral neuropathy, ileus, inappropriate antidiuretic hormone (ADH) secretion, and convulsions have been associated primarily with vincristine or vinblastine administration.

6. Nephrotoxicity. Renal tubular impairment, occurring secondary to hyperuricemia, is caused by rapid cell destruction and the release of nucleotides. The treatment of leukemias and lymphomas often results in rapid tumor destruction with a consequent high uric acid level. Allopurinol (Zyloprim) is routinely administered before the initiation of a regimen of antineoplastic agents to prevent hyperuricemia.

7. Immunosupression. Immune deficiency may occur, resulting in an enhanced susceptibility to infection or a second malignancy, since many antineoplastic agents have an immunosuppressant effect.

8. Germ cells. Inhibition of spermatogenesis and oogenesis is frequent, at least temporarily. Mutations within the germ cells may occur. The menstrual cycle may also be inhibited. Recovery occurs after discontinuation of the drug.

9. Oral effects. Adverse effects on the oral tissue are primarily those of discomfort, sensitivity of the teeth and gums, mucosal pain and ulceration, gingival hemorrhage, and dryness and im-

---

Table 21-4. Oral care protocol for patients receiving chemotherapy

A. Rinses

1. Rinse with a warm dilute solution of baking soda every 2 hours to control oral acidity, especially if frequent emesis is present.
2. If pain is present, rinse with 5 ml of diphenhydramine (low alcohol content, such as Benylin) liquid before meals.
3. For dry mouth, sip cool water or dissolve ice chips in mouth all day long. Artificial saliva (e.g., Moi-Stir, Salivart, Xerolube, Orex) can be used frequently. Lubricate the lips with lanolin or cocoa butter. Avoid commercial mouthwashes, coffee, tea, and cola drinks, which tend to dry the mouth.
4. If oral infection develops, appropriate antibacterial or antifungal medication can be prescribed by the physician or dentist.
5. Newer commercial mouthrinses with high alcohol concentration will need to be evaluated. They may prove to be beneficial in spite of their high alcohol content because of other properties they possess, such as antibacterial action.

B. Care of teeth and gums

1. Neutropenic (absolute granulocyte count <1500) or thrombocytopenic (platelet count <60,000) patients:
   a. To reduce the risk of oral complications during chemotherapy, the patient should have a complete oral examination to eliminate any areas of infection and irritation, before the induction of chemotherapy, if possible.
   b. Prophylactic antibiotics must be given in certain situations such as the use of an indwelling Hickman catheter or when there are abnormal blood counts.
2. Patients with adequate white blood cell and platelet counts:
   a. Carefully floss the teeth after each meal and avoid snacking, unless it is necessary to maintain weight.
   b. Brush the teeth after each meal using a soft brush and a fluoride toothpaste or sodium bicarbonate paste.
   c. If the patient experiences xerostomia, frequent emesis, or thick saliva it may be advisable to apply a fluoride gel (0.4% stannous fluoride or 1.0% sodium fluoride) for 5 minutes once daily.
   d. Remove dentures while sleeping, clean them by brushing, and store them in water.

C. Nutrition

Liquid dietary supplements may be needed for adequate nutrition.

D. Maintenance

Oral prophylaxis should be performed at appropriate intervals when the patient is not immunocompromised to achieve and maintain a plaque-free status.

---

paired taste sensation. Infection from leukopenia and bleeding from thrombocytopenia can occur. Appropriate maintenance of the oral cavity should be undertaken even before and certainly during antineoplastic therapy (Table 21-4).

REVIEW QUESTIONS

1. Describe the different stages in the reproductive cycle of a cell. State their importance to antineoplastic drug therapy.
2. State the major classifications of the antineoplastic agents, and give one example of each.

3. Explain the adverse effects associated with the antineoplastic agents, and state the symptoms associated with each effect.
4. Explain the oral care for patients receiving chemotherapy. Explain the importance of factors such as white blood cell level. State agents to avoid or use to alleviate oral discomfort.
5. Describe two or three cancers that are amenable to drug treatment. State two that are usually not.

Chapter **22**

Respiratory and gastrointestinal drugs

Because diseases of the respiratory and gastrointestinal tracts are not uncommon, patients taking drugs for these diseases will be seen for dental treatment. Because medications given to treat these diseases can affect dental treatment, the dental hygienist needs to be aware of the effects of these drugs on the patient and how these drugs can alter the dental treatment plan.

RESPIRATORY DRUGS

Diseases that are treated with respiratory drugs include chronic obstructive pulmonary disease (COPD), asthma, and upper respiratory tract infections. Respiratory drugs include a wide range of drug groups, from adrenergic drugs for bronchodilation and nasal decongestion to corticosteroids for reducing inflammation. Drugs that increase expectoration and reduce coughs are also included here. Inhalers are a useful dosage form for administration of a variety of drugs to the respiratory tree.

The most common respiratory disease is asthma. It is characterized by reversible airway obstruction and is associated with reduction in expiratory airflow. It may be precipitated by allergens, exercise, and stress. In **status asthmaticus** patients have persistent life-threatening bronchospasm despite drug therapy. The dental hygienist should treat patients with asthma so that minimal stress is induced. Signs of asthma include shortness of breath and wheezing. The adrenergic agonists, xanthines, cromolyn, and the corticosteroids are used to treat this disease.

Chronic obstructive pulmonary disease (COPD), characterized by irreversible airway obstruction, occurs with either chronic bronchitis or emphysema. Chronic bronchitis is a result of chronic inflammation of the airways and excessive sputum production. Emphysema is characterized by alveolar destruction with air-space enlargement and airway collapse. The adrenergic agonists and xanthines are used to produce bronchodilation in these patients. Both conditions are associated with an increase in the incidence of bronchospasm, as well as fixed airway obstruction. Patients with upper respiratory tract infections frequently take adrenergic agonists for nasal congestion, antihistamines for their ability to reduce secretions, expectorants to thin sputum, and antitussives to control coughing. Each drug group is discussed separately.

Sympathomimetics (adrenergic agonists)

Sympathomimetic or adrenergic agonists produce bronchodilation by stimulation of the β_2-receptors in the lungs. β_2-receptor activation results in accumulation of cyclic adenosine monophosphate (cAMP) in the smooth muscles, producing a reduction in cytoplasmic calcium concentration thereby relaxing the smooth muscle. Chapter 5 discussed the presence of β_1-receptors in the heart (tachycardia) and β_2-receptors in the lungs (bronchodilation). With the development of selective β_2-agonists, bronchodilation with fewer cardiac side effects could be achieved. This group of selective β_2-agonists, used orally, by inhalation, and parenterally, is currently one of the mainstays of respiratory therapy.

Nonspecific adrenergic agonists

Both epinephrine, an α- and β-agonist, and iso-proterenol, a nonspecific β-agonist, can produce bronchodilation by stimulation of the β_2-receptors in the lungs. Parenteral epinephrine is still used to treat acute asthmatic attacks. Isoproterenol has been used orally, parenterally, and by inhalation, but selective β_2-agonists are preferred because they produce fewer side effects.

Selective β_2-agonists

The selective β_2-agonists have some specificity for the respiratory tree. Although, like epinephrine, they can still produce side effects, they do so to a lesser extent. Side effects include nervousness, tachycardia, and insomnia. β_2-agonists may be administered either orally (tablet or liquid), parenterally (intramuscularly or intravenously), and by inhalation (metered dose or by nebulization with

an air compressor). They differ in their duration of action and preparations available. Table 22-1 lists some selective β_2-agonists and their routes of administration.

Methylxanthines

The methylxanthines consist of theophylline, caffeine, and theobromine. Theophylline, used as a bronchodilator, can be complexed with ethylenediamine producing aminophylline, which is more soluble.

Some brands of theophylline and aminophylline are listed in Table 22-1. Theophylline is used to treat chronic asthma and the bronchospasm associated with chronic bronchitis and emphysema. Bronchodilation is the major therapeutic effect desired. The mechanism of action of the xanthines is complex. It involves antagonism of receptor-mediated action of adenosine, inhibition of cyclic

Table 22-1. Bronchodilators

Drug group (example)	Routes*				
Adrenergic-agonists					
Selective β_2-agonists					
Terbutaline (Brethine, Bricanyl)	PO	IH	SC		
Metaproterenol (Alupent, Metaprel)	PO	IH			
Albuterol (Proventil, Ventolin)	PO	IH			
Isoetharine (Bronkosol, Bronkometer)		IH			
Nonselective β-agonists					
Epinephrine		IH	SC	IM	
Ephedrine	PO		SC	IM	IV
Xanthine derivatives					
Theophylline (Theo-Dur, Slo-bid, Slo-Phyllin)	PO				IV
Aminophylline (Theophylline with ethylenediamine) (Somophyllin)	PO				IV
Anticholinergics					
Ipratropium bromide (Atrovent)		IH			
Cromolyn (Intal, Nasalcrom Nasal Solution)		IH			N

*IH, Inhalation; IV, intravenously; N, intranasally; PO, orally; SC, subcutaneously.

nucleotide phosphodiesterase (an enzyme that metabolizes cAMP), mobilization of intracellular calcium pools, and inhibition of prostaglandins. Side effects associated with the methylxanthines include central nervous system (CNS) stimulation, cardiac stimulation, increased gastric secretion, and diuresis. Patients often complain of nervousness and insomnia. Erythromycin can increase the serum levels of theophylline into the toxic range.

Intravenous aminophylline and rapidly absorbed oral preparations are used to manage acute asthmatic attacks and status asthmaticus. To manage chronic asthma, the sustained-release preparations in tablet or capsule form are used. The products designed for once-a-day dosing are not able to maintain adequate serum levels of theophylline over a 24-hour period. Patients on chronic theophylline often have blood levels drawn to determine if the dose they are taking is appropriate.

Anticholinergic drugs

Atropine is an old remedy for asthma, although its side effects limit its usefulness. Newer anticholinergic drugs have been produced that have fewer side effects. An example is ipratropium bromide (Atrovent) available for inhalation. It has several advantages over atropine. Its low lipid solubility limits its bioavailability and makes it bronchoselective with minimal side effects. Side effects including dry mouth and bad taste are minimized by using it by inhalation. Its bronchodilating effect is additive with that of the β_2-agonists. Studies suggest that it will be useful for the long-term management of COPD, for poorly controlled asthmatics, or for those who do not tolerate the side effects of the β_2-agonists.

Cromolyn

Cromolyn (Intal) is unusual because it is effective only for the prophylaxis of asthma and not for treatment of an acute attack. It has no intrinsic bronchodilator, antihistaminic, or antiinflammatory action. Cromolyn prevents the antigen-induced release of histamine, leukotrienes, and other substances from sensitized mast cells. It appears to do this by preventing the influx of calcium provoked by immunoglobulin E (IgE) antibody-antigen interaction on the mast cell. Cromolyn is the least toxic of all asthma medications. The most common adverse effects include bronchospasm, wheezing, coughing, nasal congestion, and pharyngeal irritation. These effects must be due to the irritant effect of the inhaler, since they do not occur with the use of the solutions. Cromolyn was originally available in a capsule form that was dispersed into the respiratory tree. It is currently available in a metered dose form like the other inhalation agents.

The advantage of cromolyn is its safety. It may be used prophylactically by chronic asthmatic patients or taken before exercise-induced asthma. It is not effective for treatment of an acute attack. Theophylline is usually more effective, but cromolyn may be useful when theophylline is poorly tolerated because of its side effects. It is also used intranasally (Nasalcrom Nasal Solution) and in ophthalmologic preparations (Opticrom) for allergic manifestations.

Miscellaneous bronchodilators

Several drugs are under clinical investigation as bronchodilators. They include members of the calcium channel blockers and newer histamine type I (H_1) receptor blockers, and ketotifen (Zaditen).

Corticosteroids

First used for the treatment of arthritis, the corticosteroids were soon employed for the treatment of asthma. Their large and varied number of side effects soon became evident (see Chapter 19) and physicians began limiting corticosteroid therapy to only those patients who were refractory to other treatments. In 1975, however, aerosol preparations containing corticosteroids were introduced. The typical side effects associated with corticosteroid therapy occur much less frequently with topical aerosol administration.

Several aerosolized corticosteroids are marketed in the United States for the therapy of asthmatic patients. The most common are beclomethasone dipropionate (Beclovent, Vanceril) and triamcinolone acetonide (Azmacort). Patients taking these corticosteroids have a significant improvement in pulmonary function with a decrease in wheezing, tightness, and cough. The use of an aerosolized corticosteroid combined with a β_2-agonist improves therapeutic action. In some severe asthmatic patients, oral steroids may still be necessary.

The aerosolized corticosteroids are useful in the treatment of asthmatic patients refractory to β_2-agonists. Although they have no immediate benefit in an acute asthmatic attack, they may hasten recovery and decrease morbidity in these patients.

The side effects of the steroids vary depending on the route of administration, frequency of intake, the duration of intake, the total dose, and the preexisting diseases a patient may have. Prolonged use can result in adrenal suppression, poor wound healing, and immunosuppression. Supplemental steroids should be considered, as discussed in Chapter 19. Oral candidiasis that requires discontinuation of therapy may occur with the inhalation corticosteroids. The dental hygienist in oral examination of the patient should pay careful attention to symptoms of candidiasis.

Nasal decongestants

Nasal decongestants are α-adrenergic agents that act by constricting the blood vessels of the nasal mucous membranes. Some examples include phenylpropanolamine (in Entex LA, in Naldecon, Tavist-D), pseudoephedrine (Sudafed, Sucrets, in Actifed), and phenylephrine (Neo-Synephrine, Sinex, Allerest). Many nasal decongestants are available over the counter (OTC) for both local as well as systemic use (see also Table 5-5). Chronic use of decongestants may result in rebound swelling and congestion. Unwanted side effects of adrenergic stimulation may occur. Phenylephrine (Neo-Synephrine) is used topically, whereas phenylpropanolamine is used systemically as a decongestant (α-agonist action). Ephedrine, both an α- and β-agonist, is sometimes used as a nasal decongestant when an oral action is desired.

Expectorants and mucolytics

Expectorants are drugs that promote the release of exudate or mucus from the respiratory passages. Liquefying expectorants are drugs that promote the ejection of mucus by decreasing its viscosity. Mucolytics destroy or dissolve mucus.

Expectorants act by their ability to cause reflex irritation of the stomach, resulting in stimulation of bronchial secretions. Guaifenesin, the most popular expectorant, is contained in a variety of OTC products mixed with other active ingredients. Robitussin is available as guaifenesin alone, as well as with an antitussive, for example, dextromethorphan (Robitussin DM), a decongestant and an antitussive. Other expectorants include iodinated glycerol, terpin hydrate, ammonium chloride, and ipecac syrup.

Mucolytics are enzymes that are able to digest mucus, decreasing its viscosity. Examples include acetylcysteine (Mucomyst) and pancreatic dornase (Dornavac).

Antitussives

Antitussives may be opioid or related agents used for the symptomatic relief of nonproductive cough. Opioids are the most effective, but because of their addicting properties, other agents are often used. Codeine-containing cough preparations are commonly employed, but their histamine-releasing properties may precipitate bronchospasm.

Dextromethorphan, an opioid relative, suppresses the cough reflex by its direct effect on the cough center. It does not cause the release of histamine. It may potentiate the effects of CNS depressants. It is available both alone and in combination with other ingredients. By impairing expectoration, dextromethorphan may increase airway resistance.

Dental concerns

Since about 10% of the population has some pulmonary disease, patients taking medications for asthma, emphysema, or chronic bronchitis are frequently encountered. With severe COPD, a patient can develop pulmonary hypertension, increasing the risk for cardiac arrhythmias. Stress in these patients should be minimized and adrenal supplementation instituted if the patients are taking steroids. Patients prone to developing respiratory failure, if given oxygen, either alone or with nitrous oxide, or CNS depressants, may manifest acute respiratory failure. Aspirin should be avoided in asthmatics and erythromycin may alter the metabolism of theophylline. Emergency equipment and medications should be available when treating these patients.

Metered-dose inhalers

The metered-dose inhaler (MDI), developed in the 1950s, provides a useful method to administer certain medications to the respiratory tree. Its advantages include the following:

1. It delivers the medication directly to the bronchioles, thereby keeping the total dose low and side effects minimal.
2. The bronchodilator effect is greater than a comparable oral dose.
3. The inhaled dose can be accurately measured.
4. The onset of action is rapid and predictable (versus unpredictable response with orally administered agents).
5. MDIs are compact, portable, and sterile, making them ideal for the ambulatory patient.

The disadvantages of the MDIs are that they are difficult to use properly (poor for children and handicapped) and they can be abused with a resultant decrease in response. Medications currently available in the MDIs include the β-agonists, both specific and nonspecific, the corticosteroids, and cromolyn.

GASTROINTESTINAL DRUGS
Antacids

Antacids are used to treat a variety of gastric conditions, both by self-medication and by recommendation of the patient's prescriber. Both acute gastritis and ulcers are sometimes treated with antacids. Acute gastritis, the most common type of gastric distress, is termed heartburn or upset stomach. The symptoms include epigastric dis-

comfort or "burning." Gastric ulcers can also occasionally be treated with antacids.

Antacids are drugs that partially neutralize the hydrochloric acid in the stomach. By raising the pH to 3 or 4, the erosive effect of the acid is decreased and pepsin's activity is reduced. The antacids are classified as systemic or nonsystemic, depending on the amount of absorption from the gastrointestinal tract (Table 22-2).

Sodium bicarbonate, the only systemic antacid, rapidly neutralizes gastric acid. Its major disadvantage is that alkalosis can occur. It also contains sodium and is contraindicated in cardiovascular patients who are to minimize sodium intake. For these reasons it is not recommended, although it is still used by the lay public.

The active ingredients in nonsystemic antacids, the preferred antacids, include calcium carbonate, aluminum and magnesium salts, and magnesium-aluminum hydroxide gels. Calcium salts may result in acid-rebound, constipation, or hypercalcemia. Aluminum salts can produce constipation. Magnesium salts produce osmotic diarrhea. Hypermagnesemia has been reported in patients with renal disease. Drug interactions with the antacids include altering the absorption of other drugs from the gastrointestinal tract. Drugs whose absorption is inhibited include tetracyclines, digitalis, iron, chlorpromazine, and indomethacin. Conversely, levodopa's absorption is increased because stomach emptying time is shortened. By mixing aluminum and magnesium salts in a single preparation the effects on the bowel can be balanced out.

Sucralfate

Sucralfate (Carafate), a complex of aluminum hydroxide and sulfated sucrose (a polysaccharide with antipeptic activity), is used to treat duodenal ulcers. In the stomach, the aluminum ion splits off, leaving an anion that is essentially nonabsorbable. Sucralfate combines with proteins forming a complex that binds preferentially with the ulcer site. It inhibits the action of pepsin and absorbs the bile salts. Its acid-neutralizing capacity does not contribute to its antiulcer action. Constipation is the most frequent side effect reported (2.2%).

Table 22-2. Gastrointestinal drugs

Antacids
Systemic
Sodium bicarbonate

Nonsystemic
Magnesium aluminum hydroxide (Maalox)
Calcium carbonate (Tums)
Dihydroxyaluminum sodium carbonate (Rolaids)
Sucralfate (Carafate)

H₂ Receptor antagonists
Cimetidine (Tagamet)
Ranitidine (Zantac)
Famotidine (Pepcid)

Laxatives
Milk of magnesia
Bisacodyl (Dulcolax)
Dioctyl sodium sulfosuccinate (Colace)
Psyllium seed (Metamucil)

Antidiarrheals
Adsorbents
Kaopectate

Opioids
Paregoric
Diphenoxylate (Lomotil)
Loperamide (Imodium)

Antiemetics
Anticholinergics
Dimenhydrinate (Dramamine)
Cyclizine (Marezine)
Scopolamine (Transderm-Scop)
Hydroxyzine (Atarax)
Trimethobenzamide (Tigan)

Phenothiazines
Prochlorperazine (Compazine)

Other
Metoclopramide (Reglan)
Benzquinamide (Emete-Con)
Diphenidol (Vontrol)

Cannabinoids
Dronabinol (Marinol)
Nabilone (Cesamet)

Other side effects (less than 0.3%) include dry mouth, nausea, rash, and dizziness.

H₂ Receptor antagonists

The histamine type 2 (H₂) receptor antagonists competitively block the release of gastric acid produced by histamine. The three members of this group of drugs are cimetidine (Tagamet), ranitidine (Zantac), and famotidine (Pepcid). This group of drugs is the most effective and most commonly used ulcer therapy.

The side effects of cimetidine include bradycardia, cholestatic hepatitis, pancytopenia, confusion, hallucinations, and fever. Because it binds with the androgen receptors it also produces gynecomastia and sexual dysfunction, for example, impotence. Unlike cimetidine, neither ranitidine nor famotidine has been found to possess antiandrogenic activity. Cimetidine inhibits certain liver enzymes responsible for the hepatic metabolism of some drugs (P-450 oxidase system) resulting in a delay in elimination and an increase in serum levels of some drugs. A few examples of drugs that are metabolized by the P-450 pathway include warfarin, phenytoin, theophylline, diazepam, and carbamazepine.

Metoclopramide (Reglan)

Metoclopramide stimulates the motility of the upper gastrointestinal tract without stimulating secretions. It is indicated in the relief of symptoms associated with diabetic gastroparesis (gastric stasis) and improves delayed gastric emptying time. Another indication is short-term therapy for gastroesophageal reflux with symptoms. CNS side effects including restlessness, drowsiness, and fatigue are the most common side effects occurring in 10% to 25% of patients. Parkinson-like reactions can occur in up to 10% of patients. Gastrointestinal side effects include nausea and diarrhea. Additive CNS depression may occur when other CNS depressants are used concomitantly.

Laxatives

Self-medication with laxatives is common practice by the lay public. Although a few indications for

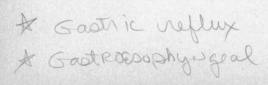

the use of laxatives exist, overuse is common and habituation can result. The myth that "regular" bowel habits are essential has led to this practice. Abuse of these substances occurs in bulimic patients. Short-term, occasional use for constipation and use before diagnostic procedures (barium enema) are legitimate indications. Types of laxatives are the following:

1. Bulk laxatives. These laxatives are preferred because they are the safest and act most like the normal physiology. They contain polysaccharides or cellulose derivatives that combine with intestinal fluids to form gels. This increases peristalsis and facilitates movement through the intestine.

2. Lubricants. Mineral oil, a lubricant that used to be frequently used, is no longer recommended. It can be absorbed if used over a long period of time and can interfere with the absorption of the fat-soluble vitamins (A, D, E, K).

3. Stimulants. These laxatives act by producing local irritation of the intestinal mucosa. Because of their potent effect, intestinal cramping can result. Bisacodyl, a member of this group, is frequently used before bowel surgery or radiologic examinations, but should not be used for simple constipation.

4. Stool softeners (emollients). Dioctyl sodium sulfosuccinate (Colace), an anionic detergent, wets and softens the stool by accumulating water in the intestine. These agents should be limited to short-term use, even though they are termed nontoxic.

5. Osmotic (saline) laxatives. Magnesium sulfate or phosphate produces its laxative effect by osmotically holding water. It should be used with caution in patients with renal impairment.

Antidiarrheals

Drugs used to treat diarrhea are either adsorbents or opioid-like in action. Antidiarrheals are used to minimize fluid and electrolyte imbalances. In certain poisonings or infections, antidiarrheals are contraindicated. The most common adsorbent combination used to treat diarrhea is kaolin and pectin (Kaopectate). The opioids, such as diphenoxylate with atropine (Lomotil) and loperamide

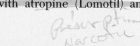

(Imodium) (now OTC), are the most effective antidiarrheal agents. They decrease peristalsis by acting directly on the smooth muscle of the gastrointestinal tract.

Antiemetics

Vomiting may occur because of a variety of situations such as motion sickness, pregnancy, drugs, infections, or radiation therapy. Choice of the drug to treat vomiting depends, to some extent, on the cause of the vomiting.

Anticholinergics can be used for the nausea and vomiting associated with motion sickness and labyrinthitis. Both dimenhydrinate (Dramamine) and meclizine (Bonine) possess antiemetic, antivertigo, and anti–motion sickness action. Because they have antihistaminic action, sedation is a side effect. Diphenhydramine (Benadryl), an antihistamine with antiemetic properties, commonly produces sedation. Hydroxyzine (Atarax) is used in dentistry as an antiemetic or antianxiety agent. Scopolamine is recently available in a transdermal patch (Transderm-Scop) that is placed postauricularly and releases medication over a 3-day period. It is contraindicated whenever anticholinergics are. Idiosyncratic reactions, dry mouth, blurred vision, sedation, and dizziness have been reported. Trimethobenzamide's (Tigan's) antiemetic effect is mediated through the chemoreceptor trigger zone (CTZ).

Phenothiazines like chlorpromazine (Thorazine) and prochlorperazine (Compazine) are used to control severe nausea. Their side effects include sedation and extrapyramidal symptoms including tardive dyskinesia (see Chapter 17). Promethazine (Phenergan), a phenothiazine with antihistaminic and anticholinergic properties, is used in dentistry to treat nausea and vomiting associated with surgery and anesthesia. It also has sedative and antisialogogue action. It is sometimes used concurrently with opioids to minimize their nausea.

Metoclopramide (Reglan) can control the nausea and vomiting of patients receiving cancer chemotherapeutic agents. It acts both centrally (dopamine antagonist) and peripherally (stimulates release of acetylcholine). It is also indicated for the management of gastric motility disorders, for example, diabetic gastric stasis.

Miscellaneous antiemetics

Benzquinamide (Emete-Con) is used to treat nausea associated with anesthesia given during surgery. Both dry mouth and salivation have been reported with its use. It can potentiate the pressor effects of epinephrine.

Diphenidol (Vontrol) acts on both the CTZ and the vestibular apparatus. Hallucinations, disorientation, and confusion limit its use to hospitalized patients.

Cannabinoid antiemetics

Dronabinol (Marinol) and nabilone (Cesamet) are psychoactive substances derived from *Cannabis sativa* L. (marijuana). They produce effects similar to marijuana. These agents are highly abusable. Tolerance and both physical and psychologic dependence can occur. These agents are indicated to treat the nausea and vomiting associated with cancer chemotherapy in patients who have failed to respond to conventional antiemetic therapy. Close supervision is required when these agents are administered. Side effects include drowsiness and dizziness. Perceptual difficulties, muddled thinking, and elevation of mood can also occur.

REVIEW QUESTIONS

1. State the two major types of respiratory diseases and state their differences.
2. Name the autonomic drug group used for bronchodilation and state the most specific agent and route.
3. State the drug group often used for bronchodilation in addition to the response to question 2, above. Describe two of their side effects.
4. State one drug that cannot be used prophylactically for asthma and explain why not.
5. Describe the use of inhalers including their advantages and types of drugs dispensed in this fashion.
6. State the drug group for the nasal decongestants.
7. Define the term "expectorants," "mucolytics," and "antitussives" and give one example of each.
8. What drug group is most commonly prescribed for treatment of ulcers and stomach ailments? Describe its mechanism of action.
9. Name a laxative and state an indication for its use.
10. Describe the use of the antidiarrheals and name one.
11. State two antiemetic agents in different groups and describe their mechanism of action. State their appropriate and inappropriate use.

Chapter 23

12/1/93

Emergency drugs

More and more patients who are older or are taking multiple drug therapies are seeking dental treatment. Dental offices are administering more complicated drug regimens, as well as utilizing longer dental appointments in the dental office. With these changes, the chance of an emergency occurring in the dental office is increasing. The dental hygienist needs to become familiar with the most common emergency situations, their management, and the drugs used to treat these conditions. Many emergency situations can be handled correctly with adequate knowledge. Lack of this knowledge can cause everyone in a dental office to panic in an emergency. If the office is prepared for an emergency, handling one will be easier.

To prepare the **dental office** for an emergency the following steps should be taken:

1. Practice emergency procedures before an emergency occurs. Train all office personnel. *CPR yearly*
2. Post the telephone number of the closest physician, emergency room, and ambulance service (often 911).
3. Update the office's emergency kit, including the drugs and the devices. *meds, O₂!*

To minimize the chances of an emergency each **patient** should have these procedures performed:

1. Observe the patient's stature, build, gait, coloring, age, facies, and respiration.
2. Record the amount of anxiety.
3. Take the patient's blood pressure and pulse rate, and perform any necessary laboratory examination.

4. Take a complete patient history, including drug therapy, past dental and anesthetic experiences, restrictions on physical activity, diseases, and present condition.
5. Request medical consultations as needed.
6. Prescribe premedication and avoid drug interactions.

The following preliminary steps should be taken when an emergency occurs:

1. Recognize the abnormal occurrence.
2. Make a proper diagnosis.
3. Note the time.
4. Position the patient properly.
5. Maintain an airway.
6. Administer oxygen.
7. Monitor vital signs.
8. Provide symptomatic treatment while awaiting help.

GENERAL MEASURES

It is easier to prevent a medical emergency in the dental office than to treat one that has already occurred. One way of preventing an emergency is by taking an adequate medical and health history. A medical history can determine if dental treatment can be administered safely or if a medical consultation is indicated.

Preparation for treatment

Before emergency treatment can be administered, the patient's signs and symptoms must lead to a diagnosis of the problem. In most cases the maintenance of respiration and circulation is of primary importance. The use of drug therapy in

241

these situations is **only** ancillary to the primary measures of maintaining adequate circulation and respiration.

Every dental professional, including the dental hygienist should be certified and current in cardiopulmonary resuscitation (CPR). The legal implications of lack of CPR training could be serious.

This chapter discusses the signs, symptoms, and treatment of the most common emergency situations, dividing them into cardiovascular, central nervous system (CNS), respiratory, endocrine, and other emergencies. The most commonly used drugs and the choice of drugs and equipment for a dental office emergency kit is also discussed.

CARDIOVASCULAR SYSTEM EMERGENCIES

The emergency situations involving the cardiovascular system include cardiac arrest, angina pectoris, myocardial infarction, acute congestive heart failure, arrhythmias, hypertensive crisis, cerebrovascular accident, and hypotension. The primary concern in any cardiovascular emergency is the maintenance of adequate circulation. CPR, calling emergency personnel, and administration of oxygen are appropriate for most emergencies. The drugs used in cardiovascular emergencies are discussed individually later in the chapter.

Cardiac arrest

When cardiac arrest occurs, generally there is sudden circulatory and respiratory collapse. Without immediate therapy, cardiac arrest is fatal. Permanent brain damage occurs in 4 minutes. Pulse is absent and blood pressure is unobtainable. After a few minutes the patient becomes cyanotic and the pupils are fixed and dilated. The first and most important treatment is immediate, adequate CPR.

Other medications used in a hospital setting for cardiac arrest include epinephrine for cardiac stimulation and lidocaine for arrhythmias. Defibrillation is used to treat asystole.

Angina pectoris

Without a previous history of angina, diagnosis of this condition can be difficult. It often begins as substernal chest pain that radiates across the chest, to the left arm, or to the mandible. It may also produce a feeling of heaviness in the chest. The pulse becomes rapid, and tachypnea can occur. An anginal attack can be brought on by stress from pain, trauma, or fear, especially in a dental situation.

Premedication with sublingual nitroglycerin before a stressful dental situation can frequently prevent an acute anginal attack. Treatment of an acute attack (see Chapter 15) is with sublingual nitroglycerin. Opioids or diazepam are used in hospitalized patients.

Acute myocardial infarction

⟶ Nitro: doesn't help

An acute myocardial infarction (heart attack) often begins as severe pain, pressure, or heaviness in the chest that radiates to other parts of the body. Sweating, nausea, and vomiting can occur. The pain is persistent and unrelieved by rest or nitroglycerin. In this way a myocardial infarction can be differentiated from an anginal attack. An irregular rapid pulse, shortness of breath, diaphoresis, and indigestion can occur. Treatment includes administration of oxygen and an opioid analgesic agent and transfer to a hospital.

Hospitalized patients who have suffered a myocardial infarction are given lidocaine for arrhythmias and vasopressor agents to maintain adequate blood pressure.

lidocaine - arrythmias

Other cardiovascular emergencies

Arrhythmias, another cardiovascular emergency, depend on an electrocardiogram for diagnosis before treatment. A cerebrovascular accident (stroke), resulting in weakness on one side of the body or speech defects, is treated with oxygen administration. Hypertensive crisis is treated with antihypertensive agents given intravenously (see Chapter 15). Hypotension, sometimes caused by medications administered in the dental office, is treated by positioning (modified Trendelenburg), oxygen, methoxamine (a vasopressor), and hydrocortisone.

CENTRAL NERVOUS SYSTEM EMERGENCIES

With cardiovascular emergencies, such as syncope and seizures, consciousness is often lost. The treatment depends on the specific situation and is primarily symptomatic. The CNS emergencies include convulsions (for example, epilepsy), toxic reactions to local anesthetics, syncope, and extrapyramidal reactions.

Convulsions

Convulsions are most commonly associated with epilepsy, especially the grand mal type (see Chapter 16), but can also result from a toxic reaction to a local anesthetic agent. Convulsions are abnormal movements of parts of the body in either clonic or tonic contractions and relaxations. The patient may become unconscious. Generally convulsions are self-limiting, and the treatment should include protecting the patient from self-harm, moving any sharp objects out of the patient's reach, and turning the patient's head to prevent aspiration. In some situations diazepam may be administered intravenously (IV), but observation of the patient is often sufficient.

Toxic reactions to local anesthetics

Toxic reactions to local anesthetic agents usually result from excessive plasma levels of the anesthetic. Both CNS stimulation and CNS depression can occur. The stimulation is exhibited as excitement or even convulsions (see Chapter 9). Following stimulation, depression can occur with symptoms of drowsiness, unconsciousness, or even cardiac and respiratory arrest. The treatment of this toxic reaction is symptomatic. If convulsions are a predominant feature, diazepam can be administered. If hypotension is predominant, a pressor agent can be given. In the presence of reflex bradycardia, atropine may be administered. Usually patients who have a toxic reaction to local anesthetics must be watched closely, but drug administration is rarely needed.

Syncope

The most common emergency encountered in the dental office is syncope (fainting) or transient unconsciousness. Because of a loss of normal motor tone and a pooling of blood peripherally, there is a sudden fall in blood pressure, severe bradycardia, and diaphoresis. These effects are brought about by anxiety, fear, or apprehension, all common in a dental situation. The treatment involves placing the patient in the Trendelenburg position (head down), causing blood to rush to the head, which has the effect of giving the patient a transfusion of whole blood. Spirits of ammonia can be administered by inhalation.

The most important component in the treatment of syncope is for the dental hygienist to exhibit confidence. If the hygienist shows control over the situation, the patient will be less anxious and apprehensive and less likely to repeat the syncopal attack.

Extrapyramidal reactions

The antipsychotic agents (see Chapter 17) can produce extrapyramidal reactions. Parkinson-like movements such as uncoordinated tongue, muscular movements, and grimacing can occur. Diphenhydramine intravenously is the treatment of choice.

RESPIRATORY EMERGENCIES

The respiratory emergencies involve difficulty in breathing and exchange of oxygen. They include asthma, anaphylactic shock, apnea, acute airway obstruction, hyperventilation, and pulmonary embolism. An allergic reaction may also be manifested by difficulty in breathing.

Asthma

Normally patients who have acute asthmatic attacks have a history of previous attacks and carry their own medication. The most common sign of an asthmatic attack is wheezing with prolonged expiration. The patient's own medication (multiple-dose inhalers containing a β_2-agonist such as metaproterenol, as well as a steroid such as betamethasone) should be used first. If response to these agents does not occur, hospitalization for administration of aminophylline (parenteral or oral) and parenteral corticosteroids and epinephrine should be considered. Oxygen should also be administered.

Anaphylactic shock

The most common cause of anaphylactic shock is an injection of penicillin, although anaphylactic reactions have also been caused by many other agents. Usually, a weak, rapid pulse and a profound decrease in blood pressure occur. There is dyspnea and severe bronchial constriction.

Parenteral epinephrine is the drug of choice. It must be administered immediately in severe anaphylactic shock. Diphenhydramine, corticosteroids, metaproterenol inhalers, and aminophylline may also be used.

Apnea

The use of an opioid analgesic agent in the dental office can depress respiration or even induce respiratory arrest. Treatment consists of administration of the opioid antagonist naloxone (Narcan) parenterally.

Acute airway obstruction

Acute airway obstruction or aspiration (such as of vomitus) is usually due to a foreign body (crown preparation) in the pharynx or larynx; laryngospasm may be drug induced. Gasping for breath, coughing, gagging, acute anxiety, and cyanosis are signs and symptoms of acute airway obstruction. Treatment begins by placing the patient in a Trendelenburg position on the right side, and encouraging coughing. Do not allow the patient to sit up. Clearing the pharynx and pulling the tongue forward before performing the Heimlich maneuver (external subdiaphragmatic compression) should be attempted next. Finally, the

Heimlich maneuver should be performed and repeated if needed. A cricothyrotomy or tracheotomy, hardly dental office maneuvers, are indicated if the object cannot be dislodged by the other methods. For aspiration, the use of suction, intubation, and ventilatory assistance are suggested. Steroids, antibiotics, and aminophylline are also administered. When laryngospasm is present (drug induced), succinylcholine, a neuromuscular blocking agent, and positive pressure oxygen are the agents of choice. The operator must have training and equipment to artificially breathe for the patient before succinylcholine is administered. Prevention of "swallowed" objects can best be attained by the use of the rubber dam and throat packing, when appropriate.

Hyperventilation

Hyperventilation is one of the most common dental emergency situations. The increased respiratory rate is often brought on by emotional upset associated with dental treatment. Tachypnea, tachycardia, and paresthesia (tingling of the fingers and around the mouth) have been reported. Nausea, faintness, perspiration, acute anxiety, lightheadedness, and shortness of breath can also occur. The treatment is calm reassurance. Encourage patients to hold their breath or "rebreathe" in a paper bag or an unconnected face mask.

Pulmonary embolism

Pulmonary embolism occurs when a clot, fat, or air travels from the legs, typically, through the circulation to lodge in the lungs. Pleuritic pain, suffocation, tight chest, dyspnea, and cough can result. A sudden blood pressure drop, collapse, weakness, sweating, syncope, apprehension, and hemoptysis can occur. The treatment includes opioids and heparin.

ENDOCRINE EMERGENCIES

The most common emergency associated with the endocrine system is hypoglycemia following an overdose of insulin. Adrenal crisis and thyroid storm are also endocrine emergencies.

Hypoglycemia

The most common cause of hypoglycemia is an excessive dose of insulin in a diabetic patient. The medical history in this case is important to determine the dose of insulin and the intake of food before the dental appointment. Often patients inject their usual daily dose of insulin but fail to eat before coming to the dental office. Patients should be asked to eat before most dental procedures are begun.

The patient with hypoglycemia has a rapid pulse and decreased respiration. Hunger, dizziness, weakness, and occasionally tremor of the hands can occur. Diaphoresis, nausea, and mental confusion are other signs of hypoglycemia. If the signs of hypoglycemia are recognized before they become severe, the patient can be given a sugary drink or glucose orally or by other means. If the patient lapses into unconsciousness, dextrose must be given intravenously.

Diabetic coma

Less common than hypoglycemia, the diabetic coma is caused by elevated blood sugar. Symptoms of frequent urination, loss of appetite, nausea, vomiting, and thirst are seen. Acetone breath, hypercapnia, warm, dry skin, rapid pulse, and a decrease in blood pressure can occur. Treatment is undertaken only in a hospitalized setting and includes insulin after proper laboratory readings are obtained (blood sugar).

Acute adrenocortical insufficiency

Adrenal crisis usually occurs in patients who are taking steroids and are then subjected to stress without increasing their steroid dose. Unable to respond to the stress, the patient has an adrenal crisis. Nausea, vomiting, abdominal pain, and confusion may result. Cardiovascular collapse and irreversible shock may result in a fatality. The treatment is corticosteroids, for example, hydrocortisone parenterally and oxygen by inha-

lation. Hospitalized patients receive fluid replacement and vasopressor agents if symptoms dictate.

Thyroid storm

Thyroid storm is a condition in which hyperthyroidism is out of control. Signs and symptoms include hyperpyrexia, increased sweating, hyperactivity, mental agitation, shaking, nervousness, and tachycardia. Congestive heart failure and cardiovascular collapse may follow. Temperature is controlled by tepid baths and aspirin. β-blockers are given to control the cardiovascular symptoms. Other agents that may be used include reserpine, guanethidine, and hydrocortisone. Sodium iodide and propylthiouracil are given to inhibit the action of the thyroid gland. Severely hyperthyroid patients should not be given atropine or epinephrine because these agents may precipitate a thyroid storm.

OTHER EMERGENCIES
Malignant hyperthermia

Malignant hyperthermia is a genetically determined reaction that is triggered by inhalation general anesthetics or skeletal muscle relaxants. The most notable symptom is a rapidly rising temperature. Baths and aspirin are used to control the elevated temperature. Prompt treatment with dantrolene (Dantrium) can control acidosis and body temperature by reducing calcium released into the muscles during the contractile response. Fluid replacement, steroids, and sodium bicarbonate may be used.

EMERGENCY KIT FOR DENTAL OFFICE

Although the choice of drugs for a dental office emergency kit will depend on individual circumstances, experience, and personal preference, the dental hygienist should make sure there is an emergency kit in the dental office. Table 23-1 lists some emergency drugs, their therapeutic uses, and usual adult doses. Drugs that may be included if the office personnel is trained in advanced cardiac life support (ACLS) include so-

Table 23-1. Emergency kit drugs, their uses and adult dose

Drug	Drug group	Therapeutic uses	Dose (mg)*	Route†
Epinephrine (Adrenalin)	Allergy	Acute allergic reactions; asthmatic attacks; cardiac arrest	0.3	IV,IM,SC
Diphenhydramine (Benadryl)	Antihistamine	Allergic reactions; extrapyramidal reactions to phenothiazines	50	IV,IM,PO
Diazepam (Valium)	Anticonvulsant	Seizures; thyroid storm	5	IV
Naloxone (Narcan)	Opioid antagonist	Opioid overdose with respiratory depression	0.4	IV,IM
Morphine	Opioid analgesic	Severe pain; myocardial infarction	10	IV,IM
Methoxamine (Vasoxyl)	Vasopressor	Hypotension; acute adrenal insufficiency	10	IV,IM
Hydrocortisone sodium succinate (Solu-Cortef)	Corticosteroid	Adrenal crisis; allergic reactions; cardiac arrest	100	IV
Dextrose 50%	Antihypoglycemic	Hypoglycemia	50 ml	IV
Glucose	Antihypoglycemic	Hypoglycemia		PO
Oxygen		Respiratory distress; **not** with COPD	100%	IH
Nitroglycerin	Vasodilator	Angina pectoris	0.4	SL
Aromatic spirits of ammonia	Respiratory stimulant	Syncope	0.3 ml	IH
Metaproterenol (Alupent)	Bronchodilator	Asthma; bronchospasm	2 puffs	IH

*Usual adult dose in milligrams, unless otherwise stated.
†IH, inhalation; IM, intramuscular; IV, intravenous; PO, orally; SC, subcutaneous; SL, sublingual.

dium bicarbonate, atropine, lidocaine, and calcium chloride.

Equipment

An oxygen mask, manual resuscitation bag, and oxygen tank with a flow gauge are needed to administer positive pressure oxygen. A sphygmomanometer and stethoscope are used to take a patient's blood pressure. Disposable syringes, needles, and a tourniquet are used to administer

medications. A laryngeal suction cannula can suction the throat if aspiration occurs. Nasal and oral airways are used to maintain an unobstructed airway. Endotracheal tubes and a laryngoscope are required for intubation. Intravenous solutions, tubing, butterfly needles, and adhesive tape are used for administering drugs intravenously. A cricothyrotomy kit can be used for acute airway obstruction when other measures fail.

Many dental offices will have no person trained

to use the equipment listed above. Without training, attempting to use this equipment may be more harmful than using simple measures.

Drugs

Table 23-1 lists the drugs that should be considered for inclusion in an emergency dental kit. These may vary, depending on the preference and experience of the practitioner. Some equipment and drugs that are not used by dental office personnel are kept in the emergency kit for use by a physician or for those with ACLS training in an emergency. The following individual drugs are commonly used in emergency situations.

Epinephrine. It is mandatory to include epinephrine in the dental office emergency kit for the treatment of cardiac arrest, anaphylaxis, or an acute asthmatic attack. It should not be used in the treatment of shock because it can cause decreased venous return with increased ischemia and it can precipitate ventricular fibrillation. The rationale for the use of epinephrine for cardiac arrest is the β-stimulation of the myocardium. In the treatment of severe anaphylaxis and acute asthmatic attacks, it acts as a physiologic antagonist to the massive release of histamine that occurs in these conditions. Without epinephrine, this histamine leads to bronchoconstriction and decreased oxygen exchange. Because epinephrine's cardiac effects are diminished in the presence of acidosis, adequate mechanical resuscitation and external cardiac massage accompany its administration. Epinephrine may be administered by the intravenous or intracardiac routes (by trained personnel). Dental personnel may find injection into the frenulum under the tongue more convenient.

Diphenhydramine. Diphenhydramine (Benadryl), an antihistamine, is used in the treatment of some allergic reactions. Since the antihistamines compete with histamine for tissue receptor sites, a rapid reversal of allergic symptoms cannot be expected. For this reason epinephrine and diphenhydramine are used together in severe allergic reactions or anaphylaxis.

Diazepam. Diazepam (Valium) is the drug of choice for the treatment of most convulsions if a drug is needed. However, in the majority of cases convulsive episodes are self-limiting and require only supportive care in the form of protecting the patient from physical harm and administering oxygen.

One cause of convulsions in the dental office is a toxic reaction to a local anesthetic from an overdose or an idiosyncrasy (see Chapter 9). Anticonvulsant drugs should be used conservatively because they may enhance the CNS depression of the local anesthetic.

Naloxone. Naloxone (Narcan), a pure opioid antagonist, is the drug of choice for opioid-induced apnea. Its use is extremely safe, but more than one administration may be needed because of its short duration of action. The initial dose is 0.4 mg (1 ml) intravenously, but it can also be given subcutaneously or intramuscularly. The onset of action is approximately 2 minutes by the intravenous route. Naloxone is effective in reversing the respiratory depression caused by the opioid drugs; if no response occurs, other causes for the respiratory depression must be considered.

Morphine. Morphine or meperidine are opioid analgesics administered to a patient who has suffered an acute myocardial infarction. These agents relieve pain and allay apprehension. They are used in pulmonary embolism and angina for the same reasons.

Methoxamine. Although epinephrine, a vasopressor, has already been included in the emergency kit, methoxamine may also be included. It is an adrenergic agonist with almost exclusively α-adrenergic agonist properties. By peripheral vasoconstriction, it produces a mild increase in blood pressure. There is no concomitant stimulation of the myocardium; in fact, a reflex bradycardia results. It is indicated in the treatment of drug overdose reactions, acute adrenal insufficiency, and allergic reactions. Phenylephrine (Neo-Synephrine), also an α-adrenergic agonist, is used like methoxamine. Dopamine, an α- and β-adrenergic agonist, is used for certain kinds of shock. One advantage of dopamine is that it increases renal and splanchnic blood flow and cardiac output.

Hydrocortisone. Hydrocortisone sodium succinate (Solu-Cortef) is a corticosteroid used for allergic reactions, anaphylaxis, and adrenal crisis. Even given intravenously, hydrocortisone has a slow onset of action. Epinephrine is still the drug of choice for anaphylaxis and serious allergic reactions because it acts immediately as a physiologic antagonist.

Dextrose and glucose. Both dextrose and glucose are used to manage hypoglycemic episodes. These most commonly occur when the diabetic patient's insulin and food intake are out of balance. Oral glucose, or any available liquid carbohydrate, is given if the patient is conscious. Only with unconsciousness and a lack of the swallowing reflex is intravenous dextrose used to treat hypoglycemia. In the dental office, all patients should be diagnosed before consciousness is lost.

Oxygen. Oxygen is probably the most important drug in the emergency kit. It is indicated in most emergencies, especially if respiratory difficulty is a problem. Patients with chronic obstructive pulmonary disease should be given oxygen only with great caution, since apnea may result. Every dental office personnel should know how to administer inhalation oxygen.

Nitroglycerin. Sublingual nitroglycerin tablets or nitroglycerin spray (see Chapter 15) should be kept in the dental office emergency kit to manage an acute anginal attack.

Aromatic ammonia. Containers of aromatic ammonia spirits, designed to be crushed, can be used to treat syncope. Aromatic ammonia acts by irritating the membranes of the upper respiratory tract, resulting in stimulation of respiration and blood pressure. A dental office should have one (unexpired) container taped to each dental chair for easy access.

Metaproterenol. Metaproterenol is a β_2-adrenergic agonist useful in the management of bronchoconstriction. Although most asthmatic patients carry their own supply, it is possible that they may not bring their bronchoconstrictor to every dental appointment. If bronchoconstriction is severe, parenteral epinephrine is still the drug of choice.

REVIEW QUESTIONS

1. State what general measures the dental hygienist should be familiar with in order to respond to any emergency situation.
2. For each of the following common emergencies, state the signs, symptoms, and treatment (including drugs):
   a. Cardiac arrest
   b. Angina pectoris
   c. Acute myocardial infarction
   d. Convulsions
   e. Syncope
   f. Asthma
   g. Anaphylactic shock
   h. Apnea
   i. Hypoglycemia
3. List the equipment required to treat the emergencies in question 2 and explain the rationale for the inclusion of each item.
4. Give the names and potential uses of the drugs required in an emergency kit for the dental office.
5. Concoct an imaginary emergency kit for the office in which you will work.

Chapter 24

12/1/93

Pregnancy and breast-feeding

The dental treatment of the pregnant or nursing woman is always of special concern to the dental hygienist. On one hand, the pregnant woman often needs additional dental treatment during her pregnancy; on the other hand, her treatment plans need to be carefully planned. Many questions about drug therapy for the pregnant or breast-feeding patient arise. The literature, unfortunately, does not provide all the answers. This chapter attempts to offer guidelines for determining the relative risk when prescribing drugs either for the pregnant woman or for the nursing mother. No unnecessary drug should be administered to the pregnant woman. If a drug is to be administered, the risk to the fetus must be weighed against the benefit to the pregnant woman. An adequate health history, including whether a woman may be pregnant, should be taken at each dental appointment. Close coordination with the patient's obstetric health-care professional when questions about her dental treatment arise is recommended. Any consultations should be documented in the patient's chart.

GENERAL PRINCIPLES

There are two main concerns when considering whether to give a drug to a pregnant woman. The first is that the drug may be teratogenic. Teratogenic is derived from the Greek work *terato*, meaning "monster." The second is that the drug can affect the fetus near-term causing the newborn infant to have an adverse reaction, such as respiratory depression. A relatively new concern is the long-term (physiologic and psychologic) consequences of in utero exposure to agents.

History

In 1941, a relationship between German measles during pregnancy and blindness, deafness, and death of the offspring was noted. Scientists recognized that exogenous agents could affect the unborn fetus, producing congenital abnormalities. Again in 1961, this lesson was still being taught. A "harmless" sedative, thalidomide, available over the counter in Europe, was taken by pregnant women. An increase in a rare birth defect, phocomelia (short or absent limbs), occurred shortly thereafter. Thalidomide later was implicated in these birth defects.

PREGNANCY
Pregnancy trimesters

Pregnancy involves three trimesters, each three months long. The **first** trimester is the time that the organs in the fetus are forming. This is considered the most critical time for teratogenicity. Often a woman is unaware that she is pregnant for at least one half of this trimester. Dental prophylaxis with detailed instructions and a visual examination of the oral cavity without x-rays should be performed if the patient is pregnant. Since this is the time when the woman may feel nauseated in the morning (morning sickness), other elective dental treatment should be avoided during this time.

The **second** trimester is an excellent time for the patient to receive both oral health instructions and another dental prophylaxis, if needed. The patient's periodontal status should be carefully evaluated during this time. The patient is most comfortable during this trimester.

The **third** trimester is that closest to delivery. The woman is beginning to feel uncomfortable

249

and it is difficult for her to lie prone for any length of time. If dental treatment is needed, she may feel more comfortable in the sitting position. Also, this is the time when premature labor is most likely to begin. Drugs that may affect the newborn child should not be given during this trimester.

Teratogenicity

It is very difficult to prove that a drug is teratogenic in humans. Some of the reasons include the following: different animal species vary among themselves and differ from humans in their responses to drugs; timing of the drug exposure varies with each drug; one drug can produce a variety of abnormalities and different drugs can produce the same abnormality; drugs that are teratogenic are not uniformly so; a drug's effect on the fetus may be different from its effect on the mother; and the adverse effects of a certain drug on the fetus may not be evident for many years. Before a drug can be proved to be easily teratogenic, it must be highly teratogenic. Drugs that are known teratogens include drugs such as isotretinoin, antineoplastic agents, oral anticoagulants, some antiepileptic agents, the tetracyclines, and ethyl alcohol.

FDA pregnancy categories

The United States Food and Drug Administration (FDA) has developed pregnancy categories A, B, C, D, and X. Each drug that is the subject of FDA regulation for pregnancy labeling is given a category based on its known potential for risk. Table 24-1 gives a summary of the criteria for the different categories. Note that availability of animal or human studies is a criterion. Category A is the safest, whereas category X should not be used in pregnant women. Categories B, C, and D fall in between these two criteria.

BREAST FEEDING

Questions about the safety of a certain drug given to a nursing mother are appearing more frequently as nursing is becoming more "fashionable." As during pregnancy, the risk-to-benefit ratio should be carefully considered before drugs

are given to the nursing mother. Drugs without strong indications for use should not be taken. Almost all drugs given to the mother can pass into the breast milk in varying concentrations. While nursing, the baby ingests the drug, which may produce an effect in the infant. The amount of drug that appears in the milk depends on the plasma concentration of the drug, its lipid solubility, degree of ionization, and binding to plasma proteins.

For a few drugs, nursing is clearly contraindicated. If these drugs must be given, then breastfeeding should be discontinued or the milk expressed and discarded until the mother stops taking the contraindicated drug. For drugs that are not contraindicated, the timing of nursing can further reduce the dose to which an infant is exposed. For example, taking a dose of drug around the time of nursing will allow the peak concentration in the mother's plasma to occur during a time when the infant is not nursing. Table 24-2 summarizes the available data on the use of dental drugs for nursing mothers.

DENTAL DRUGS

Questions relating to drug administration in conjunction with dental treatment refer to whether a specific drug may be safely given to the pregnant woman. In general, a drug should be used in a pregnant woman only if the benefits to the pregnant woman outweigh the risks to the fetus and a definite indication exists. Table 24-3 summarizes the information about whether dental drugs should be used in pregnant women.

Local anesthetics

No drug is used more frequently in the dental office than local anesthetic agents. Local anesthetic amides have been reported to produce fetal bradycardia and neonatal depression when given in very large doses near-term. High doses may produce uterine vascular constriction leading to fetal heart rate changes. Lidocaine, prilocaine, and etidocaine have been tested in animals without teratogenic effects (category B). Bupivacaine has been shown teratogenic in rats and rabbits (category C), whereas mepivacaine and procaine

Table 24-1. FDA pregnancy categories for prescription drugs

Description	Example
A. Adequate and well-controlled studies have failed to demonstrate a risk to the fetus in the first trimester of pregnancy (and there is no evidence of risk in later trimesters). The possibility of fetal harm appears remote.	A. Potassium chloride
B. Animal reproduction studies have failed to demonstrate a risk to the fetus and there are no adequate and well-controlled studies in pregnant women, or animal studies do show an adverse effect on the fetus but well-controlled studies in pregnant women have failed to demonstrate a risk to the fetus.	B. Narcotic analgesic agents,* erythromycin, pentobarbital, penicillins, cephalosporins, acetaminophen, antihistamines (B or C), prednisone, caffeine, nonsteroid antiinflammatory agents,† sulfonamides†
C. Animal reproduction studies have shown an adverse effect (teratogenic or embryocidal) on the fetus and there are no adequate and well-controlled studies in humans, or no studies are available in either animals or women. Potential benefits may warrant use of the drug in pregnant women despite potential risks.	C. Epinephrine, phenylpropanolamine, trimethobenzamide, aspirin,† atropine, phenothiazines, promethazine, theophylline, antidepressants (B or C), beta blockers
D. There is positive evidence of human fetal risk based on adverse reaction data from investigational or marketing experience or studies in humans, but potential benefits in certain situations (serious) may warrant use of the drug in pregnant women despite potential risks.	D. Oral anticoagulants, tetracycline, cortisone, diazepam, oral hypoglycemic agents, thiazide diuretics, phenytoin
X. Studies in animals or humans have demonstrated fetal abnormalities or there is positive evidence of human fetal risk based on adverse reaction data from investigational or marketing experience, and the risks involved in use of the drug in pregnant women clearly outweigh any potential benefits.	X. Trimethadione, phencyclidine (PCP), disulfiram, diethylstilbestrol

*High-dose, near-term; prolonged use = D.
†Near-term = D.

have not been tested (category C). Small doses used by careful, slow injection have not been associated with any problems in the fetus. Lidocaine is the local anesthetic of choice for the pregnant woman since it is category B and is not associated with methemoglobinemia (prilocaine) and not highly lipid soluble (etidocaine).

Epinephrine

Small doses of epinephrine, administered with appropriate care, are similar to those produced endogenously. Large doses could produce adverse effects in the fetus, including anoxia from vasoconstriction. If procedures are to be short, then local anesthetics without epinephrine are preferred. These comments also apply to other vasoconstrictor substances contained in local anesthetic solutions.

Analgesics

Analgesics should be given in the lowest possible dose and for the shortest duration possible to control pain. In dentistry, adjunctive therapy (inci-

Table 24-2. Dental drug usage by nursing mothers*

Dental drug	Acceptable for nursing	Watch infant for symptoms of:
Local anesthetics		
Amides (lidocaine, and mepivacaine)	Yes	CNS changes; avoid bupivacaine (high lipid solubility and long action)
Vasoconstrictors		
Epinephrine	Yes	Hyperactivity or irritability
Analgesic agents		
Aspirin	Yes	Chronic high-dose use may present problems
Nonsteroidal antiinflammatory agents	Yes; caution	Use ibuprofen, whose concentration in milk is not detectable; others, small % in milk
Acetaminophen	Yes	Present in milk; no documented problems
Opioids	Yes	Sedation; poor feeding; constipation
Antiinfective agents		
Penicillin	Yes	Allergic symptoms
Erythromycin	Yes	Concentrated in milk
Cephalosporins	Yes	Allergic symptoms
Tetracycline	No	Tooth staining
Clindamycin	Yes; caution	Diarrhea?; pseudomembranous colitis?
Metronidazole	No	Carcinogenic in animals; express and discard milk if must use (not for dental use)
Aminoglycosides	Yes	Not absorbed when administered orally
Nystatin	Yes	Not absorbed into the systemic circulation from the mouth or gastrointestinal tract
Clotrimazole	Yes; caution	Excreted in milk; use nystatin first
Ketoconazole	No	Express and discard milk
Antianxiety agents		
Nitrous oxide (with oxygen)	Yes	Excreted through mother's lungs
Benzodiazepines	No	Sedation; infants metabolize more slowly
Barbiturates	No	Only for anticonvulsant action

*Use no unnecessary agents. Check the current literature. Remember that differences of opinion exist. Check with patient's health care provider before using if questionable.

sion, drainage, and curettage) should be used first.

Aspirin. Studies in animals have shown that aspirin can cause a variety of birth defects involving the eyes, CNS gastrointestinal tract, and skeleton. In humans, controlled studies have not been able to demonstrate that aspirin use during pregnancy increases the incidence of birth defects. During the third trimester, aspirin can pro-

long gestation, complicate delivery, decrease placental function, or increase the risk of maternal or fetal hemorrhage. Premature closure of the patent ductus arteriosus may occur. These effects have been reported with chronic high-dose aspirin use. **Abuse** of aspirin may increase stillbirths or neonatal death.

Nonsteroidal antiinflammatory agents. Since the nonsteroidal antiinflammatory agents produce

Table 24-3. Dental drug usage during pregnancy,* and their FDA categories

Dental drug	1st trimester	2nd/3rd trimester	FDA risk factor	Comments
Local anesthetics				
Lidocaine	Yes	Yes	B	First choice anesthetic; fetal bradycardia near-term (all amides)
Mepivacaine	Yes	Yes	C	No animal testing
Bupivacaine	No	No	C	Embryocidal in rabbits; high lipid solubility
Vasoconstrictors				
Epinephrine	Yes	Yes	C	Vasoconstriction can produce hypoxia; use sparingly
Analgesic agents				
Aspirin	No	No	C/D†	Near-term dystocia and prolonged parturition; bleeding; premature closure of patent ductus arteriosus
Nonsteroidal antiinflammatory agents	No	No	B/D	See aspirin
Acetaminophen	Yes	Yes	B	Teratogenic at overdose levels
Opioids	Yes	Yes	C-D/D†	Respiratory depression near-term; high doses contraindicated; use lowest dose, shortest duration
Antiinfective agents				
Penicillin	Yes	Yes	B	Safe, especially penicillin V
Erythromycin	Yes	Yes	B	Safe, except **estolate** form (cholestatic hepatitis)
Cephalosporins	Yes	Yes	C	Use only if above options fail
Tetracyclines	No	No	D	Stains teeth; affects bones
Clindamycin	No	No	C?	Only if other alternatives do not exist
Aminoglycosides	No	Yes; caution	C	Cranial nerve VIII toxicity (hearing and balance); nephrotoxicity
Metronidazole	No	No	D?	Carcinogenic and mutagenic in animals
Nystatin	Yes	Yes	B?	Not absorbed into systemic circulation from gastrointestinal tract (or mouth)
Clotrimazole	No	Yes; caution	C?	Abnormal liver function tests in adult can occur
Ketoconazole	No	No	C	Embryotoxic in rat
Antianxiety agents				
Nitrous oxide (with oxygen)	No	Yes; caution	D?	Ensure adequate O_2 intake; female operators avoid chronic exposure
Benzodiazepines	No	No	D-X	Cleft lip; neural tube defects; few strong indications
Secobarbital	No	No	C	No dental use now

*Administer no unnecessary drugs to a pregnant woman. The potential risk to the fetus may be weighed against the benefit to the woman. Consult with patient's health care provider before using drugs, if needed.
†Refers to during the third trimester, or near-term.
?,FDA category derived from literature; drug has not been given an FDA category.

effects similar to aspirin, the outcome on the fetus if they are given near-term would be expected to be the same. They can delay and make delivery more difficult, as well as constrict the ductus arteriosus. They also potentiate vasoconstriction if hypoxia exists. All carry a warning to avoid use during pregnancy. For ibuprofen and naproxen, studies in animals have not shown adverse effects on the fetus. Diflunisal (category C), but not naproxen (category B), has been shown to be teratogenic in rabbits in large doses. Ibuprofen is the NSAIA of choice for the nursing mother.

Acetaminophen. Acetaminophen is generally considered to be safe in pregnancy, although no controlled studies in humans have been done. In large doses, it may be associated with fetal renal changes similar to that in adults.

Opioids. Doses used by addicts have been demonstrated to produce problems. The opioids, with the exception of codeine, have not been associated with teratogenicity. Retrospective studies have associated the use of codeine during the first trimester with fetal abnormalities involving the respiratory, gastrointestinal, cardiac and circulatory systems, as well as inguinal hernia and cleft lip and palate. These studies suggest that codeine or other opioids should not be used indiscriminately during the first trimester. Whether the birth defects associated with codeine are related to its ubiquitous use or to some difference it possesses is not known. Near-term administration can produce respiratory depression in the infant. If the mother is addicted, the infant will experience withdrawal symptoms. The use of codeine in limited quantities for a limited duration of time is common in clinical practice. Although opioids appear in breast milk when analgesic doses are administered, the small amounts appear to be insignificant. By properly timing the doses of analgesic, the dose the infant receives is reduced further. The infant should be observed for signs of sedation and constipation.

Antiinfective agents

Antiinfective agents should only be used when a definite indication for their use exists. Prophylactic use, use when no indication exists, or use when an infection can be locally treated are inappropriate.

Penicillin. The most common antiinfective agent used in dentistry is penicillin. It is generally agreed that the penicillins are safe to use during pregnancy. Using penicillin V for a dental infection that is not controlled by local measures and is indicated would be acceptable. Penicillins appear in breast milk and infants should be observed for signs of diarrhea, candidiasis, and allergic reactions.

Erythromycin. Erythromycins, other than the estolate form, also appear to be safe for use during pregnancy. The estolate form (Ilosone) should not be used in pregnant women because it has been associated with reversible hepatic toxicity in the mother. Erythromycin is concentrated in breast milk but has not been documented to produce problems.

Cephalosporins. The cephalosporins have not been associated with teratogenicity, but the newer cephalosporins (third generation) have not been studied. Cephalosporins should be used in dentistry only if a specific indication exists.

Tetracyclines. Tetracycline, doxycycline, and all tetracyclines are contraindicated during pregnancy because of the potential for adversely affecting the fetus. They cross the placenta and are deposited in the fetal teeth and bones. Deciduous teeth may become stained and fetal bone growth inhibited. Hepatotoxicity can occur in the pregnant woman treated with large doses of tetracycline. Whether the amount excreted in milk, after it is complexed with the calcium in milk, can produce problems in the nursing infant is not known.

Clindamycin. Clindamycin should be used during pregnancy only for susceptible *Bacteroides* species not sensitive to penicillin. No adverse fetal problems have been reported. Since clindamycin is excreted in breast milk, it should not be prescribed for nursing mothers.

Metronidazole. In animals, metronidazole can produce birth defects. Even for *Trichomonas* infection, metronidazole is contraindicated during the first trimester. It would be difficult to encounter a dental situation in which the risk to the fetus would not be greater than the benefit to the mother. Because animal studies have shown metronidazole to be carcinogenic, the nursing mother should only be given metronidazole if the breast milk is expressed and discarded during treatment and for 48 hours after the last dose.

Aminoglycosides. Some aminoglycosides have been associated with congenital deafness. They should not be administered during the first trimester. Ototoxicity in the fetus has been associated with relatively low doses given early in pregnancy. Fetal nephrotoxicity may be a possibility. The amount of aminoglycoside that appears in breast milk varies, but since oral absorption is poor, it is unlikely that it would present a problem for the infant.

Nystatin. Nystatin is safe to use during pregnancy to treat oral candidal infections. When applied topically or taken orally it is not absorbed into the systemic circulation. It may also be used by either the pregnant woman or the nursing infant to treat thrush.

Clotrimazole. Small amounts of clotrimazole are absorbed from topical administration of this agent. No occurrences of abnormality have been reported, but nystatin is probably safer.

Ketoconazole. Ketoconazole has been shown to be teratogenic in rats, producing an abnormal number of digits (syndactyly and oligodactyly). Dystocia during delivery has been demonstrated in animals. It appears in breast milk and may increase the chance of kernicterus (jaundice) occurring in the nursing infant. If it must be used, breast milk must be expressed and discarded during therapy and for 72 hours after cessation of therapy.

Antianxiety agents

Nitrous oxide. Operating room personnel exposed to trace amounts of nitrous oxide have a significantly higher incidence of spontaneous abortion and birth defects in their children, regardless of whether a man or woman was exposed. These data suggest that methods for reducing the environmental exposure, especial-

ly chronically, should be explored and implemented. Pregnant dental hygienists should have knowledge of the levels of nitrous oxide that are present in the dental offices in which they practice.

Benzodiazepines. First-trimester use of the benzodiazepines (chlordiazepoxide and diazepam) has been reported to increase the risk of congenital malformations. Cleft palate and lip and neural tube defects have been seen. Other benzodiazepines may be associated with this increase in risk also. Temazepam and triazolam are FDA pregnancy category X, whereas alprazolam, halazepam, and lorazepam are category D. Benzodiazepines are indicated during pregnancy only for the treatment of status epilepticus.

Chronic ingestion of the benzodiazepines can produce physical dependence in the infant. Floppy infant syndrome, or neonatal flaccidity, has been seen at birth with inadequate sucking reflex or apnea. Use of the benzodiazepines in the nursing mother, which may accumulate in the neonate because of slower metabolism, may cause sedation and feeding difficulties. Therefore they are not recommended for the nursing mother.

Barbiturates. Phenobarbital has been implicated as a teratogen. It induces hepatic enzymes and can treat hyperbilirubinemia. It also increases the rate of steroid and vitamin D metabolism. Vitamin K–dependent clotting factors have altered clotting in neonates when mothers have ingested phenobarbital. Withdrawal can be seen in neonates. Nursing mothers can take barbiturates without problems; look for signs of sedation in the infant.

Alcohol. Although alcohol is not a dental drug, the evidence for the teratogenicity of alcohol is very strong. Fetal alcohol syndrome (FAS) is the name associated with the changes that occur in an infant exposed to excessive alcohol intake by the mother. FAS involves abnormalities in these three areas: growth retardation (prenatal or postnatal), CNS abnormalities (neurologic or intellectual), and facial dysmorphology (such as microcephaly, microophthalmia or short palpebral fissures, and flat maxillary area or a thin lip). Infants born to those mothers who drank throughout pregnancy showed more tremors, hypertonia, restlessness, crying, and abnormal reflexes compared with control groups after birth.

Pregnant dental patients should be encouraged to abstain from or minimize the ingestion of alcohol. No threshold level that is safe for the pregnant woman is known. Well-documented studies show that adverse effects of the fetus are dose related and can extend for years after the birth of the baby. As a health care professional, the dental hygienist is in a position to remind the pregnant woman not only to care for her oral cavity health, but also her baby's development.

REVIEW QUESTIONS

1. Describe the proper method for the dental hygienist to obtain information about possible pregnancy or breast-feeding patients. State the information to be obtained.
2. Explain the three trimesters and the special risks for each one.
3. Define teratogenicity and describe why identifying drugs that produce it is so difficult.
4. Explain the FDA pregnancy categories and state their significance.
5. Determine the factors that are important when a woman is breast-feeding and to receive drugs. Describe the method of timing drug intake to minimize exposure to the infant.
6. For the commonly used dental drugs, such as local anesthetics, antibiotics, and analgesics, rank the agents available from safest to least safe.
7. Describe two activities that the dental hygienist should perform before giving a pregnant woman any medications to minimize future legal problems.

Chapter 25

Drug interactions

A drug interaction is defined as the action of an administered drug on the effectiveness or toxicity of another drug administered earlier, simultaneously, or later. This phenomenon often results in undesired drug effects. It is a problem of growing concern to the health professions and is directly related to an increase in multiple drug therapy. Since many dental patients are regularly using a greater number of drugs, the possibility for drug interactions is increasing. As more studies are done, the importance of these drug interactions is elucidated.

The dental hygienist can encounter a drug interaction in several situations. First, a patient may already be taking drugs that interact with each other. Second, drugs prescribed or suggested for use in the dental office may interact with drugs prescribed by the patient's physician. It is important to remember that many patients who seek dental treatment are already taking medication, either self-prescribed in the form of over-the-counter medication or prescribed by their physicians.

A complete medical history is necessary to minimize the problems of drug interactions. This chapter discusses some of the possible mechanisms for drug interactions and a list of the drug interactions most commonly encountered in dental practice (Table 25-1). In many instances these drug interactions are discussed in the chapters on individual drug groups and will be only briefly mentioned here.

MECHANISM OF INTERACTIONS

When two or more drugs interact, the result may be potentiation or enhancement of the pharmacologic effects or antagonism between the agents.

By understanding the mechanism of a drug interaction, one can often predict the results. Although the mechanism of many drug interactions is poorly understood, the more commonly known mechanisms will be discussed. The types of drug interactions may be pharmacologic (same or opposite actions), pharmacodynamic (receptor sites), or pharmacokinetic (alteration in absorption, distribution, metabolism, or excretion).

Pharmacologic

Similar action. Drug interactions that result in enhanced activity are caused by combinations of drugs having similar actions. For example, the respiratory depression produced by opioid analgesics is potentiated by other agents, such as phenothiazines, which in themselves cause respiratory depression.

Opposite action. For example, theophylline given to an asthmatic for bronchodilation causes insomnia and counteracts the benzodiazepine given for sleep.

Pharmacodynamic

Both the adrenergic (sympathetic) nervous system and the cholinergic (parasympathetic) nervous system possess sites for drug interactions to occur.

The enzyme monoamine oxidase (MAO) normally destroys only a small amount of the norepinephrine produced at the synapse. Drugs called monoamine oxidase inhibitors (MAOIs) cause an accumulation of norepinephrine at the neuroeffector junction. Since certain sympathomimetic agents such as ephedrine and phenylpropanolamine produce their pressor effects by releasing norepinephrine, administration of these agents can

Table 25-1.　Drug interactions

Dental drug	Medical drug	Potential outcome
Analgesics		
Salicylates (aspirin)	Oral anticoagulants (warfarin [Coumadin])	Hemorrhage
	Probenecid (Benemid), sulfinpyrazone (Anturane)	Acute attack of gout
	Ammonium chloride	Decreased aspirin excretion
	Oral antacids	Altered salicylate levels
	Oral hypoglycemic agents (antidiabetic agents)	Hypoglycemia
	Corticosteroids	Ulcers
	Ethyl alcohol	Increased gastrointestinal irritation
	Methotrexate	Increased methotrexate toxicity
Acetaminophen	Anticoagulants	No significant effect
Opiods		
General	Monoamine oxidase inhibitors	CNS depression
	CNS depressants	Enhanced CNS depression
Meperidine	Monoamine oxidase inhibitors	Excitation, hypertension, coma Hypotension and coma
Antibiotics		
Penicillin	Tetracycline, erythromycin, kanamycin	Inhibition of penicillin
	Probenecid	Enhanced effect of penicillin
	Oral anticoagulants	Hemorrhage
Erythromycin	Penicillin	Inhibition of penicillin
	Clindamycin (Cleocin), lincomycin (Lincocin)	Antagonism
Tetracycline		
General	Oral antacids	
	Dairy products	
	Iron (oral)	Decreased absorption and effect of tetracycline
	Zinc	
	Penicillin	Inhibition of penicillin
	Barbiturates	Decreased effect of tetracycline
	Diuretics	Increased effect of tetracycline
	Oral anticoagulants	Hemorrhage
Doxycycline	Ethyl alcohol, barbiturates, carbamazepine (Tegretol), phenytoin (Dilantin)	Enhanced metabolism; decreased effect of doxycycline
Oxytetracycline	Antidiabetic agents	Enhanced hypoglycemic effect
Cephalosporins	Aminoglycosides, furosemide	Additive nephrotoxicity
	Probenecid	Inhibition of renal excretion of cephalosporins

Table 25-1. Drug interactions—cont'd

Dental drug	Medical drug	Potential outcome
Antianxiety agents		
Barbiturates	Oral anticoagulants	Intravascular clotting
	Phenytoin	Decreased effect of phenytoin
	Alcohol	Enhanced sedation
	CNS depressants	Enhanced sedation
	Tetracycline	Decreased effect of tetracycline
	Tricyclic antidepressants	Decreased blood levels of tricyclic antidepressants
	β-Adrenergic blockers	Reduced plasma concentration of β-blockers
	Corticosteroids	Reduced effect of corticosteroids
	Griseofulvin	Decreased effects of griseofulvin
	Monomine oxidase inhibitors	Prolonged activity of the barbiturate
	Quinidine	Decreased plasma quinidine levels
	Sulfonamides	Less thiopental required for surgery
Benzodiazepines	Cimetidine	Enhanced benzodiazepine effect
	Levodopa	Deterioration of parkinsonism
		Enhanced CNS depression and hypotension
		Transient delirium
CNS depressants	Other CNS depressants	
	Tricyclic antidepressants	
	Monoamine oxidase inhibitors	Enhanced CNS depression
Parasympatholytics (anticholinergics)		
Atropine, propantheline (Pro-Banthine), methantheline (Banthine)	Tricyclic antidepressants	Additive anticholinergic effects; xerostomia, constipation, blurred vision
	Phenothiazines	
	Quinidine	Increased heart rate
	Amantadine	Potentiated anticholinergic effects
	Methotrimeprazine	Extrapyramidal symptoms
	Many drugs	Increased or decreased gastrointestinal absorption
Sympathomimetics		
Epinephrine (Adrenalin)	Digitalis glycosides, digoxin (Lanoxin)	Cardiac arrhythmias
	Monoamine oxidase inhibitors	Hypertension
	β-Adrenergic blockers (propranolol [Inderal])	Hypertension and bradycardia
	Anticholinergics	Enhanced mydriasis and bronchial relaxation
	Cyclopropane, halogenated hydrocarbon anesthetics	Cardiac arrhythmias
	Oral hypoglycemic (antidiabetic) agents	Hyperglycemia
	Insulin	Hyperglycemia
	Tricyclic antidepressants	Hypertension
Norepinephrine (Levarterenol)	Guanethedine (Ismelin), methyldopa (Aldomet)	Hypertension
	Monoamine oxidase inhibitors	Increased response to norepinephrine
	Halothane	Cardiac arrhythmias
	Tricyclic antidepressants	Increased pressor response to norepinephrine

result in severe hypertension in patients taking MAOIs. Even tyramine, an agent found in cheeses and wines, can produce a hypertensive crisis in patients being treated with MAOIs.

The tricyclic antidepressants block the reuptake of norepinephrine. The antihypertensive agent guanethidine must be taken up to exert its effect. Since the tricyclic antidepressants prevent the uptake of guanethidine, they antagonize its effect.

In the parasympathetic nervous system the anticholinergic drugs block the action of the cholinergic nervous system. Other agents, including the phenothiazines and the tricyclic antidepressants, also possess anticholinergic activity. Used concomitantly, agents with anticholinergic action can produce excessive anticholinergic activity. This can cause dry mouth, constipation, tachycardia, urinary retention, and mydriasis.

Pharmacokinetic

The majority of drug interactions are pharmacokinetic. This involves an alteration in absoption, distribution, metabolism and/or excretion.

Absorption. The absorption of a drug may be decreased if an inactive or insoluble derivative is formed in the intestinal tract. For example, calcium can chelate with tetracycline resulting in decreased effectiveness. If the gastrointestinal motility is slowed by anticholinergic agents the absorption of certain drugs may be decreased because they are broken down in the stomach acid. With increased motility, slowly absorbed drugs may pass through the gastrointestinal tract before absorption is complete. Disintegration and dissolution are the rate-limiting steps for the absorption of some drugs. If the pH is altered, the dissolution may be reduced thereby reducing the absorption. Ionization of weak acids and bases is pH dependent. Altering the pH may alter the proportion of drug in the ionized form leading to a change in absorption. Bacterial flora are involved in the synthesis of vitamin K. If antibiotics reduce the flora, the concentration of vitamin K

will be reduced exaggerating the oral anticoagulant action.

Distribution. After drugs are absorbed, they become reversibly bound to the plasma proteins. The amount of this binding varies with the particular drug. The free drug exerts the pharmacologic effect, and the bound portion is biologically inactive. Since many weak acids are bound to the same site on the plasma proteins, an acidic drug can displace a bound acidic drug from its plasma protein binding site. This increases the plasma concentration of the displaced drug and indirectly increases its pharmacologic effect and toxicity. For example, warfarin (Coumadin), a very highly bound drug, is displaced from the plasma protein binding sites by aspirin, another acidic drug that is bound. This can result in an increase in the free warfarin and also an increase in its pharmacologic effect and toxicity producing hemorrhage. Because the coumarin-type anticoagulant agents are highly bound to plasma proteins, they interact with many drugs.

Metabolism. The metabolism of one drug may be enhanced or inhibited by another drug. Before drugs can be excreted by the kidney, they must be metabolized into more water-soluble derivatives in the liver. Certain drugs can induce the hepatic microsomal enzymes that normally metabolize many drugs. If there is an increase in these enzymes, then drugs metabolized by these enzymes would have less effect. Phenobarbital and carbamazepine are two common enzyme inducers. Interference with metabolism of a drug would increase its pharmacologic effect. Cimetidine inhibits hepatic microsomal drug metabolism and enhances the action of many drugs metabolized by that system.

Excretion. Glomerular filtration removes a portion of the free drug from the plasma. If another bound drug is administered it could displace a drug already bound so that the amount of free drug is increased. With active tubular secretion, two or more drugs may compete for the same site of excretion. Administering one drug, for example, probenecid, would interfere with the excretion of another drug, for example, penicillin, excreted by the same mechanism. Tubular reabsorption is one method whereby the body retains some drugs. The pH of the urine determines the amount of a drug that is ionized passing through the urine, and therefore the amount of tubular reabsorption. In this way, changes in the pH may produce changes in the excretion of both weak acids and bases.

DENTAL DRUG INTERACTIONS

Although there are many drug interactions documented in the literature, this discussion centers on those most likely to be encountered in dentistry. The drugs included in this section are analgesics, antiinfectives (antibiotics), antianxiety agents (benzodiazepines), anticholinergics, and epinephrine. These are the agents most frequently used in dentistry. Table 25-1 lists their most common interactions and should be available in the dental office for easy reference. This is only a guide; the actual clinical effect can be determined only by considering the individual patient. Just because a drug interaction is listed does not mean the two drugs cannot be used together. What it does mean is that caution should be exercised if using two interacting drugs concomitantly.

Analgesics
Aspirin

Probably the most important drug interaction between a dental drug and a medical drug occurs between aspirin and the orally administered anticoagulant, warfarin.

Given alone, the salicylates, can produce hypoprothrombinemia and decreased platelet adhesiveness, thereby prolonging the prothrombin time. Both the salicylates and the oral anticoagulants are bound to the same plasma protein binding sites. When salicylates are given to patients taking warfarin, the salicylates displace the warfarin from the binding sites and increase the level of free (unbound) warfarin. When the unbound warfarin concentration is increased, the therapeu-

tic effect is also increased and severe hemorrhage can occur. Patients taking orally administered anticoagulants should not be given aspirin or aspirin-containing products.

The salicylates also interact with probenecid (Benemid). Probenecid, used alone, increases the excretion of uric acid and is employed in the treatment of gout. When salicylates are administered to patients taking probenecid, the uricosuric effect of the probenecid is blocked. This can result either in increased uric acid concentrations in the blood or in precipitation of an acute attack of gout. An occasional analgesic dose of salicylate may be insufficient to interact with probenecid, but large doses can inhibit probenecid uricosuria. An alternative analgesic should be prescribed for patients taking probenecid.

The excretion of methotrexate appears to be blocked by the salicylates. Methotrexate, an antimetabolite, is used to treat various malignancies and severe psoriasis. Patients taking methotrexate should be given aspirin with caution, if at all.

The salicylates interact with corticosteroids and alcohol to cause an additive ulcerogenic effect. Since all these agents can cause gastrointestinal irritation and exacerbate ulcers, their concomitant use should be avoided.

In diabetic patients the salicylates tend to produce hypoglycemia. In patients taking oral hypoglycemic agents (sulfonylureas), salicylates may contribute to hypoglycemic coma. In these patients moderate to large doses of the salicylates should be given with caution. An occasional small dose of salicylate does not seem to be a problem. The effect of salicylates on patients taking insulin is unpredictable.

Aspirin also interferes with the blood levels of ibuprofen, potentially reducing its effectiveness. It also has similar side effects and theoretically would offer no advantage.

Ibuprofen

Ibuprofen can reduce the antihypertensive effects of β-adrenergic blockers, furosemide, and captopril. The mechanism of interaction involves both retention of fluids by the nonsteroidal antiinflammatory agents and possibly by inhibition of prostaglandins. It has been reported to increase the effects of phenytoin and digoxin. Cimetidine can increase ibuprofen's effects, but short-term treatment should not be of concern.

Opioids

The most important drug interaction associated with the opioids occurs with other central nervous system (CNS) depressants. The primary outcome of this interaction is additive CNS depression leading to respiratory depression. Other CNS depressants include the sedative-hypnotic agents, minor tranquilizers, major tranquilizers (phenothiazines), antihistamines, and alcohol.

In patients taking MAOIs the administration of meperidine (Demerol) has produced a severe reaction including sweating, hypertension, excitation, and rigidity. In some patients hypotension and coma have also developed. Meperidine should be avoided in patients receiving MAOIs. Other narcotics may be given with caution, preferably in a decreased dosage.

Antibiotics

Some antibiotics, when used in combination, may have an additive, synergistic, or antagonistic effect. The concentration of each antibiotic, the order in which the antibiotics are administered, the particular pathogen being treated, and the number of microorganisms affect the outcome. Typically bacteriostatic and bactericidal antibiotics, for example, penicillin and tetracycline, would demonstrate antagonism. An example of synergism is the combination of sulfonamides and trimethoprim. Because these two agents act at different steps in the production of folic acid, resistance to the combination would require resistance at two different steps.

A relatively new interaction to become generally known is that between the antiinfective agents and the oral contraceptives. Rifampin, the most documented, and also amoxicillin and tetracyclines have been shown to reduce the effectiveness of the oral contraceptives. Although ex-

tremely uncommon considering the widespread use of oral contraceptives, the seriousness of the interaction requires informing every woman taking birth control pills of the remote possibility of this occurrence and documenting this fact.

Penicillin

The bactericidal penicillin and the bacteriostatic tetracycline antagonize the action of each other. Probenecid can prolong the action of the penicillins by interfering with its absorption. This can be used to therapeutic advantage for difficult infections.

Erythromycin

Erythromycin inhibits the hepatic metabolism of several drugs, for example, theophylline, warfarin, digoxin, and carbamazepine. The outcome may be enhancement of these drugs' effects or even toxicity.

Tetracycline

The absorption of tetracycline itself is inhibited by divalent and trivalent cations. It should be given at least 1 hour before or 2 hours after the use of dairy products, oral antacids, or sucralfate. Doxycycline, less affected by dairy products or food, is affected by inhibitors of metabolism leading to a buildup of doxycycline.

Metronidazole

The possibility of a disulfiram-like reaction with metronidazole makes it important for the patient to be warned against drinking alcohol while taking this medication. Alcohol-containing mouthwashes should also be avoided.

Antianxiety agents
Benzodiazepines

The benzodiazepines, CNS depressants themselves, are additive with other CNS depressants. With chronic use, such as for muscular relaxation to treat temporomandibular joint problems, the benzodiazepines may accumulate if their metabolism is blocked by cimetidine or valproic acid.

Barbiturates

The barbiturates, now used infrequently in dentistry, can stimulate liver microsomal enzymes increasing the metabolism of themselves and other drugs. Phenobarbital, by enzyme induction, can reduce the effectiveness of oral anticoagulants, phenytoin, and tricyclic antidepressants, to name a few. This induction requires several doses over a few days.

Autonomic drugs
Anticholinergics

Anticholinergic drugs are used in dentistry as antisialagogues for occlusal analysis or impression taking. Additive anticholinergic effects with the tricyclic antidepressants or phenothiazines can lead to xerostomia, constipation, urinary retention, blurred vision, hot dry skin, and tachycardia.

Epinephrine

Epinephrine, a vasoconstrictor, is commonly added to local anesthetic agents to reduce systemic toxicity and prolong duration of action. The two epinephrine drug interactions most carefully documented are with β-adrenergic blocking agents and the tricyclic antidepressants. Both can produce hypertension, and the β-blockers also produce reflex bradycardia (unopposed α-agonist action). Diabetic patients given epinephrine may need an increase in either sulfonylurea or insulin. Short-term administration of epinephrine should have little effect unless the diabetic patient is in poor control or is very brittle. Epinephrine reacts little with MAOIs, although this interaction is much publicized.

SUMMARY

The recognition of the possibility of drug interactions is the first step toward preventing problems from these interactions. The dental hygienist should make sure that an adequate drug interaction chart is posted in the dental office for easy reference. Many reference books are available on the subject of drug interactions. Only with a high level of suspicion and adequate reference material available can the dental health care team give the patient the complete care deserved.

REVIEW QUESTIONS

1. Describe the mechanism by which tetracycline and calcium interact.
2. Explain the mechanism(s) of action by which warfarin and aspirin interact to produce hemorrhage.
3. Describe the mechanism of a drug interaction that involves enzyme induction, and give one example of a drug that acts in this fashion.
4. Name four common medical drugs with which the salicylates interact. For each of these drug interactions, state the potential outcome.
5. Describe the type of drug with which ibuprofen may interact. State a potential outcome.
6. Explain the interaction between two different CNS depressants, and state specific groups of drugs that would be classed as CNS depressants.
7. Describe the interaction between the barbiturates and the oral anticoagulants and the potential outcome.
8. Explain the interactions between epinephrine and the β-adrenergic blocking agents and between epinephrine and the tricyclic antidepressants.
9. State what the dental hygienist should have in the dental office to keep alert about drug interactions.

Chapter 26

Drug abuse

The dental hygienist may encounter drug abuse in either patients seen in the office or professionals working there. Friends or relatives may also abuse drugs. For this reason, the dental hygienist should be familiar with the various types of drugs commonly abused and their patterns of abuse. Appointment management of the patient who abuses drugs will also be mentioned. Since drug abuse is also a community issue, the hygienist should have a heightened awareness of the potential for problems. The concept of using drugs to produce profound effects on mood, thought, and feeling is as old as civilization. Only the kinds of substances used for this purpose have changed.

Agents used for their psychoactive properties (capability of changing behavior or inducing psychosis-like reactions or both) can be divided into those that also have therapeutic value (narcotics and sedative-hypnotics) and those that have no known therapeutic value (psychedelics). Some agents may move from one category to the other. For example, marijuana, an agent previously considered to be worthless, is now used to treat the nausea associated with cancer chemotherapy.

GENERAL CONSIDERATIONS

Abuse of a drug is defined as the use of a drug for nonmedical purposes, almost always for altering consciousness. In contrast, the misuse of a drug means using the drug in the wrong dose or for a longer period of time than prescribed. The difference between these two usages is subtle.

Definitions

The following terms are used in this chapter:

drug abuse Excessive drug use inconsistent with acceptable medical practice.

misuse Use of the drug for a disease state in a way considered inappropriate.

drug dependence A state, either physical or psychologic, that occurs as a consequence of the interaction between a drug and a patient. It is characterized by a compulsion to take the drug to obtain its effects or to prevent the abstinence syndrome. Tolerance may be present.

physical dependence The state in which the drug is necessary for continued functioning of certain body processes. In a dependent person, withdrawal of the drug produces the abstinence syndrome.

psychologic dependence A state in which, following withdrawal of the drug, there are manifestations of emotional abnormalities and drug-seeking behavior.

addiction This vague term, although still used, should be replaced with "dependence."

tolerance The necessity for increasing the dose of a drug to produce the same effect.

abstinence syndrome A combination of both physical and psychologic manifestations occurring in a drug-dependent person when the drug is removed.

Psychologic dependence

Psychologic dependence is a state of mind in which a person believes that he or she is unable to maintain optimum performance without having taken a drug. Psychologic dependence can vary in severity from mild desire (as for a morning cup of coffee) to compulsive obsession (as for the next heroin dose). With prolonged self-administration, a person can often develop tolerance to, and physical dependence on, the drug.

Tolerance

Tolerance is characterized by the necessity to increase the dose continually to achieve the desired effect, or when a continually diminishing effect is obtained with the same dose. The type of tolerance referred to in this discussion of the abuse of psychoactive drugs is central (functional or behavioral) tolerance, that is, a definite decreased response of brain tissue to constantly increasing amounts of a drug. Tolerance of metabolic origin (dispositional or metabolic tolerance) is caused by an accelerated rate of metabolism of the drug and is excluded in this discussion. Metabolic tolerance is an insignificant factor in the tolerance observed in humans to most of the psychoactive drugs.

Physical dependence

Physical dependence refers to the altered physiologic state resulting from constantly increasing drug concentrations. The presence of physical dependence is established by the **withdrawal** or **abstinence syndrome,** a combination of many drug-specific symptoms that occurs on abrupt discontinuation of drug administration. The degree of physical and psychologic dependence as well as tolerance is listed in Table 26-1.

Addiction, habituation, and dependence

Addiction and habituation are terms that have been misused almost as much as the drugs they attempt to characterize. Any use of these terms must be preceded by adequate definitions. In both addiction and habituation the desire to continue using the drug is present, but in addiction, tolerance and physical dependence also are present. Habituation and addiction are really only degrees of misuse or abuse of drugs. It has been recommended that these terms be replaced by the term "dependence," a state of psychologic or physical desire to use a drug.

Drugs that produce tolerance and physical dependence are grouped according to their ability to be substituted for one another. For example, different opioids can be administered to obtain a desired effect with no withdrawal syndrome; however, a barbiturate cannot be substituted for a narcotic and vice versa. Therefore the opioids and barbiturates are separate groups of dependence-producing drugs. The phenomenon of substitution to suppress withdrawal between different drugs is called **cross-tolerance** or **cross-dependence.** It is observed among members of the same drug group but not among different drug groups. Cross-tolerance may be either partial or complete and is determined more by the pharmacologic effect of the drug than by its chemical structure.

Most characteristics of drug abuse are determined by the individual drug involved, but the following generalizations can be made:

1. When comparing drugs in the same group, the time required to produce physical dependence is shortest with a rapidly metabolized drug and longest with a slowly metabolized drug.

2. The time course of withdrawal reactions is related to the half-life of the drug. The shorter the half-life, the quicker the withdrawal.

Drugs too numerous to mention in this chapter have been abused extensively. At various times glue sniffing, propellant inhalation, smoking of banana peels, and ingestion of morning glory seeds have been attempted. The problem and treatment of drug abuse are related less to the drugs themselves, although they cause definite problems, than to the persons involved in this type of behavior. A multifactorial approach is needed to reduce or treat this problem. Specific types of agents abused and the problems with each group of drugs is discussed in this chapter.

OPIOID ANALGESICS

Heroin, methadone (Dolophine), morphine, hydromorphone (Dilaudid), meperidine (Demerol), oxycodone (Percodan), and pentazocine (Talwin) are currently the most popular abused opioids. The present discussion focuses on the pharmacology of the opioids themselves, although it should be noted that opioids sold illegally on the street may be adulterated.

In addition to being analgesics, the opioids produce a state described as complete satiation of all drives. The opioids elevate the user's mood, cause euphoria, relieve fear and apprehension,

Table 26-1. Drugs that produce tolerance and dependence*

Group	Tolerance	Physical dependence	Psychologic dependence
Opioid analgesics	+ + + +	+ + +	+ + +
Sedative-hypnotics, tranquilizers and alcohol	+ +	+ + +	+ +
CNS stimulants	+ + + +	+	+ + + +
Cocaine	0	0	+ + + +
Hallucinogens (LSD)	+ +	0	+
Marijuana	0	+	+ +
Tobacco	+	±	+ + +

*Graded from + to + + + +; 0, absent; ±, inconclusive.

and produce a feeling of peace and tranquility. They also suppress hunger, reduce sexual desire, and diminish the response to provocation. Undoubtedly, initial abuse is reinforced by this "positive" experience. Other effects include slowed respiration, constipation, urinary retention and peripheral vasodilation.

With the development of physical dependence, however, the driving motivation to obtain the drug becomes more and more negative. The fear of the withdrawal syndrome begins to override other motivation. At this point the addict resorts to criminal activity and violence to support the drug habit. These activities are not direct actions of the drug but are related to opioid dependence.

Pattern of abuse

Heroin is the opioid most commonly administered parenterally. The signs and symptoms of an acute overdose consist of fixed, pinpoint pupils, depressed respiration, hypotension and shock, slow or absent reflexes, and drowsiness or coma. Tolerance does not develop to the miosis and constipation associated with the use of narcotics (see Chapter 7). However, it does develop to the other pharmacologic effects, including the euphoric, analgesic, sedative, and respiratory depressant actions. The symptoms and time course of the withdrawal syndrome are determined by

the specific drug abused, usually beginning at the time of the abuser's next scheduled dose.

The first signs of withdrawal from heroin are yawning, lacrimation, rhinorrhea, and diaphoresis, followed by a restless sleep. With further abstinence, anorexia, tremors, irritability, weakness, and excessive gastrointestinal activity occur. The heart rate is rapid, the blood pressure is elevated, and chills alternate with excessive sweating. Without treatment, symptoms disappear about the eighth day after the last dose of heroin.

Management of acute overdose and withdrawal

If the triad of narcotic overdose (respiratory depression, pinpoint pupils, and coma) is present, naloxone (Narcan) should be administered immediately. If there is no response, it is unlikely that the depressed respiration is caused by opioid overdose.

The immediate withdrawal reaction from an opioid sold on the street is only moderately distressing to the patient because of the poor quality of these drugs. Patients can be made comfortable with methadone, a long-acting opioid that can be gradually withdrawn. A phenothiazine or benzodiazepine is often administered for relief of tension. In long-term rehabilitation programs the approaches can include: substitution of a physiologically equivalent drug, and/or gradual weaning from the substitute. Methadone, a long acting opioid, or naltrexone, an antagonist, are used to manage opioid abusers (see Chapter 7).

Dental implications

The following should be considered when treating a dental patient who abuses narcotic opioids:

1. Pain control. Because an opioid abuser develops tolerance to the analgesic effects of any opioid, treating pain can be difficult. It is best to alleviate the cause of the pain first and prescribe nonsteroidal antiinflammatory agents for analgesia.

2. Prescriptions for opioids. Opioid abusers often come to the dental office requesting an opioid analgesic agent for severe pain ("shopping"). Frequently the drug abuser suggests the name of a specific opioid or states allergies to several less potent agents.

3. Increased incidence of disease. Certain diseases that can be transmitted by use of needles for injections have a higher incidence in opioid abusers. These include hepatitis B, human immunodeficiency virus (HIV) producing acquired immune deficiency syndrome (AIDS), and sexually transmitted diseases. Infections caused by the use of nonsterile solutions and instruments can produce osteomyelitis, and abscesses in the kidneys and heart valves. As in rheumatic heart disease, prophylactic antibiotics should be given before dental treatment (see Chapter 8).

Opioid street drugs

Opioids available on the street change with time and are different in various parts of the country. The dental hygienist should be aware of the fact that most abusers misuse more than one substance and that street drugs are very often adulterated. One of the most dramatic demonstrations of this fact is MPTP. MPTP is a powerful neurotoxic contaminant of an illicitly produced meperidine derivative that induces classic opiod symptoms. The contaminant MPTP has a toxicity

independent of opiod effects; it produces a classic and permanent (irreversible) Parkinson's disease by destroying the cells in the substantia nigra within a very short time. This contaminant has become a valuable research tool in inducing Parkinson's disease in animals.

SEDATIVE-HYPNOTICS AND ALCOHOL

This group of abused drugs includes the barbiturates, alcohol, glutethimide (Doriden), meprobamate (Miltown), methaqualone (Quaalude), and all the benzodiazepines, with chlordiazepoxide (Librium) and diazepam (Valium) as their best-known examples. Although there is great variation in their chemical structures, their pharmacologic actions and pattern of abuse are similar.

Initial symptoms resemble the well-known symptoms of alcohol intoxication: loss of inhibition, euphoria, emotional instability, quarrelsomeness, difficulty in thinking, poor memory and judgment, slurred speech, and ataxia. With increasing doses, drowsiness and sleep will occur, respiration is depressed, cardiac output is decreased, and gastrointestinal activity and urine output are diminished. **Paradoxical** reactions can range from elation to excessive stimulation.

Pattern of abuse

The CNS depressant drugs are generally administered orally, often in combination with other drugs of abuse. With an acute overdose, respiratory and cardiovascular depression occur, leading to coma and hypotension. The pupils may be unchanged or small, and lateral nystagmus is seen. Confusion, slurred speech, and ataxia are always present. In comparison to the opioids, the CNS depressants have a slower onset of tolerance and physical dependence. Tolerance to the sedative effect is **not** accompanied by a comparable tolerance to the lethal dose. With prolonged misuse, emotional instability, hostile and paranoid ideations, and suicidal tendencies are common.

Although the withdrawal syndrome for all CNS

depressants is similar, its time course depends on the half-life of the drug abused. The first signs of withdrawal are insomnia, weakness, tremulousness restlessness, and perspiration. Often nausea and vomiting, together with hyperthermia and agitation occur. Delirium and convulsions may culminate in cardiovascular collapse and loss of the temperature-regulating mechanism. When alcohol is the abused agent, withdrawal is termed delirium tremens (DTs).

Management of acute overdose and withdrawal

The most important consideration with an acute overdose of a CNS depressant is support of the cardiovascular and respiratory systems. An airway must always be established and maintained. Early gastric lavage after intubation and dialysis can assist in removal of some drugs. CNS stimulants are harmful and should not be given.

In contrast to withdrawal from opioids, withdrawal from CNS depressants can be life-threatening and the patient should be hospitalized. The principles of treatment of withdrawal from any CNS depressant include (1) replacement of the abused drug with an equivalent drug, and (2) gradual withdrawal of the equivalent drug.

The drug usually substituted for the abused drug is a benzodiazepine such as chlordiazepoxide or diazepam. The substitute drug is then gradually withdrawn over a period of weeks; during this time the patient receives psychotherapy.

An approach to managing alcoholism is to prescribe disulfiram (Antabuse). This drug, an aldehyde dehydrogenase inhibitor, blocks the metabolism of alcohol after it has become acetaldehyde. Accumulation of this intermediate metabolite produces undesirable symptoms including flushing, throbbing headache, nausea, vomiting, sweating, hypotension, and confusion. It is used in conjunction with other behavioral therapies. Drugs containing alcohol (mouthwashes) should be avoided in patients taking disulfiram. Other drugs, for example, metronidazole, may produce disulfiram-like reactions.

SYMPATHOMIMETIC CENTRAL NERVOUS SYSTEM STIMULANTS

The widely abused member of this class is cocaine. Other drugs that are abused include methamphetamine (Methedine), dextroamphetamine (Dexedrine), diethylpropion (Tenuate), methylphenidate (Ritalin), and phemetrazine (Preludin). The sympathomimetic CNS stimulants are abused for their ability to produce a euphoric mood, a sense of increased energy and alertness, together with a feeling of omnipotence and self-confidence. Other effects include mydriasis, increased blood pressure and heart rate, anorexia, and increased sweating.

CNS stimulants are taken orally, parenterally, intranasally, or by inhalation (smoking). With prolonged use, tolerance develops to the euphorigenic effect and toxic symptoms appear including anxiety, aggressiveness, stereotyped behavior, hallucinations, and paranoid fears. Of special note to the dental hygienist is the occurrence of xerostomia and bruxism.

Symptoms and signs of an acute overdose include dilated pupils, elevated blood pressure, rapid pulse, and cardiac arrhythmias. The patient has xerostomia, diaphoresis, and hyperthermia. Fine tremors may be present, and often the patient exhibits hyperactive behavior.

Although tolerance develops to the central sympathomimetic effect, no tolerance develops to the tendency to induce toxic psychoses at higher doses. Modest levels of abuse over a long period do not produce withdrawal reactions except fatigue and prolonged sleep, but very large doses can precipitate a withdrawal syndrome consisting of aching muscles, ravenous appetite with abdominal pain, and long periods of sleep. This is followed by profound psychologic depression, sometimes even suicidal. During this period abnormal electroencephalographic results have been recorded.

Management of acute overdose and withdrawal

Treatment of an overdose of a CNS stimulant may include a phenothiazine for CNS symptoms, a short-acting sympathomimetic-blocking agent if hypertension is severe, and a tricyclic antidepressant if a severe depression occurs.

The most serious sociologic problem with stimulant abuse is the induction of mental abnormalities, especially in young abusers. Experimental evidence suggests that amphetamine psychoses can be induced in previously unaffected volunteer subjects. Psychoses are dose-related and can be reproduced.

Cocaine

Cocaine is a CNS stimulant with local anesthetic properties when applied topically. It is used primarily for its stimulant action by "sniffing," "snorting," or intravenous injection. The most recent variant is a free-base form that is smoked and goes by the street name of "crack" or "rock." It is more pure and potent and the resultant intoxication is far more intense than that of snorted cocaine, much quicker, and much more euphoric and addicting. Cocaine induces intense euphoria, a sense of total self-confidence, and anorexia. The effects last only a few minutes because of its short duration of action. Paranoid feelings and extreme excitability cause cocaine users to perform violent acts while under its influence. Psychologic dependence becomes intense, but neither tolerance nor withdrawal has been shown. Cocaine's main medical use is in nose operations, where it causes local anesthesia and produces vasoconstriction to reduce hemorrhage.

PSYCHEDELICS (HALLUCINOGENS)

The psychedelic agents are capable of inducing states of altered perception and generally do not have any medically acceptable therapeutic use. The drugs in this section include lysergic acid diethylamide (LSD) and phencyclidine (PCP), but many other agents, including psilocybin, dimethyltryptamine (DMT), 2,5-dimethoxy-4-methylamphetamine (STP), methylene dioxyamphetamine (MDA), and mescaline (peyote), also fall into this class. Clearly, the agents discussed in this section represent only a fraction of those released on the illicit drug market. These hallucinogens are often mislabeled or adulterated with substances such as strychnine.

Psychedelics affect perceptions in such a way that all sensory input is perceived with heightened awareness; sounds are brighter and clearer, colors are more brilliant, and taste, smell, and touch are more acute. Psychedelic-induced dependence is psychologic and tolerance develops within a short time. These two characteristics combined with the unpredictable nature of the response favor periodic rather than continuous abuse of psychedelic drugs. Prolonged use, however, can cause long-lasting mental disturbances varying from panic reactions to depression to schizophrenic reactions.

LSD. LSD is the most potent of these agents with only micrograms required for an effect. In addition to its psychogenic actions, LSD has sympathomimetic effects including tachycardia, rise in blood pressure, hyperreflexia, nausea, and increased body temperature.

An overdose of LSD produces symptoms including widely dilated pupils, flushed face, elevated blood pressure, visual and temporal distortions, hallucinations, derealization, panic reaction, and paranoia ("bad trip"). Since the user does not lose consciousness and is highly suggestible, treatment is to provide reassurance ("talking down"). Rarely chlorpromazine has been used to treat the situation in an emergency. Experiences ("flashbacks"), commonly precipitated by marijuana, can occur years after ingesting LSD.

Phencyclidine. Phencyclidine (PCP, or angel dust), originally developed as an animal tranquilizer, was very popular in the 1970s. It is a powerful CNS stimulant with dissociative properties. Users may exhibit sweating and a blank stare. Changes in body image and disorganized thought have led to bizarre behavior. Elevation of blood pressure and pulse, and muscle movement and rigidity occur. It is abused alone or as an adulterant to other street drugs.

Marijuana. Marijuana (marihuana, cannabis) is derived from the hemp plant, and its active ingredient is tetrahydrocannabinol (THC). Marijuana can be administered orally or by inhalation (smoking) and its effects include an increase in pulse rate, reddening of the conjunctivae (bloodshot eyes), and some behavioral changes. Slight changes in blood pressure and pupil size as well as hand tremors have been noted. With normal doses, euphoria and enhanced sensory perception occur. This is followed by sedation and altered consciousness—a dreamlike state.

Studies of the influence of marijuana on driving have concluded that the drug impairs motor and mental abilities required for safe driving. For example, the perception of time and distance is distorted and reflexes are decreased. A more common adverse reaction is apprehensive, nervous, and panic-stricken feelings that the user is losing his or her mind. This reaction responds to friendly reassurance. Psychologic dependence on marijuana is determined by the frequency of use. Physical dependence, tolerance, and withdrawal symptoms are very rare.

Of particular interest to the dental hygienist is the fact that a high level of marijuana abuse may be manifested by xerostomia. It has been noted anecdotally that some marijuana users develop gingivitis. In these patients the gingival tissue was inflamed, and various leukoplakias with hyperkeratosis and perakeratosis with pseudoepitheliomatous hyperplasia were identified.

THC is known to reduce intraocular pressure and has been used in the treatment of resistant glaucoma. It may also be effective as an antiemetic to treat the nausea associated with cancer therapy (see marabinol, Chapter 22).

NICOTINE AND TOBACCO

Awareness of the toxicity from chronic smoking and chewing of tobacco has increased dramatically over the last 2 decades. The CNS-active component of tobacco is nicotine, but a large number of components of the gaseous phase of tobacco smoke contribute to its undesirable effects: carbon monoxide, nitrogen oxides, volatile nitrosamines, nitriles, volatile hydrocarbons, and many others.

Pattern of abuse

Smokers claim that the most desirable effects of smoking are an increased alertness, muscle relaxation, facilitation of concentration and memory, and decreases in appetite and irritability. These are consistent with the effect of nicotine on the CNS. In addition, nicotine produces an increase in blood pressure and pulse rate and induces nausea, vomiting, and dizziness as a result of stimulation of the chemoreceptor trigger zone.

Smokers are tolerant to these latter effects, but such tolerance is not of long duration. The first cigarette of the day may induce a certain degree of dizziness and nausea.

Chronic use of tobacco is causally related to many serious diseases, ranging from coronary artery disease to lung cancer.

Smokeless tobacco. An increase in the use of chewing tobacco in college students is alarming (22%). Oral mucosal changes include chronic gingivitis, leukoplakia, and precancerous lesions. In these patients, an extremely thorough oral examination should be done at each prophylaxis. Education concerning the oral health hazards that smokeless tobacco poses should also be included.

Management and withdrawal

The withdrawal syndrome that occurs after cessation of chronic tobacco smoking varies greatly from person to person. The most consistent symptoms are anxiety, irritability, difficulty in concentrating, and a craving for a smoke. Drowsiness, headaches, increased appetite, and sleep disturbances are also common. The syndrome is rapid in onset (within 24 hours after the last cigarette) and can persist for months. The syndrome of withdrawal from tobacco can be suppressed to some extent by administration of nicotine chewing-gum (Nicorette). It does reduce the irritability and difficulty in concentrating but appears to be less effective in controlling insomnia, hunger, and craving for tobacco. The most important side effect of nicotine gum to the dental profession is due to excessive gum chewing dislodging dental fillings and adhering to dentures.

NITROUS OXIDE

Nitrous oxide, a general anesthetic, is readily available in many dental offices (see Chapter 11). Misuse often begins as "therapeutic," only becoming abusive or "recreational use" at a later stage. The dental hygienist has the responsibility to encourage professionals in the office to seek help for this behavior before serious consequences occur. Dentists self-administering nitrous oxide have been found dead in their dental chairs.

REVIEW QUESTIONS

1. Define the following terms:
   a. Psychologic dependence
   b. Tolerance
   c. Physical dependence
   d. Withdrawal syndrome
   e. Addiction
2. Describe the symptoms of withdrawal from a narcotic analgesic agent such as heroin.
3. State the treatment of the withdrawal syndrome and an overdose of a narcotic analgesic agent.
4. Explain the concept of a methadone maintenance program.
5. State diseases that are more common in opioid abusers.
6. Explain the rationale for the inclusion of alcohol in the discussion of the sedative-hypnotics.
7. Describe the withdrawal syndrome from the sedative-hypnotic agents and explain its potential severity.
8. Define delirium tremens and discuss its treatment.
9. Describe the symptoms of an overdose of a CNS stimulant.
10. State the current therapeutic use(s) of the amphetamines.
11. Name three psychedelic or hallucinogenic agents.
12. State the danger(s), if any, of phencyclidine (PCP).
13. Discuss the adverse reactions associated with marijuana use.
14. Describe a therapeutic use of marijuana.
15. Describe the long-term problems associated with cigarette smoking.
16. Compare and contrast the terms "addiction" and "habituation."
17. State the major adverse effects associated with the use of cocaine ("crack").
18. State oral changes that can occur with smokeless tobacco.

Appendix

Top 200* prescribed drugs in 1987 new and refill combined listed in alphabetic order by rank and chapters

Drug name	Generic name constituents	Pharmacologic class	1987 rank	Chapter no.†
Acetaminophen/codeine (Lemmon)	Acetaminophen	Nonopioid analgesic	173	6
	Codeine	Opioid analgesic		7
Acetaminophen/codeine (Rugby)	Acetaminophen	Nonopioid analgesic	54	6
	Codeine	Opioid analgesic		7
Acetaminophen/codeine (URL)	Acetaminophen	Nonopioid analgesic	112	6
	Codeine	Opioid analgesic		7
Achromycin-V	Tetracycline	Antibiotic	75	8
Aldomet	Methyldopa	Antihypertensive	46	15
Aldoril	Hydrochlorothiazide	Diuretic; antihypertensive	141	15
	Methyldopa	Antihypertensive		15
Alupent	Metaproterenol	Bronchodilator (adrenergic)	35	5,22
Amcill	Ampicillin	Antibiotic	83	8
Amitriptyline (Rugby)	Amitriptyline	Tricyclic antidepressant	117	17
Amoxcillin (Warner-Chilcott)	Amoxicillin	Antibiotic	70	8
Amoxil	Antibiotic	Amoxicillin	2	8
Anaprox	Naproxen	Nonsteroidal antiinflammatory	96	6
Anusol-HC	Hydrocortisone plus misc. ingredients	Anorectal; corticosteroid	172	19
Atarax	Hydroxyzine	Antihistamine; antipruritic	153	18
Ativan	Lorazepam	Antianxiety (benzodiazepine)	42	10
Augmentin	Amoxicillin	Antibiotic	50	8
	Clavulanate	Beta-lactamase inhibitor		
Bactrim DS	Trimethoprim	Antibacterial	135	8
	Sulfamethoxazole	Antibacterial (sulfa)		8
Beepen VK	Penicillin VK	Antibiotic	113	8
Bentyl	Dicyclomine	Anticholinergic	167	5
Brethine	Terbutaline	Antiasthmatic; adrenergic	140	5,22
Bumex	Bumetanide	Diuretic (loop)	191	15
Calan	Verapamil	Calcium channel blocking agent	60	15
Capoten	Captopril	Antihypertensive	23	15
Carafate	Sucralfate	Antiulcer	76	22
Cardizem	Diltiazem	Calcium channel blocking agent	17	15
Catapres	Clonidine	Antihypertensive	65	15
Ceclor	Cefaclor	Antibiotic (cephalosporin)	18	8
Clinoril	Sulindac	Nonsteroidal antiinflammatory	44	6

*American Druggist **197:**36-52, Feb. 1988.
†Refers to chapter in text where drug is mentioned.

Drug name	Generic name constituents	Pharmacologic class	1987 rank	Chapter no.†
Compazine	Prochlorperazine	Antipsychotic; antiemetic	142	17
Corgard	Nadolol	Beta-adrenergic blocker	58	5,15
Cortisporin Otic	Hydrocortisone	Corticosteroid	124	19
	Neomycin	Antibiotic		8
	Polymixin B	Antibiotic		8
Coumadin	Warfarin	Anticoagulant	59	15
Dalmane	Flurazepam	Antianxiety (benzodiazepine)	58	10
Darvocet-N	Propoxyphene napsylate	Opioid analgesic	15	7
	Acetaminophen	Nonopioid analgesic		6
Deltasone	Prednisone	Corticosteroid	177	19
Demulen	Ethynodiol diacetate	Oral contraceptive; progestin	78	20
	Ethinyl estradiol	Oral contraceptive; estrogen		20
Desyrel	Trazodone	Antidepressant	88	17
DiaBeta	Glyburide	Oral hypoglycemic	87	20
Diabinese	Chlorpropamide	Oral hypoglycemic	84	20
Diazepam (Rugby)	Diazepam	Antianxiety (benzodiazepine)	125	10
Dilantin	Phenytoin	Anticonvulsant	27	16
Dipyridamole (Rugby)	Dipyridamole	Antiplatelet	64	15
Dolobid	Diflunisal	Nonsteroidal antiinflammatory (salicylate)	114	6
Donnatal	Atropine	Anticholinergic	103	5
	Hyoscine	Anticholinergic		5
	Hyoscyamine	Anticholinergic		5
	Phenobarbital	Sedative		10
Doxycycline (Rugby)	Doxycycline	Antibiotic (tetracycline)	196	8
Duricef	Cefadroxil	Antibiotic (cephalosporin)	89	8
Dyazide	Hydrochlorothiazide	Diuretic, antihypertensive	1	15
	Triamterene	K-sparing diuretic		
E.E.S.	Erythromycin ethylsuccinate	Antibiotic	38	8
Elavil	Amitriptyline	Tricyclic antidepressant	110	17
Empirin/codeine	Aspirin	Nonopioid analgesic	184	6
	Codeine	Opioid analgesic		7
E-Mycin (UpJohn)	Erythromycin base	Antibiotic	37	8
Entex LA	Phenylpropanolamine	Decongestant	71	5,22
	Guaifenesin	Expectorant		22
Eryc (Parke Davis)	Erythromycin base	Antibiotic	47	8
Erythromycin base (Abbott)	Erythromycin base	Antibiotic	163	8
Erythrocin stearate	Erythromycin stearate	Antibiotic	73	8
Estraderm	Estradiol	Estrogen	185	20
Feldene	Piroxicam	Nonsteroidal antiinflammatory	32	6

Continued.

Drug name	Generic name constituents	Pharmacologic class	1987 rank	Chapter no.†
Fiorinal	Aspirin	Nonopioid analgesic	80	6
	Butalbital	Sedative		10
	Caffeine	Xanthine derivative		22
Fiorinal/codeine	Aspirin	Nonopioid analgesic	98	6
	Butalbital	Sedative		10
	Caffeine	Xanthine derivative		22
	Codeine	Opioid analgesic		7
Flexeril	Cyclobenzaprine	Muscle relaxant	57	10
Furosemide (Rugby)	Furosemide	Diuretic (loop)	77	15
Glucotrol	Glipizide	Oral hypoglycemic	86	20
Halcion	Triazolam	Antianxiety (benzodiazepine)	22	10
Haldol	Haloperidol	Antipsychotic	133	17
Hydrochlorothiazide (Rugby)	Hydrochlorothiazide	Diuretic; antihypertensive	41	15
Hydrochlorothiazide (United Research)	Hydrochlorothiazide	Diuretic; antihypertensive	100	15
Hydrochlorothiazide (Geneva)	Hydrochlorothiazide	Diuretic; antihypertensive	170	15
HydroDiuril	Hydrochlorothiazide	Diuretic; antihypertensive	159	15
Hydroxyzine (Rugby)	Hydroxyzine	Antihistamine, antipruritic	198	18
Hygroton	Chlorthalidone	Diuretic; antihypertensive	186	15
Ibuprofen (Boots)	Ibuprofen	Nonsteroidal antiinflammatory	105	6
Ibuprofen (Rugby)	Ibuprofen	Nonsteroidal antiinflammatory	97	6
Imodium	Loperamide	Antidiarrheal	161	7,22
Inderal	Propranolol	Beta-adrenergic blocker	7	15
Indocin	Indomethacin	Nonsteroidal antiinflammatory	67	6
Intal	Cromolyn	Antiasthmatic, antiallergic	182	22
Isoptin	Verapamil	Calcium channel blocker	181	15
Isordil	Isosorbide dinitrate	Antianginal vasodilator	72	15
Isosorbide dinitrate (Rugby)	Isosorbide dinitrate	Antianginal vasodilator	119	15
Keflex	Cephalexin	Antibiotic (cephalosporin)	26	8
Klotrix	Potassium chloride	Electrolyte (potassium)	123	15
K-tab	Potassium chloride	Electrolyte (potassium)	81	15
Lanoxin	Digoxin	Cardiac glycoside	3	15
Lasix	Furosemide	Diuretic; antihypertensive	13	15
Ledercillin VK	Penicillin VK	Antibiotic	111	8
Lidex	Fluocinonide	Corticosteroid (topical)	149	19
Lomotil	Diphenoxylate	Antidiarrheal	157	7,22
	Atropine	Anticholinergic		5
Lo/Ovral	Norgestrel	Oral contraceptive; progestin	33	20
	Ethinyl estradiol	Oral contraceptive; estrogen		20
Lopid	Gemfibrozil	Antihyperlipidemic	145	15
Lopressor	Metoprolol	Beta-adrenergic blocker	24	15
Lorazepam (Rugby)	Lorazepam	Antianxiety (benzodiazepine)	164	10
Lotrimin	Clotrimazole	Antifungal	121	8
Lotrisone	Clotrimazole	Antifungal	118	8
	Betamethasone	Corticosteroid		19

Drug name	Generic name constituents	Pharmacologic class	1987 rank	Chapter no.†
Lozol	Indapamide	Diuretic; antihypertensive	179	15
Macrodantin	Nitrofurantoin	Antibacterial	94	8
Maxzide	Triamterene	K-sparing diuretic	31	15
	Hydrochlorothiazide	Diuretic; antihypertensive		15
Meclomen	Meclofenamate	Nonsteroidal antiinflammatory	192	6
Medrol	Methylprednisolone	Glucocorticoid	165	19
Mellaril	Thioridazine	Antipsychotic	152	17
Micro-K	Potassium	Electrolyte (potassium)	36	15
Micronase	Glyburide	Oral hypoglycemic	56	20
Minipress	Prazosin	Antihypertensive	43	15
Minocin	Minocycline	Antibiotic (tetracycline)	129	8
Moduretic	Hydrochlorothiazide	Diuretic	69	15
	Amiloride	K-sparing diuretic		
Monistat 7	Miconazole	Antifungal	29	8
Motrin	Ibuprofen	Nonsteroidal antiinflammatory	16	6
Naldecon	Phenylpropanolamine	Decongestant	134	5
	Phenylephrine	Decongestant		5
	Chlorpheniramine	Antihistamine		18
	Phenyltoloxamine	Antihistamine		18
Nalfon	Fenoprofen	Nonsteroidal antiinflammatory	108	6
Naprosyn	Naproxen	Nonsteroidal antiinflammatory	14	6
Nasalcrom	Cromolyn	Antiasthmatic, antiallergic	180	22
Nasalide	Flunisolide	Corticosteroid	144	19
Navane	Thiothixene	Antipsychotic	199	17
Nicorette	Nicotine	Smoking deterrent	82	26
Nitro-Bid	Nitroglycerin	Antianginal	158	15
Nitro-Dur	Nitroglycerin	Antianginal	156	15
Nitrostat	Nitroglycerin	Antianginal	61	15
Nordette	Levonorgestrel	Oral contraceptive; progestin	99	20
	Ethinyl estradiol	Oral contraceptive; estrogen		20
Norinyl	Norethindrone	Oral contraceptive; progestin	62	20
	Mestranol	Oral contraceptive; estrogen		20
Normodyne	Labetalol	Alpha & beta-adrenergic blocker	169	15
Norpramin	Desipramine	Tricyclic antidepressant	139	17
Omnipen	Ampicillin	Antibiotic	101	8
Ortho-Novum	Norethindrone	Oral contraceptive; progestin	11	20
	Mestranol	Oral contraceptive; estrogen		20
Ortho-Novum 7/7/7	Norethindrone	Oral contraceptive; progestin	28	20
	Ethinyl estradiol	Oral contraceptive; estrogen		20
Ovcon	Norethindrone	Oral contraceptive; progestin	143	20
	Ethinyl estradiol	Oral contraceptive; estrogen		20
Ovral	Norgestrel	Oral contraceptive; progestin	91	20
	Ethinyl estradiol	Oral contraceptive; estrogen		20
PCE	Erythromycin base	Antibiotic	127	8

Continued.

Drug name	Generic name constituents	Pharmacologic class	1987 rank	Chapter no.†
Pediazole	Erythromycin ethylsuccinate	Antibiotic	107	8
	Sulfisoxazole	Antibacterial (sulfa)		8
Penicillin VK (Warner-Chilcott)	Penicillin VK	Antibiotic	85	8
PenVee K	Penicillin VK	Antibiotic	95	8
Percocet	Oxycodone	Opioid analgesic	90	7
	Acetaminophen	Nonopioid analgesic		6
Percodan	Oxycodone	Opioid analgesic	106	7
	Aspirin	Nonopioid analgesic		6
Persantine	Dipyridamole	Antiplatelet	63	15
Phenergan	Promethazine	Antihistamine	190	18
Phenergan/codeine	Promethazine	Antihistamine	175	18
	Codeine	Opioid analgesic (antitussive)		7
	Potassium guaiacolsulfonate	Expectorant		22
Phenobarbital (Lilly)	Phenobarbital	Sedative-hypnotic; anticonvulsant	137	10,16
Prednisone (Rugby)	Prednisone	Corticosteroid	92	19
Prednisone (URL)	Prednisone	Corticosteroid	154	19
Premarin	Conjugated estrogens	Estrogen	10	20
Premarin Vaginal	Conjugated estrogens	Topical estrogen	197	20
Procan	Procainamide	Antiarrhythmic	200	15
Procardia	Nifedipine	Calcium channel blocker	25	15
Propine	Dipivefrin	Sympathomimetic (glaucoma)	194	5
Propoxyphene Nap w/ APAP (Barr)	Propoxyphene napsylate	Opioid analgesic	162	7
	Acetaminophen	Nonopioid analgesic		6
Propoxyphene Nap w/ APAP (Rugby)	Propoxyphene napsylate	Opioid analgesic	151	7
	Acetaminophen	Nonopioid analgesic		6
Propranolol (Rugby)	Propranolol	Beta-adrenergic blocker	131	5,15
Proventil	Albuterol	Beta$_2$-adrenergic (bronchodilator)	40	5,22
Provera	Medroxyprogesterone	Progestin	52	20
Questran	Cholestyramine	Antihyperlipidemic	193	15
Reglan	Metoclopramide	GI stimulant	122	22
Restoril	Temazepam	Antianxiety (benzodiazepine)	79	10
Retin-A acne	Tretinoin	Antiacne (antiwrinkle)	130	13
Ritalin	Methylphenidate	CNS stimulant (attention deficit disorder)	174	5
Rufen	Ibuprofen	Nonsteroidal antiinflammatory	146	6
Seldane	Terfenadine	Antihistamine	20	18
Septra	Sulfamethoxazole	Antibacterial (sulfa)	138	8
	Trimethoprim	Antibacterial (sulfa)		8

Drug name	Generic name constituents	Pharmacologic class	1987 rank	Chapter no.†
Septra DS	Sulfamethoxazole	Antibacterial (sulfa)	150	8
	Trimethoprim	Antibacterial		8
Serax	Oxazepam	Antianxiety (benzodiazepine)	171	10
Sinequan	Doxepin	Tricyclic antidepressant (antianxiety)	115	17
Slo-Bid	Theophylline	Xanthine; bronchodilator	116	22
Slow-K	Potassium chloride	Electrolyte (potassium)	30	15
Stuartnatal 1 + 1	Vitamins A, D, E, B_1, B_2, B_3, B_6, B_{12}, C, FA, Ca, Fe, I, Mg	Prenatal vitamins and minerals	183	13
Sumycin	Tetracycline	Antibiotic	120	8
Synthroid	Levothyroxine	Thyroid hormone	12	20
Tagamet	Cimetidine	H_2-antagonist (antiulcer)	5	22
Talwin NX	Pentazocine	Opioid agonist-antagonist	188	7
	Naloxone	Opioid antagonist		7
Tavist-D	Clemastine fumarate	Antihistamine	102	18
	Phenylpropanolamine	Decongestant		5,22
Tegretol	Carbamazepine	Anticonvulsant	93	16
Tenoretic 50	Atenolol Chlorthalidone Diuretic	Beta-adrenergic blocker	176	15
Tenormin	Atenolol	Diuretic	8	15
		Beta$_1$-adrenergic blocker	21	15
Theo-Dur	Theophylline	Xanthine; bronchodilator		22
Thyroid (USV)	Thyroid	Thyroid hormone	74	20
Timoptic	Timolol	Beta-adrenergic blocker (glaucoma)	49	5
Tolectin DS	Tolmetin	Nonsteroidal antiinflammatory	160	6
Topicort	Desoximetasone	Corticosteroid	166	19
Transderm-Nitro	Nitroglycerin	Antianginal	53	15
Tranxene	Clorazepate	Antianxiety (benzodiazepine)	45	10
Trental	Pentoxifylline	Hemorrheologic (for intermittent claudication)	104	15
Triavil	Perphenazine	Antipsychotic	128	17
	Amitriptyline	Tricyclic antidepressant		17
Trimethoprim-sulfamethoxazole (Rugby)	Trimethoprim	Antibacterial	132	8
	Sulfamethoxazole	Antibacterial (sulfa)		8
Trimox	Antibiotic	Amoxicillin	39	8
Trinalin	Pseudoephedrine	Decongestant	148	5
	Azatadine maleate	Antihistamine		18
Tri-Norinyl	Norethindrone	Oral contraceptive; progestin	155	20
	Ethinyl estradiol	Oral contraceptive; estrogen		20
Triphasil-28	Levonorgestrel	Oral contraceptive; progestin	51	20
	Ethinyl estradiol	Oral contraceptive; estrogen		20

Continued.

Drug name	Generic name constituents	Pharmacologic class	1987 rank	Chapter no.†
Tussi-Organidin	Iodinated glycerol	Expectorant	168	22
	Codeine	Opioid analgesic (antitussive)		7
Tussi-Organidin DM	Iodinated glycerol	Expectorant	187	22
	Dextromethorphan	Antitussive		7,22
Tylenol/codeine	Acetaminophen	Nonopioid analgesic	6	6
	Codeine	Opioid analgesic		7
Tylox	Oxycodone	Opioid analgesic	136	7
	Acetaminophen	Nonopioid analgesic		6
Valium	Diazepam	Antianxiety (benzodiazepine)	19	10
Vanceril	Beclomethasone dipropionate	Corticosteroid	195	19
Vasotec	Enalapril	Angiotensin converting enzyme inhibitor	34	15
V-Cillin-K	Penicillin VK	Antibiotic	178	8
Veetids	Penicillin VK	Antibiotic	55	8
Ventolin	Albuterol	Beta$_2$-adrenergic (bronchodilator)	48	5,22
Vicodin	Hydrocodone	Opioid analgesic	66	7
	Acetaminophen	Nonopioid analgesic		6
Visken	Pindolol	Beta-adrenergic blocker	189	15
Wymox	Amoxicillin	Antibiotic	109	8
Xanax	Alprazolam	Antianxiety (benzodiazepine)	4	10
Zantac	Ranitidine	H$_2$-antagonist (antiulcer)	9	22
Zovirax	Acyclovir	Antiviral	147	8
Zyloprim	Allopurinol	Antigout	126	6

Index

A

Abbreviations, 27, 28
Abokinase; *see* Urokinase
Absorption, 12-14
Abstinence syndrome, 264, 265
Abuse, drug, 264-271
Accepted Dental Therapeutics, 2
Accutane; *see* Isotretinoin
ACE inhibitors; *see* Angiotensin-converting enzyme
    inhibitors
Acebutolol, 184t
Acetaminophen, 54t, **55-57**, 272a, 276a, 278a
    breast feeding and, 254
    pregnancy and, 254
Acetaminophen/codeine, 272a
Acetohexamide, 223t
Acetone sodium bisulfite, 113
N-Acetyl para-aminophenol; *see* Acetaminophen
Acetylcysteine, 236
Achromycin-V, 272a; *see also* Tetracycline
Acids, weak, 13
Acidulated phosphate fluoride, 148, 150
ACT, 150
ACTH; *see* Adrenocorticotropic hormone
Actidil; *see* Triprolidine
Actifed; *see* Pseudoephedrine
Actinic lip, 168
Actinomycin D; *see* Dactinomycin
Activase; *see* Alteplase
Acute necrotizing ulcerative gingivitis, 168
Acyclovir, **101-102,** 278a
Adalat; *see* Nifedipine
Adapin; *see* Doxepin

Boldface type indicates a primary discussion of a drug; "t" indicates
that a name appears in a table; "a" indicates that a name appears in
the appendix.

Addiction, 264
Addison's disease, 213, 214
Adrenal corticosteroids, 212
Adrenalin; *see* Epinephrine
Adrenergic, definition of, 34
Adrenergic agents, 40-45
    α-, **44**
    α- and β-, **44-45**
    β-, **44**
Adrenergic agonists, 233
    nonspecific, 234
Adrenergic blocker(s), 183-184
    α-, 184
    α- and β-, 184
    β-, 177, 184
Adrenocortical insufficiency, acute, 245
Adrenocorticosteroids, 212-217
    administration of, 213
    adverse reactions to, 214
    as antineoplastics, 230t
    classification of, 212
    definitions with, 212-213
    dental implications for, 215-216
    mechanism of action of, 213-214
    pharmacologic effects of, 214
    release mechanism of, 212
    uses of, 214-215
Adrenocorticotropic hormone, 212, 213, 218
Adriamycin; *see* Doxorubicin
Adverse reactions; *see* Reactions, adverse
Advil; *see* Ibuprofen
Affective disorders, 199
Afrin; *see* Oxymetazoline
Aftate; *see* Tolnaftate
Agencies, federal regulatory, 4-5
Agonists, 15-16
$β_2$-Agonists, selective, 234
Aim, 149

279